Removing the Barriers to Global Health Equity

Removing the Barriers to Global Health Equity

Théodore H MacDonald PhD, MD, FRSM
*Professor (Emeritus) and Member of Research Institute for Human Rights
and Social Justice, London Metropolitan University
Former Director of Postgraduate Studies in Health, Brunel University
Consultant to the World Health Organization, International Development
Agency and various NGOs in developing countries*

Forewords by

Professor Amiya Kumar Bagchi
*Director
Institute of Development Studies, Calcutta*

and

Dr Ann Wylie PhD
*Senior Tutor, Medical Educator and Health Promoter
King's College London, School of Medicine*

Radcliffe Publishing
Oxford • New York

Radcliffe Publishing Ltd
18 Marcham Road
Abingdon
Oxon OX14 1AA
United Kingdom

www.radcliffe-oxford.com
Electronic catalogue and worldwide online ordering facility.

British Library Cataloguing in Publication Data

A catalogue record for this book is available from the British Library.

ISBN-13: 978 1 84619 308 8

Typeset by Pindar NZ, Auckland, New Zealand
Printed and bound by TJI Digital, Padstow, Cornwall, UK

Contents

Foreword

I have been engaged in research into the economic development of India and the Third World (euphemistically called 'developing countries') all my life. Starting out with establishing the roots of the low rate of industrial investment and growth in South Asia in the colonial and the immediate post-independence period, I tried to determine the social and political structures forcing Third World countries into a condition of 'underdevelopment'. I was aware of the human costs of growth in advanced capitalist countries and wrote a dissenting note to the presidential address (given by Edmond Malinvaud) of the International Economic Congress, held in Tokyo in 1977.

I was aware that lack of health and education were both causes and effects of underdevelopment. In my *Political Economy of Underdevelopment* (Cambridge University Press, 1982), I devoted a chapter to population and the quality of life. In the meantime, like many of the social scientists and activists in South Asia, Latin America and Africa, along with like-minded social scientists and activists in Western Europe, North America and Australia, I became involved in fighting neoliberalism, which had many allies among the upper classes of the Third World nations. I became an adviser to the longest-serving democratically elected left-wing government in the world, namely the Government of West Bengal, and had first-hand experience of how neoliberalism was reversing the few gains that had been made by ordinary people in India until the 1980s.

The formal onset of neoliberalism can be dated from June 1991, when the Government of India accepted an IMF loan with many conditionalities, although the shadow of its influence was already darkening the policy space from the mid-1980s. All this time, I was also engaged in writing the history of India's oldest and largest commercial bank, which had started its life as a handmaiden of British imperialism in India. Concurrently I was also writing on the neoliberal impact on banking and fiscal policies in South Asia.

In the 1990s I became interested in tracing the history of human development and traced it in both advanced capitalist countries and in the Third World. I showed how capitalism thwarted the possibilities of universalisation of education and healthcare, even as scientific advances rendered those possibilities reachable for all human beings. That history, together with the recent depredations of armed capitalism (it has never been unarmed!) has been related in my *Perilous Passage: mankind and the global ascendancy of capital* (Rowman & Littlefield Publishers, 2005).

In view of all of the above, it was a real pleasure for me to discover how relentlessly and with how much expertise at his command Professor Théodore MacDonald has been fighting for the cause of equality among all human beings, irrespective of race, ethnicity, nationality, gender or class. Therefore, it has also been a great honour to be requested to write a foreword for his new book. Unlike many other analysts, who are content to ascribe the ill-health of the world to this or that programme of the World Health Organization or the World Bank – or even worse – to governance problems in Third World nations, MacDonald goes to the taproot of the poison tree, namely, imperialism fomented by unlimited profit-seeking by capitalists all over the world. The author's attention is not focused only on the deteriorating health situation in most of the Third World countries, a deterioration that has led to genocidal proportions in sub-Saharan lands. He also shows how the same capitalist drive for accumulation has led to worse nutrition and healthcare for the poor in the First World as well.

Today the world is faced with the worst food crisis since the end of World War Two. Professor MacDonald shows how this is linked not only to the inappropriate subsidy policies of the affluent countries, creating a totally lopsided trade regime, but also to the wanton privatisation of all common property resources, including the water needed for survival, the air needed for proper breathing and all the gifts of nature that have hitherto been taken by all humanists as the birth right of all the children of women. One of the principal virtues of the book is that it is not content with painting the big, unlovely picture but focuses on the nitty-gritty of local decision-making that tends to favour the plutocrats at the cost of human welfare. His case studies of the depredations of private economic and political power in Latin America are particularly illuminating in this respect.

But Théodore MacDonald is not content with simply painting the blackness of dehumanisation caused by neoliberalism. He also draws our attention to the resistance of ordinary people against the privatisation of water and other resources. He would like all right-minded people to join in fighting the demons of neoliberalism, now gone berserk over Iran, Iraq, Afghanistan, Somalia, Yugoslavia and countless other places, where the peace of death has been delivered to millions by imperialist seekers of 'peace'. He has a slew of recommendations, of which two are critical. One is to turn the United Nations into a real forum for bringing about a democratic order of global governance. The other is to re-empower states and communities to deliver universal healthcare and education on the foundations of proper nutrition and freedom of action, so readily promised by the proponents of democracy. I hope that all readers of this impassioned and scalpel-like book will feel energised to fight for the cause of rights of all human beings in all areas of human endeavour.

Professor Amiya Kumar Bagchi
Director, Institute of Development Studies, Calcutta
September 2008

Foreword

It was a privilege to be asked to write a foreword to this book, one that builds on Professor Théo MacDonald's more recent work in challenging the global structures that influence the health and wellbeing of some of the most vulnerable people and poorest countries.

The very structures set up to improve health and reduce inequality, based on worthy aspirations, and reiterated in declarations such as the Alma-Ata, have, he argues, become the main protagonists in widening rather than narrowing the health inequity gap. The more urgent need to address this is now evident, given that we have a food crisis and environmental degradation, war and conflict on a massive scale. In addition, we are beset by so-called natural disasters in politically challenging areas, hampering the response of NGOs.

He presents us with convincing and robust arguments, enabling readers, be they public health workers and medics, politicians and policy makers, bankers and corporate donors, NGOs and journalists, with ample substance and fodder for debate.

The crux of his argument centres around the economically flawed neoliberalism paradigms, which, he reminds us, are not governed by the physical laws of science but are human social constructs and this is where he offers hope. We can break free! In admiration of the achievements of the UN, and some of its agencies such as UNICEF and WHO, he avers that we have the means by which to change and it is imperative that we do so.

As a medical educator and health promoter, my daily contact with medical students also inspires me with hope – they are full of ideals, dedicating a considerable amount of their time and money to electives, whereby they will work with and for some of the poorest communities whose basic health needs are barely met. Prior to their electives they familiarise themselves with the public health issues of the countries and communities they will visit. Some will explore the macro politics to better contextualise the health problems they see and feel more able to offer contributions to the debate on global health inequalities. This book, and previous ones by MacDonald, are valuable resources for our students and their supervisors.

Examples of policies that actually tackle public health issues, such as the food crisis or drug trafficking, are presented as feasible and sustainable. Medical students may want to treat the suffering children, but are also enriched by a wider knowledge base of the contextual macro politics and how they impact at the root-and-branch level on their efforts. This will add to their experiences and foster their moral responsibilities to assist them in promoting global access to health and in reducing health inequalities.

Professor MacDonald's call to educators, intellectuals and higher education *per se* to prepare students to address questions of social justice, freedom and self-development should be well received and be compatible with the ethos by those in medical and health education faculties. What this book does is to provide us with valuable debating material, drawn from a wealth of experiences and a passion for justice. He asks us to 'enlarge our own moral parochialism' to overcome the ethical issues we face and presents us with more than mere rhetoric but with practical alternatives to achieve this. He asserts that our moral response is in the ascendancy. The hegemony of the United States, central to the rise of neoliberalism, is, he argues, itself under threat, thus opening up opportunities for reducing the global inequalities gap and thus 'rediscovers our common humanity by making the world a safer and happier place for the generations to come'.

He argues that we can remedy any defects in the UN rather than demolishing it. The inception of the 'Global Fund' should be seen as a source of optimism and, together with the work of NGOs and other stakeholders, this fund has already shown its worth in making a difference in health outcomes. In addition, the advent and growth of social entrepreneurism, fair trade initiatives and innovative and sustainable energy provision all offer ways forward, enabling the 'Health for All' ideas to be put back on the agenda. Indeed, this is a moral imperative. We in the rich countries must be agents of change and recognise, in actions as well as words, 'the worth, dignity and ineffable potential of every single one of our fellow human beings'.

Given that my son works, as he says 'with and for the poorest of the poor' in his role with Save the Children, the need to remove barriers to global health inequalities has become part of our regular discourse. It has been most satisfying to recommend this latest scholarly work from Professor Théo MacDonald as a book which adds gravitas to our own humble arguments and endeavours towards social justice, access to health and promotion of health for all.

Dr Ann Wylie PhD
Senior Tutor, Medical Educator and Health Promoter
King's College London, School of Medicine
September 2008

Preface

After nearly a lifetime of work in various Third World countries, in both medicine and education, I have had ample opportunity to ponder the question: Why have we done so poorly in securing equity in the global access to healthcare and even to health itself? And this leads to yet another rhetorical question: Should we be searching for a great medical breakthrough, a scientific advance that can give us the final victory?

As recently as the 1950s we, in the wealthy developed nations, might with some justification have claimed that we did not realise how hideously iniquitous such global access was, because we had only a short time before coming out of a dreadful war and had been concentrating on overcoming its legacy of heartbreak and destruction. However, in the five or six decades since then, we have become better informed. Newspapers, radio and TV programmes and books abound, clamouring to let the world know the truth. Moreover, the UN, especially through such of its agencies as the World Health Organization (WHO), has battled heroically (particularly in the Third World) to develop and administer vaccines, to establish health education facilities, to research and promote low-tech life-saving procedures such as oral rehydration therapies (ORT), etc. In the light of all of that, should we not have witnessed improvements?

And, indeed, we have – but largely among, say, the wealthiest 35% of the world's people. But overall, the global health inequity gap is widening.

Reflecting on this, we have perhaps gained some idea as to where to seek an answer to those two rhetorical questions. Medical breakthroughs will continue to be sought and we justifiably take pride in the fact that a great many such discoveries have bestowed their benefits on many since 1948. But, paradoxically, they have, if anything, widened the inequity gap further. For what we have witnessed is the already moderately healthy becoming healthier yet, while similar levels of progress have been far less evident among those already most deprived. In other words, it has not been through lack of knowledge, so much as through lack of wisdom (and certainly lack of morality) in applying what we know, that we have caused the problem we face now.

And to enquire as to why that wisdom has been lacking, we must go beyond the realms of biomedicine itself and consider how it has been contextualised. The issues, of course, are only partly medical, but more economic and social. That was realised in the early 1970s and was made explicit in September 1978, at a now famous meeting of the WHO at the former Soviet spa-town of Alma-Ata. There it was categorically asserted that, if most of the causes are social and economic, the solutions have to be more political than purely clinical. These insights were formalized in the Alma-Ata Declaration (ADA). This document laid out in detail what political steps had to be taken to establish a realistic basis for the achievement of global equity in health. It was agreed by the delegates (in 1982 and under the energetic and inspired leadership of Dr Halfdan Mahler – WHO's Director General at the time) that these criteria should be achieved by the turn of the millennium, in a 38-target programme called 'Health for All by 2000' (HFA2000).

Although this splendid programme was never achieved, due to externally imposed neoliberal financial constraints, the ideas of HFA2000 have initiated a sea change in the way that public health is regarded today, with the emphasis strongly oriented toward consideration of the social determinants of health. That many of the contributory problems have remained unresolved is, as this author will argue, due to the fact that, generally, advances in political thinking have not kept pace with those in public health thinking. The argument put forward will even go further and claim that political insights have not kept pace because corporate interests, through the imposition of neoliberalism, have assumed almost total hegemony over international trade. A thorough explanation of the origins of neoliberalism, and how it operates, is provided in the first chapter of this book. As the reader will see, that discourse is pivotal in addressing the rhetorical questions with which this preface began.

Succeeding chapters address some of the other barriers to the achievement of global equity in health. The list of such barriers presented here is obviously not exhaustive, but is sufficient to illustrate not only their interconnection with one another, but how neoliberalism undergirds all of them – rather like the leitmotif of a novel or of a Wagnerian opera. Thus, there are chapters on the role of transnational pharmaceutical corporations, the negative health impacts of corporate water privatisation schemes, global warming and worsening food shortages, etc.

But, in the penultimate chapter, the author addresses the philosophico-psychological issue of what he refers to as 'moral parochialism'. By this, he means that we live in an ever more insistently global community (what he refers to as 'a small global village'), but still base our reactions on much narrower terms, such as national advantage. The environmental crisis itself – greatly exacerbated by neoliberalism – urges us to allow our thinking to be governed more by the needs of that larger parish that comprises our entire planet, its biosphere and all of its people.

The final chapter summarises the problems raised in the previous chapters and considers alternative socio-political solutions to those offered by neoliberalism.

Théodore H MacDonald
Littlehampton, UK
September 2008

Acknowledgements

One cannot ever thank everyone who should be thanked or recognise all of the influences that deserve such mention in providing an author with the help and inspiration to write a book such as this. Instead, as is customary, I trust that the reader will appreciate the constraints when I narrow the field right down, only mentioning the most recent few who were pivotal to the undertaking.

In this respect, for instance, I must go on record as heartily thanking David John Holmes, who volunteered to perform the invaluable, and quintessentially tedious, task of proof-reading the typescript as it was being word-processed. His latent skills as a copy-editor really came to the fore and, in a lifetime of author-ship, I have rarely come across his match. It was also he who drew up the *List of relevant acronyms*, found at the front of the book. Many thanks must also go to Beth Archer, who word-processed the entire manuscript, heroically battling against my impenetrable handwriting.

As usual, Radcliffe Publishing, under its gracious editor Gillian Nineham, exhibited the highest degrees of efficiency and professionalism in bringing this volume to the light of day.

Above all, I cannot fail to mention the love and encouragement given me by my family, most especially my dear wife Chris, which enabled me to complete the task. It is her moral strength and idealism which is the source of much of my ability to undertake such projects.

Théodore H MacDonald
Littlehampton, UK
September 2008

List of relevant acronyms

AAD	Alma-Ata Declaration
ACT-UP	Aids Coalition to Unleash Power – USA
AI	Amnesty International
AIDS	acquired immune deficiency syndrome
ALBA	Bolivaran Alternative for the Americas
ANC	African National Congress
APF	Anti-Privatisation Forum
ARV	antiretrovirals
AT	appropriate technology
AZT	azidothymidine
B&MGF	Bill and Melinda Gates Foundation
BMJ	British Medical Journal
CARE	Cooperation for Assistance and Relief Everywhere
CCM	Country Coordinating Mechanism
CEO	chief executive officer
CIA	Central Intelligence Agency – USA
CIDA	Canadian International Development Agency
CIS	Commonwealth of Independent States
CSR	corporate social responsibility
DATA	Debt, AIDS, Trade, Africa
DFID	Department for International Development
DMAE	Departamento Municipal do Agua e Esgoto – Brazil
EARS	Early Alert and Response System
EPZ	export processing zone
EUWI	European Union Water Initiative
EU	European Union
FAO	Food and Agriculture Organization
FBW	free basic water
FDA	Food and Drug Administration – USA
FEDECOR	Federación Departmental de Regantes de Cochabambina de Regantes – Bolivia

FTAA	Free Trade Area of the Americas
GAO	Government Accountability Office – USA
GATS	General Agreement on Trade and Services
GATT	General Agreement on Tariffs and Trade
GDP	gross domestic product
GFATM	Global Fund to Fight AIDS, Tuberculosis and Malaria
GNP	gross national product
HFA2000	Health For All 2000
HIPC	Heavily Indebted Poor Countries – IMF and World Bank
HIV	human immunodeficiency virus
IAEA	International Atomic Energy Agency
IBRD	International Bank for Reconstruction and Development
ICRC	International Committee of the Red Cross
IFPRI	International Food Policy Research Institute – USA
IIRSA	Initiative for the Integration of the Regional Infrastructure of South Africa
IMF	International Monetary Fund
IMGs	international medical graduates
IP	intellectual property
IRIN	Integrated Regional Information Network
ISAPREs	private insurance entities
IT	information technology
ITUC	International Trade Union Confederation
LDCs	less developed countries
LFA	local fund agent
MAI	Multilateral Agreement on Investment
MDG	Millennium Development Goal
MIGA	Multilateral Investment Guarantee Agency
MSF	Médecins Sans Frontières – 'Doctors Without Borders'
MSP	Member of Scottish Parliament
NAFTA	North American Free Trade Agreement
NAWAPA	North American Water and Power Alliance
NGO	non-governmental Organisations
NHS	National Health Service
NIH	National Institutes of Health – USA
NPT	Nuclear Non-Proliferation Treaty
NPTREC	NPT Review and Extension Conference
OECD	Organisation for Economic Co-operation and Development
OFWAT	The Water Services Regulation Authority – UK
PAHO	Pan American Health Organization

PEPFAR	President's Emergency Plan For AIDS Relief – USA
PHM	People's Health Movement
PhRMA	Pharmaceutical Research and Manufacturers of America
PLoS	Public Library of Science
PPP	Plan Puebla Panama
PR	principal recipient
PRSP	Poverty Reduction Strategy Paper
PT	Workers Party – Brazil
PUP	public-private partnerships
R&D	research and development
SACP	South African Communist Party
SAGUAPAC	Cooperative de Servicios Publicos Santa Cruz – Bolivia
SAPs	Structural Adjustment Policy
SARS	severe acute respiratory syndrome
SEZ	special economic zone
SUV	sports utility vehicle
TINA	'There is no alternative'
TRIPS	Trade-Related Property Rights
TWN	Third World Network
UDHR	Universal Declaration of Human Rights
UK	United Kingdom of Great Britain and Northern Ireland
UN	United Nations
UNAIDS	Joint United Nations Programme on HIV/AIDS
UNCTAD	United Nations Conference on Trade and Development
UNDP	United Nations Development Programme
UNEP	United Nations Environment Programme
UNESCO	United Nations Educational, Scientific and Cultural Organization
UNICEF	United Nations Children's Fund
UN-OCHA	United Nations Office for the Coordination of Humanitarian Affairs
UNSCEAR	United Nations Scientific Committee on the Effects of Atomic Radiation
US	United States
USA	United States of America
WFP	World Food Programme – United Nations
WHO	World Health Organization
WTO	World Trade Organization
WWF	World Water Forum

To the memory of the life and work of

Martin Kelly

this book is humbly and gratefully dedicated.

Martin Kelly was well known in wealthy circles as a craniofacial reconstructive surgeon of immense ability and for his outstandingly daring and innovatory techniques in the pursuit of facial beauty. Many are the wonderful things he achieved for his patients by his inspired skill with the scalpel.

But much more wonderfully, he devoted so much of his time and talents to undertaking the same sort of work, without cost, for numerous economically deprived victims of hideous facial disfigurements in the Third World. To promote these endeavours he initiated and heavily financed the program called 'Facing the World' to make it possible for his colleagues and himself to visit such afflicted people (usually children) in parts of the world rarely visited by a doctor. Without his intervention these people could only expect to live a short and unpleasant life, marked by social rejection and economic ruin.

He even financed the passage to England of a number of children, so that he could treat them even more extensively under modern hospital conditions. His sudden and unexpected death by heart-failure was a profound shock to all who admired him.

In his devotion to his branch of surgery, he exemplified the attitudes required to make this world a better place and all of us better people.

Théodore H MacDonald

Chapter 1

Is neoliberalism compatible with global health equity?

WHAT IS NEOLIBERALISM?

Neoliberalism features prominently in the discourse of this book and hence an introductory chapter on the issue is called for. The term 'neoliberalism' has become so widely used in recent years that many users of the word have a very hazy idea of its meaning. The situation is further complicated by ideological commitments of various types and a rather severe difference between what the general public, along with the ever corporate-compliant media, mean by it on the one hand and what bankers and other corporate-type people mean by it on the other.

In the mid-seventies ordinary people started to run across the term, but generally in a rather positive context. Along with wonderful expressions such as 'wealth creation' and 'big government', neoliberalism suggested a breaking away from totalitarian restraints, leaving people free to rub exciting arguments together without over-burdensome restraints, thereby creating jobs and money-making opportunities. All off this was euphemistically referred to as 'wealth creation'. And for this magnificent flowering of talent and opportunity to take place, we had to remove obstructive legislation, including such things as health and safety rules, union rights and so on.

Back then, neoliberalism was widely promoted and presented as 'the wave of the future', the 'only way forward', virtually a guarantee of individual fulfilment and general happiness. Not only did comparatively few non-economists question the wisdom of this widespread approbation, but indeed, almost any criticism of it and/or the suggestion that government should monitor it in any way was called

1

'unrealistic'. It was as though we had somehow evolved to a high point of social development with the development of neoliberalism and it became part of our moral responsibility to help the teeming masses of Asia and Africa understand that we had discovered the Holy Grail and to encourage them to acquiesce in the globalisation of neoliberalism.

In fact, this author recalls attending a meeting in Australia of the New South Wales History Teachers Association in Sydney in 1982, where the general consensus was that, although students should be told about such totalitarian vulgarities as communism, socialism, fascism, etc., the students must realise that 'everyone accepts that neoliberalism is the only realistic solution'. Moreover, certain inalienable laws govern the give-and-take of market forces and to interfere with the self-regulation of the market is to court economic suicide. In a sense, it regards 'market forces' as being akin to the great force fields in physics, such as magnetism, thermodynamics, etc. In other words, like these other forces, humans must respond according to those 'laws' or face annihilation. But in reality humans – not some outside agencies – design their economies and markets to meet their needs. If the model they are using is not delivering the goods, they can change the market rules. That is, market forces do not control human societies. Instead human societies can adjust their market regulations to meet with their needs.

Although certain events, such as the increasing tendency to resort to war, the need to find sustainable sources of energy instead of relying on fossil fuels, global warming, international economic insecurity (especially with respect to our banking system), etc., have – since the 1970s – gradually caused some people to be suspicious of neoliberalism, not much has really changed. For instance, none of the major political parties in the First World nations have seriously threatened to actively try to develop alternatives to neoliberalism.

But, as tends to happen, if a political or social system has some flaw in its make-up – some unresolved logical contradiction, say – this flaw will become increasingly evident the harder and longer the model is pursued. For instance, in mid-April 2008, the Director of the World Food Programme warned the UN Security Council that the world, during 2008, would begin to feel the effects of a global food crisis.[1] This situation is now causing serious questioning about the merits and defects of neoliberalism.

Before proceeding further, though, with these details, we must briefly consider the economic theories behind neoliberalism and to do that, a brief résumé of its history cannot be avoided.

NEOLIBERALISM, MONETARISM AND 'THE WASHINGTON CONSENSUS'

This author has even heard economists state that neoliberalism had its origins in the monetarist arguments of Milton Friedman at the Chicago University Department of Economics in the 1960s and 70s and that it became a dominant plank of Prime Minister Margaret Thatcher's government in Britain in the 1980s. But that leaves out some of the prior twists and turns and tends to confuse monetarism (Friedman) with neoliberalism (Hayek). And to confront the Austrian conservative economist Friedrich von Hayek, we have to go back before World War Two. Von Hayek was concerned primarily with business cycles in Europe and was virulently anti-socialist.

But, before returning to von Hayek's influence on these matters, it is important – if only briefly – to indicate the differences between neoliberalism, monetarism and what later became known as 'the Washington Consensus'. The latter term was first used in 1989, by the US economist John Williamson, of the Institute for International Economics, and at a conference at which he played a principal rôle. The conference in question took place in Barcelona and he had entitled it 'From the Washington Consensus to Global Governance'. By 'Washington Consensus' he meant to refer to the increasing degree to which some Third World countries, especially in Latin America, had modernised their economies with respect to both trade and domestic policies and in line with US governmental and business views on what constituted 'sound economics'. Basically, this involved the application of monetarism in banking practices and neoliberalism at the broader levels of fiscal policy.

The author draws the reader's attention to the issue at this point because the three terms tend to be used loosely in much public commentary in the media and hence are readily confused with one another. It helps to think of the Washington Consensus as the USA's response, at the time, to the ways adopted by a number of Third World national economies in adapting to the neoliberal context increasingly imposed upon them through international trade. Monetarism fitted into the equation by providing a theoretical foundation for this process.

As for monetarism, it has had a number of incarnations since the early days of the 20th century, largely originating at Chicago University's School of Economics. The earlier versions of monetarism were found to be lacking for various reasons, but economists at the Chicago School kept working at the idea, until they felt that they could offer a workable model. Fundamentally, it involved the regulation of money supply as a means of controlling and stabilising the economy and thus avoiding sudden unanticipated swings.

But it is Milton Friedman, who became Professor of Economics at the Chicago School in the 1950s, who is widely acknowledged as the father of modern political monetarism. As a philosophical basis for national economic policy, it is largely congenial to a high degree of flexibility on the part of the banks and to an emphasis on the flow of money being determined by market forces, rather than by government diktat. In particular, the banks had to be free of ideological restrictions being placed on their lending policies.

It goes without saying that the above four paragraphs have grossly oversimplified much of the economic theory behind the phenomena described but, hopefully, they have provided an adequate basis for the reader to better understand the impact of von Hayek's thinking.

His ideological orientation against socialism deeply influenced the rest of his life's work and he saw in neoliberalism a method of removing constraints on business practice. His views gained some popularity among a few economists, but generally he was shunned. Keynes was regarded as the man to watch!

The author, in a previous book, described how John Maynard Keynes, the internationally respected British economist, had been somewhat involved in setting up the UN during the 1940s, but the UN had bigger political backers, leaving Keynes to play a more minor rôle.[2] Indeed, it was he who had suggested the creation of the International Monetary Fund (IMF) and also the International Bank for Reconstruction and Development (IBRD), known more commonly as the World Bank. But the IBRD did not develop in the way that Keynes hoped it would! He had the view that future international military conflict could be avoided if the IBRD would help the war-torn nations regain their strength through loans.

However, it was at this point that things began to go wrong and neoliberal ideas intruded. The US government, under President Roosevelt at the time, wanted to insist on three conditions for the loans:

a   They must be paid back in US dollars.
b   The loans had to be used to engage private providers for the services required. They could not come under government control.
c   The IMF would apply 'conditionalities' (Structural Adjustment Policies or SAPs) with each such loan, heavily controlling how the client country used the money, but such SAPs did not enter the scene fully until the 1970s.

What the formation of the IMF and the World Bank under these restrictions meant was that the latter – instead of representing that progressive thrust forward to world peace and international justice – became a method of imposing economic imperialism on some of the world's poorest countries. Since 1970, indeed, the World Bank and those SAPs have had a disastrous impact on global health and, since 1988, this has been widening the global health equity gap rather than diminishing it.[3] And the mechanism has been neoliberalism.

This is all described in the book cited above, but basically it worked like this:

a   Since the debtor countries were obliged to repay the debts (including compound interest) in US dollars, they were required to raise that money by selling their national resources to US markets at prices determined by them.

b   This, in turn, meant that they had to sacrifice all other internal needs of their country to creating a total infrastructure of roads, rail, etc., to the trading ports. Union rights were slashed and the workforce rendered tame. Large areas had to be deforested and rivers were poisoned by excess use of chemicals, etc. All of this had negative impacts on health.

c   In just about any government, the two main areas of government expenditures are in health and education, but the SAPs required that – instead of domestic governments administering these matters – private providers had to be used, opening the country to higher costs for these services. Of course, IMF and World Bank stockholders (living in opulence in the First World) greatly rejoiced in this as their stock values rose. This is neoliberalism in action.

POPULIST VIEWS OF NEOLIBERALISM

Looked at dispassionately, why should anyone be surprised that neoliberalism has developed in this way? Only a very modest degree of logic would persuade the average thinking person of such political 'axioms' as: People evolved government to protect the tribe, group or community. To mediate conflicts between interests in that group, the government must play a dominant rôle. That is why we invented it!

Therefore, such ideas as 'markets' being allowed to make major social and political decisions without the mediating influence of government is nonsense. The corollary is that the 'government' should acquiesce in this by 'withdrawing' and playing as small a part as possible in the economy, and that also flies in the face of logic (if not of social anthropology!).

It is these perversions that now make it seem reasonable that 'corporation' (in most national constitutions) be regarded legally as an 'individual person' and with the same constitutional rights to protection under the law, etc. This runs into sticky situations when an operative, say, a relatively lowly placed worker on a building site or whatever, employed by a corporation without due regard to that actual individual's right to health and safety protection, becomes killed or injured as a result.

Suddenly, in *that* case, the situation changes in court. Although the 'corporation' (legally protected and defined as a 'person') has injured or killed another person (an actual person, this time), no one can be held criminally responsible for it. The owners, including the chief executive officer (CEO) of the corporation, are all 'real' people, but suddenly become not legally responsible for what they did to the injured or killed 'real' person! We are truly in 'cloud-cuckoo land' here, but it is par for the course if we accept that neoliberalism is a benign social idea.

It not only implies that 'government' (which we evolved over human history to protect us) should voluntarily curtail its own rôle in the economy, but that 'corporations' (those 'persons' that are not 'real persons') should be accorded unhindered scope for their exercise of power. Not only that, but the consequence of such an idea is that trade unions (which also evolved over time to protect the human rights of workers in different trades) should be restricted in exercising their power. The end result is that 'ordinary' citizens – many of whom regarded themselves as 'apolitical' and 'not involved in the argument' – suddenly find their human rights reduced.

But all of that has already happened and is still happening and is all part of the same neoliberalism that we have been urged for the past few decades to regard as the guarantor of our human rights and of our development as people and nations. It is the same neoliberalism that remains rampant as any lion and clawing as much of our once public/community life into privatisation as it possibly can. And it makes it possible for those of us committed to health equity to appreciate how neoliberalism has gained its almost religious (and essentially 'irrational') hold over global health.

Let us now return to the sudden change in the power of the IMF and the World Bank and their increasingly malign influence on the World Health Organization (WHO), a UN agency, while all three were supposedly working in harmony to defend and promote human rights under the UN's defining Charter, the Universal Declaration of Human Rights (UDHR). It charts the gradual control of neoliberalism over global health rights – and its influence in increasing the global health inequity gap that the WHO was mandated to heal. This represents a serious conflict of interests with the objectives of the UDHR. Basic to the UDHR is the concept of 'parity of esteem' between nations, as recognised for instance in the General Assembly of the UN. But this does not apply to the IMF and the World Bank. In those two bodies, member countries do not have equal voting powers. The number of votes are determined instead by a formula based on the wealth of each individual nation concerned, and hence are heavily weighted in favour of the US and other wealthy First World nations.

NEOLIBERALISM'S GROWTH IN GLOBAL POWER

If we go back to the uncertain economic regeneration of the 1930s, we note a determined resurgence of popular appreciation of the need for greater social control over economic forces – a sort of anti-neoliberalism. In the so-called 'democratic' Western nations, it produced a welfare state mentality (as exemplified in the UK – and Europe generally – by Keynesian economies, and in the US by the New Deal and the Tennessee Valley Authority). All of this social progress was, of course, interrupted by World War Two, but the immediate post-war years saw a resurgence of these ideas.

What needs to be remembered, however, is that the power of corporate influences, especially in the USA, which also had only suffered minimal domestic damage during the war, was still very much alive and hostile to any restriction on market forces. Communism, momentarily in popular ascendancy throughout Europe and much of Asia because of the Soviet Union's magnificent rôle in smashing fascism, stood as a threat to the corporate neoliberal interests represented most potently in the USA. Conflict, therefore, between the USA and the USSR for world domination was regarded by some as inevitable.

'SAVING' THE WORLD FROM COMMUNISM

There is not much doubt that if this conflict had been allowed to express itself in military terms, the result would have been disastrous for us all. No doubt, the fact that the USA was the only nuclear power at the time played a rôle in preventing such a war. Instead the USA fought the advance of communism with the Marshall Plan, as described by the author in a previous publication.[4] The Marshall Plan created trading partnerships between the USA and most of the European nations, in that way buying off the threat of communism to corporate interests in Europe and North America.

It was not so successful in this regard in Asia, and by 1949 China came under a communist administration, while India, along with a host of other smaller countries, teetered on the edge – so to speak – as the 'non-aligned nations'.

In all sorts of ways, optimism and a sense of progress began to make itself felt worldwide. Macmillan's 'Wind of Change' speech[5] signalled an end to the British Empire's influence and, as India and various African nations, and many smaller nations in the South Pacific, gradually gained their independence, one could no longer say (supposedly) with Rudyard Kipling, 'The sun never sets on the British Empire.'[6]

NEOLIBERALISM REASSERTS ITSELF

To understand how neoliberalism made its way back after the horrors of World War Two and the establishment of the UN and WHO, we have to address such questions as: How is it that the World Bank and the IMF (both UN agencies) were allowed to intrude so violently into the economies of dozens of Third World countries to the detriment of people's health? Why do those forces which have undermined the work of WHO in the Third World now get away with attacking the welfare state (largely through privatisation) in the First World nations? Why has the wealth gap been widening globally when there has never in human history existed such usable levels of wealth?

That little nucleus of people, such as Hayek, along with his students – including Milton Friedman in the University of Chicago (School of Chicago) – were at exactly the right place (the USA) in the right time (1970s inflation caused by oil price rises) and with people at the levers of power ready to listen. Their founders endowed an international network of foundations, research centres, freedom institutes, etc., along with well-funded journals that attracted scholars from respected sectors of the academic establishment. They were surrounded by a media hungry for 'uplifting' news about the virtues of freedom and the American Way.

TACTICS FOR IMPOSING NEOLIBERALISM

It is this author's view – with the wonderful advantage of hindsight – that this was not just a happy accident for big business, but was the result of patient, prolonged and powerfully deployed financial management and planning by a comparatively small group of global power brokers.

The 'right' has been on the ascendant in the USA and in the UK since the late 1970s. Britain elected Margaret Thatcher as prime minister in 1979 and the USA elected Ronald Reagan in 1980. Both of those people espoused policies of 'reducing government input', deregulation, curtailment of union rights, privatisation of social services and active support of dictatorial regimes in Latin America and elsewhere, but especially where these regimes were being actively resisted by domestic insurgency and revolutionary movements. It was most imperative that 'client economies' of the neoliberal matrix of economic control not be allowed to break away.

In that context, Cuba was decidedly a 'bad apple' and had been since 1959. Leftist elements were destroyed by US forces in the Dominican Republic in 1965 to prevent the same thing from happening there. Then, in 1973, the Central Intelligence Agency (CIA), with the active involvement of Henry Kissinger, collaborated with the right wing in Chile to depose the first elected Marxist in the Americas (Salvador Allende), who ruled as president of Chile from 1970 to 1973. US agencies then actively collaborated in reversing the impressive number of social gains made during Allende's regime. Again, in 1983, President Reagan sent US troops into the tiny English-speaking island country of Grenada to keep it within the neoliberal orbit. It had dared to chart an independent socialist path, under its own leader, Maurice Bishop, from 1975 to 1985 – to the great glee (of course) of Cuba.

Likewise, in the UK, Margaret Thatcher not only allied herself (and UK foreign policy) with Reagan's administration, but actively supported Pinochet in Chile and committed the UK to war in the Falkland Islands in 1985. Augusto Pinochet, of course, was the dictator who, with US backing, had deposed Allende.

NEOLIBERALISM TAKES UP THE GUN

In fact, the readiness to resort to military means has increased noticeably with the strengthening influence of neoliberalism on government policy all over the world. The international arms trade, for instance, is one of the most lucrative in the world and constitutes an ideal venue for the exercise of neoliberalism. Profitability is virtually assured by the necessity of frequently upgrading military resources to take advantage of advances in technology. The old arms are then sold second-hand down the 'food chain'.

Of course, this creates more danger, insecurity and undermining of health for thousands of people already living on the edge of economic ruin – but this does not unduly worry the stockholders it enriches, who live far from the war zones. While this growth of military incidents – and their bewildering proliferation – has stimulated an increasing opposition to war in communities in both the UK and the US, the corporate media has been surprisingly efficient in trying to give the impression that these protestors/dissidents, trouble-makers, etc., 'are only a fringe element and that, on the whole, one should glory in what neoliberalism does for us.'

Naturally, these 'profitable' war adventures cost enormous sums of money, but it is not the actual dividend earners or corporate CEOs who pay. Since the tax structures in the US are not progressive, a disproportionate amount of money is taken from those at the bottom of the pile (not only as income tax but also as the gradual closing down and/or privatising of social services outlets). The same problem applies in the UK. The UK tax structure is more progressive than is the US system, but – even under a so-called 'Labour' government – every effort is made to avoid taxing the rich at a higher rate while finding various ways of making up any deficit by taxing lower down the income ladder.

But, as well as this, the vast disbursement of government funds to the military while fighting two major wars simultaneously (Iraq and Afghanistan) – and having to keep the nuclear corporate leaders happy by updating the Trident missile submarines – removes billions of pounds from the economy. If this money could be applied to the National Health Service (NHS) and to schooling programmes, it would make an immediate impact and of such a magnitude that privatisation (in either health *or* education) would have almost no rationale.

WHY HAVE WE FALLEN FOR IT?

What does it take to cause whole communities of people to voluntarily opt for such a crazy state of affairs? It obviously requires a cooperative media that keeps people agreeably misinformed, only partly informed and informed at length and in detail about trivial events and lifestyles that require wealth. This latter part is much more important than people realise because it provides a rich source of banal details, say, about the habits, dress, activities, marital conflicts, etc. of 'celebrities'. A 'celebrity' is a person who is made the object of such presentations. Many of them do not contribute in any significant way to the good of humanity. Not too many doctors or teachers, for instance, achieve celebrity status.

This is perfectly reasonable because it not only keeps audiences contented, but also induces in them a longing for wealth and public display of it. Thus it derails development of their social conscience while also making them feel that they are not really part of a community. In that way it increases their sense of loneliness, inadequacy and social alienation. The latter even induces a sense of contempt for their surroundings so that they cannot even *conceive* of achieving a sense of satisfaction in their own community and a sense that the only way out is to suddenly become rich (and respected) by winning a lottery draw – or something similar. Their own sense of worthlessness is often so great that they cannot even *begin* to see the larger picture, to empathise with people living in different countries and cultures. As for being inspired to act in such a way as to confront authorities with their questions or worries – the very idea is absurd! Life is a competition and to admit despair or loneliness is to label oneself as a 'failure'.

COMPETITION – THE RATIONALE OF NEOLIBERALISM

Margaret Thatcher, for instance, was inordinately fond of the 'competition' theme – in which we don't have 'neighbours' so much as 'rivals'. After all, the non-inflammable lady had herself been a devoted disciple of Frederick von Hayek. So convinced was she of the religion of neoliberalism that she made sure that any government policy she was planning was first of all vetted by other monetarists whom she respected. Their endorsement was enough to convince her that her proposed action was the *only* legitimate one. If people objected to a particular policy (over and above the usual rabble of unionists, social workers and liberal bishops!), she always used to reply emphatically – especially to the media: 'There is no alternative'. Media wags soon shortened this to 'TINA' and her policies were – in certain circles – often referred to by that name.

CAN TINA HELP?

That acronym, TINA, nicely sums up the philosophy of neoliberalism, which only can operate on the basis of (preferably) unregulated competition. But the apologists for neoliberalism have insisted that it is really the only fair solution. In that case, we – in public health – have been quite wrong in pushing for *decreasing* the global health-equity gap! This can lead us into a nice little logical conundrum, unless we go at solving the problem from another set of axioms.

We know that if global inequity increases, wars will also do so, and at the very time that we are facing an imminent environmental crisis and a global shortage of grain. Unless we concentrate on these issues – which will require some form of global mediation and hence international peace – we lose the candle. So we cannot let the issue go – we have to in the interests of our own survival – create systems of globalisation that will gradually *decrease* the global health equity gap.

For this, the TINA philosophy will not work. We only have to ask the question: Since the purpose of competition is to identify and honour *inequity*, how on earth could it be used to bring about *equity*?

NEOLIBERALISM AS SOCIAL EVOLUTION?

While neoliberalism apologists are ready to admit that neoliberalism is certainly 'unequal', in that it rewards the successful to the detriment of the failures, this is a good self-regulating process that should not be tampered with. The old 'keep government out of economics' argument is only a logical form of social Darwinism. We are *not* all born equal, they claim, for some are clever and some conspicuously less so, some are rich, some poor, some are physically strong and others physically disabled in various ways, etc.

The religion of neoliberalism holds out as one of its articles of faith that we interfere with this at our moral and social peril. We should stand by and let something akin to natural selection make the decisions. Again, this ignores the entire anthropological reason for the evolution of 'government'. It evolved as a means of guaranteeing the greatest good to the greatest number, thereby optimising the survival of the *community*. The 'naked struggle' model leads inevitably to the dominance of a few, or maybe even only one, and the derogation of the many. It operates *against* community survival.

THE BENEFITS TRICKLE DOWN!

A commonly expressed neoliberal answer to this is expressed in the idea of the 'trickle-down' effect. In theory, this works as follows. If one individual (or a small group) suddenly become much richer than the rest of the community, this – by definition – distorts any trend toward equity in that community. But this is not for long, and we should applaud the success of those 'winners', because they still need their community. Their exalted economic status means, for instance, that they need workers to run their estates and builders, architects, mechanics and engineers to build and service the complex infrastructure required by all that wealth to sustain itself. Therefore, everyone will eventually benefit as the rich few spend their money.

There are many obvious things wrong with the 'trickle-down effect' argument. For one thing, in real life, such winners often do *not* spend the money in the community in which they gained it, but salt it away in investments abroad. Indeed, it is not at all unknown for an inordinately wealthy individual to cut him or herself off from the community altogether and to make minimal use of the community's resources and do everything they can to alienate themselves from it.

Modern 'democratic' governments adopt a middle-of-the-road approach by taxing citizens according to how much they earn, so that the rich pay more than the poor, but the taxes so collected are used to run social services from which each member of the community benefits and to which he or she has access as required.

Under neoliberal auspices, the tax systems in the major democracies are not particularly 'transparent' and only *partly* progressive – with the rich paying more in tax than the poor. However, this is not at all proportionate, with the less well-off paying a higher proportion of their meagre income back in taxes while the well-off pay a lower proportion. But this is neoliberalism and it will – if unimpeded – become *much* worse. For increasingly our governments are privatising such social services as health, so that the less wealthy are not only having their income depleted at a higher rate than are those further up the scale, but they are also finding themselves increasingly excluded from social services which the more well-off can more easily afford. In this way, neoliberalism inexorably continues to divide our societies rather than to draw them together.

EQUITY, HEALTH AND HAPPINESS

As was certainly anticipated by the WHO in its 1978 Alma-Ata Declaration, the health of a community is much less determined by individual biomedical profiles of each of its citizens than it is by a matrix of such non-clinical measures as: sense of security with respect to employment, housing, etc., job satisfaction and social involvement.[7] Since 1978 we have received increasing empirical evidence of this, strongly suggesting that public health certainly has biomedical reference criteria, but is primarily an 'economic' and/or 'political' issue.

Large numbers of sociological studies have shown that not only do personal happiness and social confidence positively correlate with clinical health, but that the higher the level of monetary equity within a society, the higher will be its measures of health (including lower morbidity and mortality), happiness and sources of involvement in the community.[8]

HEIGHT AND HEALTH

John de Graaf's article, just cited, not only amplifies on that evidence, but also points out another interesting statistic based on adult human body height. Every society, whatever its ethnicity or state of wealth, includes people of a wide range of body heights. But the *average* height of a group is regarded in public health and epidemiology circles as a powerful indicator of the health status of that group as a whole. It indicates, for instance, how well its infants have been looked after.

This fits in with figures released by UNICEF – figures that show that the Danes and the Dutch are the healthiest societies, with the greatest average adult heights and, moreover, with the highest levels of sense of satisfaction. In this respect, how has the USA fared since neoliberalism gradually assumed hegemony over its natural life and social values system during the years 1950–2000?

Fifty years ago, Americans were the world's tallest people. But, since 2000, US citizens are shorter (on average) than most Europeans – and more than 2 inches (5 cm) shorter than those Dutch and Danes! In other words, in every European country the people have been growing faster than have the people in the USA. In fact, it gets worse, for, in February 2006, UNICEF released figures (quoted in de Graaf's article) ranking the USA 21st (out of 22 nations) with respect to provision of child welfare. The point hardly needs elaborating further.

What does it all mean with respect to whether or not neoliberalism is good for health? The answer is probably best summed up by that pithy comment – apparently made by Bill Clinton in the 1992 presidential campaign: 'It's the economy, stupid!'

HEALTH OF AMERICANS VS. NEOLIBERALISM

The rôle of neoliberalism as having a deleterious impact on the health of individuals and communities becomes absolutely clear if we take a quick look at the changes in US health statistics generally as it has become more involved with neoliberalism.

For most of the past 35 years, the United States has pursued an ideologically driven economic strategy markedly different from that of nearly all western European nations. From 1932 until 1972, the United States used government policies to increase economic opportunities for the poor, the middle-class, women and minorities. Wages kept pace with increases in productivity.

But since then, and especially since Ronald Reagan declared that 'government cannot be the solution because government is the problem', they have followed a different path, toward what has sometimes been described as 'market fundamentalism.' Increasingly, in the name of 'personal responsibility', US policies require more and more Americans to provide privately for their own economic security. For most of them, the 'ownership society' has emphasised privatisation and deregulation, but huge tax cuts for the already wealthy and of those heroes of 'wealth creation' have, in effect, penalised ordinary working people. To the average US citizen it is a message from their government that this is now a 'you are on your own society. Your problems are not ours!'

To rub salt into their wounds, their leader, President Bush, tells them that they need to do better – produce more for less pay and, above all, not grumble about tax cuts for the wealthy because it is they who make the country rich.

AND IN EUROPE?

Let us contrast this with the same time span in the northern European countries. Most of those countries since the end of World War Two have had generally liberal democratic social contract forms of government. This has been based on the assumption that markets must not be allowed to create social anarchy by running amok, but must come under strong social control through government.

For the system to work effectively in the public interest, the government must play a dominant and proactive rôle and be guided by clearly defined rules protecting consumers, employees and public health. Up until 2004, European country governments continued to strengthen social links/nets protecting the less able, offering improved unemployment compensation and better training for alternative work, old age pensions and – of course – systems of universal healthcare.

Why does the author mention the year 2004? Because since then neoliberalism's grip on the EU countries has become much stronger, rendering it difficult – illegal, in some instances – for EU countries to have normal trading relations with Cuba, for example, or to provide support for the people in the Gaza Strip of occupied Palestine or to do almost anything not completely in line with current US foreign policy.

The 'Empire' is inordinately resourceful and always seems to fight back when communities try to thwart its onward progress to global domination. But that is precisely what we must do if we are to achieve our aim of decreasing the global health inequity gap. And this brings us back to the rhetorical question raised earlier in this discussion: What are governments for, if not to protect their citizens from anarchy? One answer is that governments can organise an economy relevant to the needs of their people's security. And, in that context, we address the phenomenon of 'natural monopoly'.

NATIONAL MONOPOLIES – HOW AND WHY?

Basic to the idea of a government designed to shelter its citizens and to allow them to work together effectively has been the establishment of 'public services'. These are generally massive bureaucracies, some larger, wealthier and more powerful than entire governments elsewhere. The NHS in the UK, for instance, is such a body. It alone accounts for a significant proportion of all pharmaceutical purchases worldwide.

In terms of economic theory, a 'national monopoly' is said to exist when the minimum size to guarantee maximum economic efficiency is equal to the actual size of the market. To make this idea more understandable, consider an ordinary private company. It has to be of a certain minimum size before it can realise sufficient economics of scale to provide the best service to its customers at the lowest possible price. The 'best service' criterion has to be realised if the customers are not to drift away to a more efficient company. And the 'lowest price' criterion is necessary to prevent other companies from attracting its clients.

Public services, as well, require such enormous financial outlays at the outset (e.g. miles and miles of railway track, etc.), and this tends to cut down bidding competition. It is for this reason that public monopolies were the best solutions for these things. However, as we have seen, the confirmed convert to neoliberalism defines anything publicly owned, as opposed to privately owned, as 'inefficient'.

In that case, what happens when a public service – a natural monopoly – is privatised? The new owners are not 'public service' minded and they, and their stockholders, want fast profits. They have to impose monopoly prices on the public but – as well – make a big profit for themselves. In classical economic theory, this state of affairs would be called 'structural market failure' – because the price per item had gone up while the quality of the service had usually taken a nose-dive.

The reader will recall that 1980–85 was a pivotal time in the WHO's encounter with neoliberalism. First, of course, and as expressed in the Alma-Ata Declaration, 'health' is very much a 'political' issue, but as the majesty of that grand realisation began to fire the minds of progressive thinking, in the WHO and in the wider community, too, that logic was not lost on the neoliberals. They quickly realised that health could efficiently be 'mortgaged' very profitably in the process of gaining economic control over trade and trading infrastructures through SAPs imposed on development loans.

MORAL AND FINANCIAL ASCENDANCY OF NEOLIBERALISM

Back home, in the First World, it is therefore not surprising that the neoliberalists were anxious to apply these insights to First World contexts. Thus, starting in the early 1980s and accelerating its forward thrust to the present day, many of the segments of former social services in European countries – such as postal services, telephones, bus lines, railway systems, universities, schools – and now even primary schools – became privatised.

In the USA, the situation was not as dramatic. Neoliberalism was more easily implemented there because the private profit ethic had had a longer interaction with ordinary people and the 'community services' had never been under as much government control as they had in Europe. But in Britain, under Prime Minister Margaret Thatcher, neoliberalism came to life in a quasi-philosophic-religious sense that took masses of the electorate along with her.

In this author's view it simply is incomprehensible that in a nation like Britain, with an internationally respected health service and the NHS taken for granted as virtually unassailable, that that entire edifice of rationality and certainty should be shaken on the basis of financial considerations alone. Neoliberalism would doubtless have gained influence in the UK, as it is now doing throughout the EU, but without Margaret Thatcher it probably would not have attracted the fervent (and there is no other word for it!) mass appeal that it did. She was to neoliberalism as Saint Paul was to Christianity. The author lived in Britain during a good part of the 1980s and was amazed at the eagerness with which ordinary working people participated in the destruction of their own welfare state.

The phrase 'private enterprise' was popularly invoked, not as some arid or academic descriptor, but as something deeply spiritual, like being 'born again'.

Under the hypnotic influence of this embrace of the 'free market', crowds stood by transfixed by its splendour and majesty, as money was shifted by one law after another from 'social' to 'private' control and the adoring poor found themselves increasingly beguiled into making sacrifices for the good of the rich. It was nothing less than a wholesale change of long-cherished social values. One of Thatcher's most powerful tools in giving neoliberalism this degree of social leverage was her use of privatisation to isolate and smash the trade unions.

UNDERMINING THE UNIONS

The union movement was strongest in the public sector and she began her attack there. Between 1989 and 1994, the number of public sector posts dropped from more than seven million to five million, a decline of nearly 30%.[9] Almost all of these eliminated posts had been unionised. During that period, altogether 1.7 million jobs were lost in Britain. In neoliberal terms, however, this was regarded as a positive achievement because the fewer people there were employed, the fewer would be the demands made on shareholders' profits!

Mass privatisation also produced enormous profits for the corporations at source, even before it became general, in that the former managers of the newly privatised utilities, railways, whatever, took two- and even three-fold increases (if not more) in salary. The government (before selling off such an enterprise) used taxpayers' money to wipe out any outstanding debts and to recapitalise the enterprise. Just to give one example, the water authority was granted five billion pounds of debt relief plus 1.6 billion pounds just to make the deal more attractive to potential purchasers.[10] The whole ball game was avidly promoted by the media as a 'democratisation' process, enabling humble people to become stockholders. And, as well, the unions were vilified in much of the media as having been responsible for delaying access to the 'personal freedom' now finally enjoyed by a liberated people. The joy! The power! The freedom! Long live private ownership and blessed freedom from the dead hand of government!

IMMEDIATE IMPACTS OF NEOLIBERALISM IN THE UK

About nine million UK citizens bought shares and it was all a hugely popular topic of conversation. It reminded the author of the euphoria that greeted the start of the National Lottery later in British history. Most of these new stockholders quickly sold off their purchases while big profits thereby were to be made. This was very wise of them, as the values again fell. And, as most readers will recall, it happened to one utility or service after another.

More cautious or thoughtful people did raise the question as to what the real aim of such privatisations were. Were they to prompt economic efficiency, for instance, or improved services to the public? Whatever, the real and immediate effect was to transfer even more money from the pockets of the overtaxed and from public services into the hands of private finance. By the beginning of the second millennium, we note that most of these shares were safely in the hands – and overseas accounts – of large financial institutions and a few very wealthy individual investors.

In her account, Susan George – cited above – tells us that the employees of British Telecom bought up only 1% of the shares, while those of British Aerospace took up only 1.3%. And there were many similar examples. But it all marked a change to what had before been the prevailing pattern. Before Margaret Thatcher and her hatchet-wielding privatisations were let loose on the economy, the public sector in the UK had been profitable, on the whole. Thus, in 1989 public companies gained in excess of seven billion pounds for the UK Treasury – and this money under the more rational conditions then prevalent would have made its way into various social and community outreaches of 'big government'. But under the new dispensation of neoliberalism, much of that money was diverted to private shareholders. As is now (in 2008) widely appreciated, the people of Britain have experienced a general and noticeable decline in many of those former public services now that they are in private hands.

THE BRITISH DISEASE BECOMES GLOBAL

In many ways, Margaret Thatcher had used the UK economy as a guinea pig for neoliberal economic control. In keeping with its name, the Adam Smith Institute in London had been Thatcher's mentor and partner in creating a 'privatised' society, in which people were being encouraged to forget about community values and to find their satisfaction in self-gratification. 'Personal authenticity' became a catch word that rendered selfishness intellectually respectable.

The World Bank quickly joined in the act and soon used Adam Smith experts to promote the 'privatisation ethic' in the Third World countries. By 1991, the World Bank (largely through the IMF) had made more than 100 development loans to accelerate the rate of privatisation of various (usually health and education) services in some of the desperate less developed countries (LDCs). Since then, in its annual reports, the World Bank has shown a steady increase in the number, variety and geographical spread of privatisation initiatives in country development projects.

This author's experience, though, has been such as to recognise many of these programmes as having had disastrous impacts on the health of individual communities and people and as only further widening the global health inequity gap.

GETTING THE WORKERS TO AID THEIR BOSSES

As we have already seen, neoliberalism takes the view that governments prevent or stifle the exercise of market forces and that, in this respect, such organisations as trade unions are complicit in this because they restrict private companies in the way that the latter use labour. Neoliberalism has vigorously promoted mechanisms that remove wealth from the bottom of the social ladder and shift it to the top. In the UK, for instance – and we shall deal with the USA below – if one is in the top 20% of the income scale, one tends to gain from a neoliberal administration. Below that, one loses more and more prodigiously the further down the income scale one goes. Within that top 20%, the degree to which one profits rises sharply as one moves up the social ladder. With that in mind, let us now look at the situation in the USA, where that same 20:80 ratio also generally holds sway.

THE USA'S DALLIANCE WITH NEOLIBERALISM

As Prime Minister Thatcher was the prophet of neoliberalism in the UK, President Ronald Reagan was its eager acolyte in the USA. Almost parallel with what had happened in Britain, under Reagan's administration in the USA, the national income distribution changed consistently and dramatically from, say, 1978 to 1988. In Britain, the reader will recall, the Adam Smith Institute had been the beacon signalling that change, but in the USA it was the already mentioned Heritage Foundation.[11]

THE HERITAGE FOUNDATION

Like the Adam Smith Institute, the Heritage Foundation represents a deeply conservative viewpoint and its main function is to promote the need to get 'government' out of as much of American life as possible. It perceives 'government', and such bodies as trade unions, as having been established to imperil the freedom of the individual and the full flowering of the 'American Way of Life'. If anything, it tends to be much more doctrinaire and right wing than the Adam Smith Institute.

The Heritage Foundation played a very important rôle in promoting 'Reagonomics': loyalty to American values, privatisation and neoliberalism. It was instrumental in bringing about the following dramatic changes to life in the USA. From 1980 to 90, the top 10% of the American income distribution *increased* their average family income by 16%, while among the top 5%, incomes rose by 23%. The incomes of the top 1% increased by 50%. The annual income of that latter group rose from an already $270 000 up to $405 000. What happened to poorer US citizens? We already know that the bottom 80% (or all but the richest 20%) *lost* comparatively, but even this loss was not 'progressive'. The poorer you already were, the even poorer you became! In fact, the lowest 10% of American earners suffered a *further* reduction of 15%. Nothing this radical had happened in the UK, partly because the trade union tradition had been much stronger there at the outset of these events.

In 1997, the richest 1% of American families had 65 times as much as the bottom 10%. By 1988, a decade of neoliberalism later, the richest 1% were 115 times wealthier than the bottom 10%! As most readers can appreciate, especially in a society that has no national health service, such statistics are reflected in huge health inequities within the USA. There are two main government-run agencies in the USA that try to prevent some of the grossest impacts of such an iniquitous system, namely Medicaid and Medicare.

Medicaid is a publicly funded scheme that provides *some* of the medical costs of people below the poverty line, while Medicare is a similar scheme for those over 65 years of age. Neither scheme is in any way comprehensive and, to be sure of anywhere near adequate cover – especially for families – one has to take out private health insurance. However, private health insurance is a large and highly lucrative arena of business on its own and even a patchy sort of health insurance costs so much in premiums that about 31% of US citizens cannot afford it at all. Those people simply have to pray that they don't fall ill.

The effect is that many people who *do* fall ill merely stagger on at work, trying to make ends meet. When this author was in South Carolina in 1969, he saw spectacular examples of neglected medical needs in both children and adults and the same was true in northern California from 1962 to 1969. There exists more variation in health status in the USA than in any other developed nation.

THE PSYCHOLOGICAL HEALTH OF A DIVIDED SOCIETY

Discussion of the availability of 'healthcare' for different levels of US society leaves out the fact that a 'society' only remains recognisable as such if all of its members bear a broadly similar relationship to its institutions, means of production, housing patterns, etc. But this becomes increasingly difficult in the modern USA, where various economic sub-groups of the population diverge more widely from one another.

When the author was living in the US in the 1960s, this psychological divide was present but nowhere near to the same degree that it is now – and that is due to the relatively unchecked growth of neoliberalism in the consumer society. Until the impact of the credit crunch (in 2007) began to make itself felt, many citizens of the US had been living in a sort of 'never-never-land' where, if one did not have the cash for some 'must have' consumer item, possession of a credit card could defer the 'Home Economics Judgement Day' for a few months.

Credit cards were ridiculously easy to get, as banks and other corporate agencies chased quick profits. Of course, the people lower down the social/economic ladder have been hit the hardest, but at all levels people are left picking up the pieces of shattered dreams and asking why the government let it get to that level. Partly, of course, it was because millions of Americans had been involved for

25 years in making government as small and unobtrusive as possible while they fell hook, line and sinker for the neoliberal 'virtues' of individualism, unfettered choice and privatisation.

The psychological divide has split the people up in such a way, and so deeply, that in many cases, and especially when confronted with difficulties, communities have forgotten how to behave as such. A particularly poignant (and shocking) recent example has been provided by the tragedy arising in Louisiana – especially New Orleans – from the aftermath of the 2006 Hurricane Katrina.

On the one hand, the psychological divide there, arising from wealth discrepancies and race, led to a far higher incidence of illness than would have been the case had the community acted in concert. On the other hand, that same sense of social loss and alienation resulted in a very high incidence of mental illness.

Communities are easily beguiled by propaganda and consumerist incentives to split up and cluster at differing levels of the socio-economic scale (the sort of effect that neoliberalism encourages), but find it almost impossibly difficult to reunite. In 2006, while involved with a reconciliation programme in Bosnia, the author witnessed this at first hand and was told by many that the communities could never be healed. So it does not only happen in the United States.

But the USA, despite its financial wealth and power, is disadvantaged by the fact that, even before neoliberalism became a dominant social force, it was the most unequal society in the First World, so in many ways it constituted an almost natural cradle for neoliberalism. Its entire 'white' history – going from the first contacts of the Europeans with it – produced the ideal context for the idea. This becomes most relevant when we look at the European countries and even further abroad.

SETTING THE STAGE FOR GLOBAL NEOLIBERALISM

Some claim that in almost all countries there has been an increase in inequities and this has been paralleled by the growing influence of neoliberalism in those countries.[12] In 1997, the UN Conference on Trade and Development (UNCTAD) produced an impressive body of evidence to this effect. The reader is reminded that UNCTAD emerged in 1965 when – as the author has explained in a previous book – a group of 77 of the most economically disadvantaged nations had applied pressure on the UN to address their grievances more coherently.[13] The UN responded by establishing UNCTAD. The context was critical because, back then, the Vietnam War was in full swing and things were starting to go seriously badly for the USA. The world was, at that time, ideologically divided between Soviet spheres of influence and US spheres of influence, and the countries of the Third World were eyed by each side as potential avenues for extending superpower global influence.

The UNCTAD study of 1997, which itself was based on some 2600 separate studies of income inequities, showed that most had involved an erosion of community and social unity of purpose in favour of private developments. These trends were found not only in Western-oriented societies, like the Philippines, but across the whole spectrum – China, South East Asia, Russia and a variety of once communist/socialist countries.

What, then, is this almost lethal enchantment of the neoliberal siren call as the poor old world tries to manoeuvre a way between Scylla and Charybdis? This author would be more surprised, though, if it were otherwise, because neoliberal policies are specifically designed to give the (possibly beleaguered) rich even more wealth and hence power. This is classically achieved in two ways: decreasing taxes at the upper end of the income spectrum and reducing wages for workers at the lower end of the income scale. It seems an unbeatable formula!

NON-DOMS AND THE TRICKLE-DOWN PRINCIPLE

Arguments used to support such policies are almost all variations on the 'trickle-down' theory alluded to previously. These can be given a more sophisticated ring by arguing that higher incomes for the rich and higher untaxed profits for them will lead to more investment. This, the theory goes, will lead to a more efficient allocation of the nation's resources and hence more jobs and money for all. It is an amazingly powerful argument, presently being played out in Britain in tabloid articles about the 'Non-Doms'.

The 'Non-Doms' are people who run hugely profitable businesses in the UK but do not spend sufficient time in the country to count as 'residents'. They are British citizens but pay no taxes – either to the UK authorities or elsewhere – on their externally garnered wealth.

Probably most British taxpayers did not even know of Non-Doms, but once they had been identified, droves of overtaxed and underpaid British citizens began to call for these Non-Doms to be taxed. The justice of their argument, and the legitimacy of their grievance, would seem unanswerable, but neoliberalism is not that easily side-tracked. The media have been assiduously promoting an argument along the following lines. These people are enriching Britain (despite the fact that most of the money gets invested abroad in safe tax havens). If we complain, we might frighten them off. In fact, many of them have openly stated, 'If you threaten to tax us, we will move elsewhere.' Our leaders advise us to 'be realistic'. If we increase taxes on the rich, they will leave – and where would we be if dear old Blighty could no longer attract such clever people to live here and exercise their phenomenal 'wealth creation' skills?

But the logic behind the 'trickle-down' argument (of which the UK government's view of the Non-Dom issue is but one more variation) does not hold up and has already led us into some serious economic and financial disasters. The effect of shifting money up the income ladder has led to a number of the recent 'stock market bubbles' (recall the ones in the information technology industry in 2006), accumulation of wealth (at least on paper) for a few, but banking and other financial crises for most.

Let us look at it the other way up. Suppose that, instead of shifting money up, we shift it down to that lower 80% of the income ladder – and the lower the better. Of course, some of those Non-Doms may leave, shaking the British dust off their shoes as they do, but not all of them will. Money that thus goes downscale will be spent on foodstuffs, schooling, etc., and these will create employment and – unlike money aimed at the top 20% – it probably would not be invested abroad. It would generally be spent quickly and locally, where most of it was derived in the first place, and where the people need it.

GLOBAL NEOLIBERALISM AND HEALTH

Globally neoliberalism works in the same general way, making use of SAPs on IMF and World Bank loans and WTO regulations. Particularly powerful instruments in this regard have been the General Agreement on Tariffs and Trade (GATT) and – more sinisterly – the General Agreement on Trade in Services (GATS). These, as the reader probably knows, are the result of agreements concluded at the annual World Trade Organization (WTO) meetings, and they are designed to create conditions favourable to unrestricted free trade.[14] To sustain this level of free trade, of course, international banking transfer arrangements have been established.

The idea of the GATT was seen by some of its original proponents in much the same light as the views put forward by Keynes at Bretton Woods. Keynes' suggestion was for the establishment of an international body to mediate and regulate trade in such a way as to create a more equitable system for the poorer nations. This, as the reader probably knows, was strongly opposed by the USA, which saw it as potentially restricting its future global trading outreach. In fact, though, the GATT has aggressively pursued a very different rôle. Instead, it promotes conditionalities that enhance the power of First World neoliberal interests over those of many poorer nations. In that respect it can be seen as serving the needs of the WTO.

But these 'arrangements', and even full details of GATT and GATS operations, are not easily accessible to ordinary scrutiny. They are far from 'transparent' – a term beloved of modern politicians! But neoliberalism probably would never have become as dominant and as powerful as it is has if masses of people – especially those adversely affected by it – had known what was going on. Indeed, the philosophy of neoliberalism is that the 'economy' (as defined by the financial needs of its corporate interests) must impose its rules on society – and *not* the other way round. In other words 'democracy' is an obstacle, a barrier to the operation of neoliberalism. Neoliberalism is a philosophy for the 'winners' – not for whinging losers. Its constituency is only the top 20% of the income distribution.

From all of the above, what can we conclude first of all about neoliberalism itself and secondly about its rôle in the global health rights agenda? Neoliberalism is certainly *not* the expression of 'natural human nature'. The survival of the human race depends on cooperation much more than on competition. The latter is of fundamental value in certain 'closed' areas of social endeavour – say, in selecting players for a football team or for a string orchestra. But whenever it becomes a general governing principle in a society, it leads to anarchy, alienation, the break-down of trust and – ultimately – the collapse of society. A healthy society draws on the talent of all of its members and hence the steps it takes to protect the weakest of those members is a measure of its social strength and integrity. Competition would wipe out the weaker elements – not support them.

Thus, people in a healthy society are mindful of the human rights of all of its members. They are compassionate, open, relaxed in the company of others, positive and altruistic. These attitudes create the social health on which physical health depends. Neoliberalism undercuts physical and mental health and is ever ready to mortgage it for the financial advantages of a few. Hence, it cannot possibly be the governing principle in a world intent on closing the global health inequity gap – a world intent on survival rather than on death.

REFERENCES

1 Smith K, Edwards R. The year of global food crisis. *Glasgow Sunday Herald*. 15 Apr 2008. Available at: www.sundayherald.com/news/heraldnews/display.varr.2104849 (accessed 3 May 2008).

2 MacDonald T. *Health, Human Rights and the United Nations: inconsistent aims and inherent contradictions*. Oxford & New York: Radcliffe Publishing; 2006. pp. 16–18.

3 MacDonald T. *Sacrificing the WHO to the Highest Bidder*. Oxford & New York: Radcliffe Publishing; 2008. pp. 28–33.

4 MacDonald T. *The Global Human Right to Health: dream or possibility?* Oxford & New York: Radcliffe Publishing; 2007. pp. 22, 60–2.

5 Macmillan H. The wind of change. Speech delivered by the British Prime Minister, Harold Macmillan, to the South African Parliament. 3 Feb 1960. Available at: http://africanhistory.about.com/ed/eraindependence/a/wind (accessed 15 Apr 2008).

6 Edsitement. *Rudyard Kipling's Riki Tiki Tavi: mixing fact and fiction*. Available at: http://edsitement.neh.gov/view_lesson_plan.asp?id=584 (accessed 1 Feb 2008).

7 World Health Organization. *The Alma-Ata Declaration*. Available at: www.euro.who.int/aboutWHO (accessed 1 Feb 2008).

8 De Graaf J. *The Good ($) Life: what's the economy for, anyway?* Available at: http://seattle.consciouschoice.com/2007/09/thegoodlife0709.hmtl (accessed 2 Mar 2008).

9 Prowse P, Prowse J. A public sector model of employment in the United Kingdom. *Int J Public Sect Manage.* 2007; **20**: 42–62.

10 George S. *A Short History of Neo-liberalism.* Available at: www.globalexchange.org/campaigns/econ101/neoliberalism.htm (accessed 2 Mar 2008).

11 Heritage Foundation. Heritage Foundation official website. Available at: www.heritage.org (accessed 2 March 2008).

12 *A Short History of Neo-liberalism*, op. cit. p. 5.

13 *The Global Human Right to Health: dream or possibility?*, op. cit. p. 26

14 MacDonald T. *Health, Trade and Human Rights.* Oxford & New York: Radcliffe Publishing; 2006. pp. 26–7.

Chapter 2

Setting an optimum context for global control

COINCIDENCE OR DESIGN?

Those of us who have worked in Third World milieux over the last half century or so cannot have failed to notice a changing pattern of exploitation of the Third World by the First. In what at first seems to be a coincidence, many of these changes seem to relate to what could be considered unrelated events, such as immense natural disasters or radical shifts in politics. As an example, call to mind the tsunami of December 2004. Vast amounts of material damage and loss of human life occurred and, in a worldwide display of altruism, millions of pounds were raised from contributions by ordinary people, as well as by various governments. For a few weeks, a good feeling about our generous aid infused the First World. But it was not long before the event lost its news value and the media switched to other matters. However, what happened to all of those poor fishermen who had lost their boats, their huts close to the beaches, all of their equipment and often their families?

Millions of pounds had been raised after all, so one might suppose that their very basic resources were restored and they could get back to scraping out a subsistence living as before – but perhaps living in a stronger hut and fishing from a better boat. But no, anyone who has visited the affected areas in Indonesia, Sri Lanka, etc., will have noticed that the beaches have been cleared and an accelerated programme of hotel building, etc., has been undertaken.

The real victims have been forgotten and their misfortune turned to great profit by local entrepreneurs and the major First World banks extending 'development' loans through the IMF and World Bank. No one is suggesting that transnational corporate financial interests had somehow organised the tsunami so that they could make a profit out of it, but they were certainly ready and equipped to seize the opportunity when it arose. And likewise, the ever-compliant IMF and World Bank were ready to make those substantial 'development' loans to the governments concerned, which would, in turn, greatly enrich shareholders in the First World. There is nothing quite as good as being around and ready when disaster strikes to be able to milk it efficiently for profit. Of course, it also helps if masses of private individuals and government agencies have also been lavish in providing funds to initially prime the pumps of enterprise.

Then again, some 'natural' disasters seemed that bit more ready-made and calculated to give the profiteers a free hand. Take for instance Hurricane Katrina (2006) and the breaching of the levees in New Orleans. Meteorologists were unanimously agreed that it was a disaster waiting to happen and that it was only a matter of time before cataclysm struck. It was known that catastrophe could only be prevented by strengthening the levees and raising them. But the job was never undertaken. The poorest of the poor tended to live in the more vulnerable areas and the prophets of doom were not proved wrong when the flooding occurred. All government agencies at all levels were astonishingly slow to act and hundreds of thousands of poor (mainly black) people found themselves flooded out and their homes and modest livelihoods destroyed. Moreover, they had nowhere to go while they waited for the floods to subside. They were accommodated in refugee-style camps, many even out of state and far from 'home'. As I write these lines, a full two years or more after Hurricane Katrina, many of those displaced people have still not been able to resume a normal working life free of institutionalised 'care'. Poverty, family breakdowns, violence and degradation still characterise the lot of many of those displaced people.

But there has been no lack of money. Aid flowed even more quickly and plentifully than it had for the 2004 tsunami. Again, somehow, the money missed the victims, most of it directed to tearing down the wrecked slums and replacing them with safe flood-protected business offices and expensive apartments which only a much wealthier class of people could occupy. As with the victims of the tsunami in Indonesia, Sri Lanka and elsewhere, the victims of Hurricane Katrina have not – in the main – experienced much in the way of financial resolution. Other, already well-to-do people now profit from their disaster. Money came forward and governments rushed in to help, but somehow the funds bypassed the losers and instead fattened the bank accounts of those who didn't need it.

Obviously, natural disasters have the propensity to exacerbate existing levels of poverty, but since the 1980s the corporate interests, working hand-in-glove with the major First World banks, and relying on the IMF and World Bank Structural

Adjustment Policies (SAPs) to provide mechanisms for insuring that profits on their loans are generated, have done very well out of natural disasters. As well, they have increased the scope and power of neoliberal financial initiatives.

There are various ways of looking at these phenomena. Some would argue that neoliberalism has arisen in response to such vicissitudes as natural disasters and has solved them. Others would assert that neoliberal agencies have *used* such natural disasters to further entrench corporate power and, in doing so, have ineluctably widened the inequity gap.

THE ENVIRONMENTAL CRISIS AND NEOLIBERALISM

Part of the inequity gap is apparent in the environmental crisis confronting us all, but especially the poor. The environmental crisis is undoubtedly increasing global inequities in health, but what has been its impact on neoliberalism?

Here we run across similar convenient coincidences between corporate profits and environmental degradation. The more acute the environmental crisis is perceived to be, the greater the opportunity for huge short-term corporate profits to be made. For instance, as we desperately cast about for more carbon-free methods of creating energy, we are confronted with two broad choices: exploiting sustainable, energy sources (wind and solar power, wave power, geothermal energy, etc.) or 'going nuclear'. The only one of these of any interest to neoliberal agencies is nuclear. The nuclear option is expensive to set up and really isn't even all that 'sustainable', because there is only a finite supply of uranium. It also presents the as yet unresolved problem of how to safely decommission nuclear reactors once they are no longer needed. And the ambient temperature of seawater off coasts on which nuclear power plants are sited is affected adversely by water run-off from the reactors and this, in turn, adversely affects marine ecology. There are other obvious objections, such as that nuclear reactors would constitute ideal military targets for potential enemies, but leaving such concerns aside, there are great profits to be made by the nuclear industry and financial corporative banking – *and* they are carbon emission-free.

Again, one wonders about coincidence here. Almost all First World governments strongly favour the nuclear option and their media busy themselves relentlessly in arguing the negative side of truly sustainable sources of energy. For instance, we are constantly being told how visually unappealing ranks of wind turbines would be. As though any rational person is going to weigh that equally with problems such as how to dispose safely of spent nuclear rods! But it is promoted almost daily as an argument against wind turbines. Is this author merely being perverse in finding the forests of wind turbines in Denmark and Germany rather aesthetically pleasing? Again, just in case people cannot really be made to appreciate that wind turbines are inherently ugly and the hum they produce more annoying than traffic and aircraft uproar, we are told that sometimes migratory birds fly into them, so they represent an environmental hazard.

Really? But is it not strange that tall buildings rarely attract the same concern? When the Empire State Building was built in New York, for several years afterwards it regularly took a huge toll of migrating song birds, but now it hardly affects any. The birds learned to vary their route to avoid it. Such objections, of course, are rationalisations by government agencies against the research and enterprise necessary as a preliminary to exploiting wind, wave, sun, etc. Why? Because there is not much money to be earned by corporate power in such enterprises.

POLITICAL UNREST AND PROFITS

It is noticeable that from about 1985 until the present day, the growth of political unrest and of corporate power as expressed through globalised finance have been increasing in tandem. How much of this is coincidence and how much the product of an unhealthy nexus between governments and boardrooms? We have recently been becoming involved in various wars – Iraq, Afghanistan, Liberia, Kosova, etc. Almost all of these have involved an extensive infrastructure of corporate interests greedy for oil, diamonds, banking facilities, whatever, but the rationale for involvement in the conflict is always some high-minded assertion such as the need to defend people's human rights, to protect democracy, etc., even to prevent war! But neoliberalism is always there ready to lend a hand to the IMF and World Bank in making 'reconstruction loans', etc.

This author was particularly shocked by the series of bloody events leading to, and following, the dismemberment of Yugoslavia. Marshal Tito's administration of that large hunk of territory in the middle of Europe constituted an affront to the USSR (especially Stalin) and a growing source of irritation to salivating banks in Western Europe and the US, who could see great profit potential if Yugoslavia could be broken up.

Banking interests in West Germany (as it was then) and in Britain throughout the 1980s were encouraging Croatia to break away and all of this became easier once Marshal Tito was dead, and Serbia likewise aimed for separation under Slobodan Milosevic. CNN and other international media persistently referred to him as the 'Butcher of Belgrade' for conspiring to break up Yugoslavia, but especially after he was elected President of Yugoslavia in 1997. However, it should be noted that he only declared war on a united Yugoslavia *after* Croatia, Slovenia and Bosnia Herzegovina had already declared themselves independent in 1991 and 1992.[1]

There is not much doubt that Milosevic was a most unsavoury, totalitarian and violent character, but it is equally clear that his racist/nationalist views were unleashed by powerful foreign corporate and banking interests intent on preventing a monolithic Yugoslavia from continuing to have the high degree of financial autonomy it had gradually accumulated for its people since steering a path of independence from the old USSR, with its people year on year enjoying a much higher standard of living than elsewhere in the Soviet bloc. Especially after the collapse of the USSR, Yugoslavia represented an impediment to neoliberal financial hegemony over Europe. It was also an exceedingly pleasant place to work or to visit, and – despite the various different ethnic groups – it was characterised by a high degree of inter-ethnic humour and friendliness.

After it had been torn apart by war and robbed of much of its resources and its various ethnic groups had been reduced to mutual mistrust, it was no more the easygoing, friendly and welcoming place it had been. In 2004 I was part of an International Pathways to Reconciliation group which convened meetings for three weeks in Sarajevo. The word 'Sarajevo' in Bosniak means 'open city' and what an appropriate name that was until the early 1990s! Before that ghastly time this author, whenever he was there, would often go with friends to the main square. On one side was a Croatian Catholic church, on another a Bosniak mosque and facing it across the square was a Serbian Orthodox church. No one seemed to pay all that much attention to these ethnic or religious differences and a common source of humour was the fact that the clocks in the respective religious buildings were not synchronised. The Serbian Orthodox clock had a much slower chime than its two colleagues and started striking the midnight hour first and would not finish until the other two had gone silent. But all of that bonhomie had disappeared by 2004. Once jolly, lively and open-minded, Sarajevo was now serious and deeply suspicious. People tended to whisper a few words and then move away; making conversation was difficult.

Most of those I met blamed Milosevic and the Serbs for the overt violence but reflected a deep gut-level mistrust of American or EU banks and businesses. Therefore, once again we encounter a situation in which neoliberal finance creates a conflict and is involved in resolving it – which its advocates are quick to point out is proof of its necessity – and, as well, makes a profit out of the entire enterprise.

The author could cite numerous examples of this almost paradoxical capacity for neoliberalist development not only to parallel political upheaval but to actually benefit from it. But the best theoretical model of what has been described above is Naomi Klein's seminal book *The Shock Doctrine*, which expands on what she has appropriately termed 'disaster capitalism'.[2] By this, she refers to that nexus (alluded to above) between the growth of neoliberal influence and action and 'disaster' (such as natural disasters and wars) that have occurred recently. Her useful model of 'disaster capitalism' is worthy of the reader's attention and can be summarised as follows.

HOW DISASTER CAPITALISM WORKS

Klein argues that neoliberalism represents the counter-revolution (what this author has described previously as 'the Empire striking back') of capital and the fact that it thrives on natural disasters, banking and financial crisis, wars, etc., now occurring with increased frequency and involving more areas of the world. In a new net access journal, *Upping the Anti: a journal of theory and action,* one of that journal's reporters records a recent interview with Klein about her theories. He asked her to define 'disaster capitalism' and she answered:[3]

> Disaster capitalism the way I define it is the use of disaster, or cataclysmic events, they could be economic meltdowns or terrorist attacks or wars or natural disasters, attempts to push through a radical economic program, often a radical capitalist program, usually involving privatisation of state services. Because so much of the state has already been privatised, the last frontiers in the drive to privatise the state are the functions we think of as 'first responder' type functions, like search and rescue, fire, policing, border control, the military. So now we are not only in a situation where disasters are used to advance privatisation but the response to disasters itself is a major new privatisation frontier.
>
> What I mean by the 'shock doctrine' is a philosophy of power that holds that the best time to push through these unpopular neoliberal economic policies is in the aftermath of a shock, precisely because what large scale disasters do is they make us lose our bearings and our narratives. And when we are in a state of shock, we are more vulnerable to political manipulation, so the 'shock doctrine' is the philosophy of power, and 'disaster capitalism' is how it plays out on the ground.

This author's experiences suggest very strongly that her analysis is correct and that there is, indeed, a coherent and strategically targeted ideology of free market fundamentalism (namely neoliberalism) living in anticipation of large-scale disasters that allows it to field its forces efficiently and quickly. As will become clear in subsequent chapters of this book, the 'obstacles' to global health equity which have to be overcome not only *arise* within this context of opportunities, but are directly promoted by corporate power.

The organisational model behind this was indubitably Milton Friedman's doctrine of 'monetarism', which was so eagerly embraced by Margaret Thatcher in her union confrontation programme in the UK and, with even more terrible affect, by Augusto Pinochet in the Chilean counter-revolution.[4] In the latter case, the involvement of corporate financial interests was rendered even more transparent by the rôle of the CIA in funding the truckers strike against the Allende Government, which represented one of the critical events leading to his overthrow.

As Klein describes it, the monetarism idea provided the basis for capitalism to express itself worldwide as 'neoliberalism'. We have already seen, though, that there was nothing particularly 'liberal' about it, nor was it especially 'neo'. For instance, many have been the right-wing spokespeople who have tried to present it as a development of 'freedom' because – by commoditising as many aspects of life as possible – it gives the illusion of 'choices' being made by people. It was a view that was recognisable, after all, in the speeches of Benito Mussolini in the 1930s in Italy through to those of Barry Goldwater in the USA in the 1960s, etc. It has each time been hailed as a localised expression of freedom from such government 'oppression' as progressive tax, support of public services, profit accumulation and rendering healthcare accessible to all of a country's citizens. So Milton Friedman can hardly be credited with having 'invented' it. What he *did* do, though, was to clothe it with academic respectability in economic circles and in the social sciences.

The term 'neoliberalism' helped immensely in this propaganda exercise, and the corporate-owned media have not been slow to promote it as 'realistic' and 'the only real basis of development and progress'. It has provided a progressive-looking cover for IMF- and World Bank-funded 'development' programmes in the Third World – increasingly so since the global oil price crisis of 1973 – that have, in turn, hugely enriched First World banks and corporations and their stockholders, while steadily widening the gaps in health and other human rights inequalities in less-developed countries.

As we shall see, all of the major obstacles which we identify as preventing the achievement of global health equity are sustained by neoliberal financial control.

NEOLIBERALISM AS FINANCIAL COUNTER-REVOLUTION

Klein perceives neoliberalism, moreover, as representing a counter-revolution against Keynesian policies (especially in the First World) and, parallel to it, the development of economic nationalism (especially in the Third World). As such (and as UK governments – both Conservative and New Labour) it opposed gains in trade unions and other workers' groups. This has an important historical reso-nance, especially in the industrialised countries, for such workers' organisations arose in response to the capitalist disaster of the Great Depression of 1929–32. Examined in that light, one can see that neoliberalism is nothing more than an organised response of the moneyed classes against social gains painfully made by post-Depression social developments – union protection, government financing of public services, etc.

Thus, we see in Milton Friedman (and the Chicago School of Economics) the essential bedrock for rallying neoliberal reaction. The social reforms which were alluded to above arose in response to the naked horror of unregulated 'free' trade and competition between the economically powerful and the economically weak, and the popular groundswell of opinion that we need to confront these socially undermining forces and to demand and organise a more humane system. As Klein points out, in many countries people were demanding socialism as a rational response to the financial anarchy of the Great Depression, and these mixed economies of social democracy and Keynesian and grassroots development under local management represented a 'compromise with unregulated capitalism' – a placating sop to the rampant upsurge of left-wing ideologies and forces.

History tells us that, by and large, capitalism won that confrontation and, having emerged as the more subtle and persuasive anti-social force of neoliberalism, it is set to confront social progress again. That is, unless we do something about it! Klein explains it in the following terms.

Monetarism was really the Ground Zero of this counter-revolution, and Klein focuses on Friedman because he was the great populariser of this revolt of the elites. She was not the person who first coined the phrase but it really is rather apt. From the '30s through the '60s there were tremendous gains for workers' protection, growth of very powerful trade unions, the establishment of social pro-grammes, such as public healthcare protection, unemployment programmes and pension systems, and much else of what we think of as the welfare state. This was a period of tremendous economic growth, but it was also a period of redistribution of wealth, along with the rise of the middle class. So what that meant was that even though there was a lot of money being made, there was also a lot of money being redistributed, and the elites, not just in the US but around the world, were clearly tired of how much of what they considered to be their money was being redistributed to their workers and to the rest of society through taxes.

So what is a revolt against the gains that were made in this period, the con-struction of, for lack of a better reference, the welfare state? It represents a counter-revolution against that process. We saw that very clearly in the United States in the 'Reagan Revolution'. A large part of neoliberalism is the privatisation of those aspects of the state that were built up under these mixed economies. In an earlier era of capitalism, it was the enclosing of land and the appropriation of resources, often accompanied by high levels of violence, that fuelled an earlier stage of globalisation. Now we still have that old-school sort of colonialism, but we also have this neo-colonialism, neoliberalism, where it is the state that is the frontier and it is the state that can provide these opportunities for dramatic accumulation of wealth through privatisation.

THE RÔLE OF THE UN IN PROMOTING 'NEOLIBERALISM'

As the author has demonstrated in previous books though, the IMF and the World Bank and the WTO (a closely allied agency in enforcing loan conditionalities), have largely deflected the WHO from its mandate to promote and defend health worldwide in keeping with the UDHR (Universal Declaration of Human Rights), in order to acquiesce with neoliberal financial priorities.[5,6] Klein's concepts of 'shock doctrine' and 'disaster capitalism' endorse these findings and argue how these UN agencies fulfil a substantial rôle in imposing neoliberal policies in Argentina, Mexico, Indonesia and elsewhere. She raises the question: 'To what extent has this involved a planned policy of creating a need by demanding that IMF loans not be spent on such public services as healthcare, so that health disasters accumulate in parallel with structural developments?'

She argues tellingly that the southern core of Latin America (especially Chile), and even elsewhere (e.g. Indonesia), constituted experimental laboratories on which neoliberalism was ruthlessly tried out. Application of the doctrines of the Chicago School of Economics involved privatising everything, including all social security services, medical services and education – often on the basis of a flat, rather than a progressive, system of taxation. Such wholesale carving up of levels of access to what are recognised as 'essential services' (access to which are supposedly basic human rights) creates yawning gaps of social alienation, undermining civil society and creating a more fragile and fragmented sense of community.

In that context, in fact, we cannot really regard it as coincidental that Augusto Pinochet's senior economic advisors were graduates of the University of Chicago, where they came very much under the influence of Milton Friedman. They had been brought to the university on scholarships from the US State Department. It was considered a very extremist school at the time, and they were brought to the University of Chicago as part of an ideological battle, since there was a great concern in the State Department that Latin America was moving to the left and that many of the continent's economists were so-called 'pink-economists'. And so this was a project of ideological imperialism, of trying to interfere with, and indeed successfully interfering with, the intellectual development of the continent.

Thus it was that in this first phase, which would be the late '60s and '70s, neo-liberalism was imposed with blood and fire in Latin America, with no attempt at negotiations. It was US-backed dictators, usually with US-trained economists, in the case of Suharto and with the so-called 'Berkeley Mafia', or of the 'Chicago Boys' in the case of Pinochet. But as the dictatorships fell and as the tolerance for dictatorships around the world waned, and as the rise of the international human rights movement really took root, that's when the rôle of the IMF and the World Bank really took centre stage. In the early '80s one had what in Latin America is often discussed as the transition from military dictatorships to the dictatorship of debt. Countries went through transitions from military rule to democratic rule, but these were negotiated transitions, overwhelmingly. The terms of the transition were negotiated, and again and again it was part of the negotiations that the new governments, the post-dictatorship democracies, would agree to inherit the debts of the regimes that they had just successfully confronted. Not 'overthrown', because if they had been overthrown they would not have needed negotiation or to inherit the debts of their oppressors.

Klein points out that this was happening all over the world in the '80s, and at the same time you had something going on in Washington which was known as the 'Volcker shock', when Paul Volcker was the head of the US Federal Reserve and he dramatically increased interest rates. So at the same time as countries agreed to inherit the debts of their dictators, often very large and illegitimate debts (large amounts of the debts went to corruption and to Swiss bank accounts or buying the weaponry of military rule), the shock came from Washington, the so-called 'Volcker shock', and the effect of this was that these very large debts became unbearable debts overnight. The size of the debt in countries like Brazil or Nigeria just quadrupled in a very short period of time. And so this led to hyperinflation crises and a state of panic, and also it was the dawn of the Structural Adjustment Programme. So while there wasn't direct military rule, this was now the era of the IMF and the World Bank, and these same set of policies of privatisation, deregulation and cuts in government spending came attached to a loan in the context of a debt shock or the debt crisis.

As implied above, Klein's model matches up with the author's view of post-tsunami Sri Lanka. She visited Sri Lanka six months after the disaster. At that time the conflict between the Tamil Tigers and the Government – which had been shelved during and immediately after the disaster – had not yet resumed, but she was made aware, during interviews with academics and politicians, of an impending sense of unease. Remnants of the devastated fishing communities were already becoming highly suspicious about the way that aid money was being allocated. She noted mounting levels of anger and jealousy over the way that financial aid kept somehow missing the intended targets of need. Basically, as suggested by the author at the outset of this chapter, the element of shock and awe had been amply provided by the environment, while the local bankers (with the cooperation of the IMF) provided the 'disaster capitalism' required to keep the enterprise profitable.

DISASTER CAPITALISM APPLIED ELSEWHERE

Iraq provides an excellent example of how disaster capitalism results in the instability necessary to involve relevant UN agencies and international financial agencies, and to impose profit-making neoliberalist methods to protect the First World corporate investments in the area concerned. In the case of Iraq, the rôle of Paul Bremer has been pivotal in the neoliberal chess game. We will therefore allude briefly to his activities as a US diplomat with responsibilities to help restore civil life in post-war Iraq, while also representing corporate interests.

PAUL BREMER'S NEOLIBERAL APPROACH IN IRAQ

Various strategies were adopted by the US after Saddam Hussein's execution to restore civil order and normal 'democratic' (i.e. similar to the US) procedures for electing a government, etc. The man whom the US selected as the first US envoy to the 'new Iraq' in 2003 was Paul Bremer. But his regime quickly became associated with a rather loose accountancy of the billions of dollars of US reconstruction money pouring into Iraq. Certain US-based corporate interests flourished but there was no sustained evidence that Iraq's ruined water and electricity systems – to say nothing of its schooling or health services – were receiving much benefit from all of this money. Damien McElroy, reporting in the Daily Telegraph's net service, summarised his activities as being very much like those of old-style 19th century robber barons.[7]

He described how Bremer structured the reconstruction programmes in such a way that only certain US contractors benefited, while those of the UK (which supposedly had a 'special relationship' with the US) – along with those of all other of the Coalition partners – were completely frozen out. Bremer, of course, was supposed to reflect credit on the credentials of neoliberalism as he took up his post, but it all failed dismally. McElroy describes how expectations were high when Bremer, a protégé moreover of none other than Henry Kissinger, who had been so prominent in establishing a shrine for neoliberalism in Chile, arrived in Iraq to take charge. 'In many ways,' says McElroy, 'Mr Bremer reflected a dashing image in his desert boots and was the perfect figurehead for the ambitious project to transform Iraq.'

Klein, cited above, has been somewhat less optimistic in her analysis and argues that Bremer's rôle represented a perfect example of disaster capitalism. As she points out, in Iraq we know the story, that the 'shock and awe' invasion was used to push through this radical programme of economic shock therapy. As well attested by the media, Paul Bremer came in with cities still burning, and the theory was that Iraqis would be too shocked and focused on the daily emergencies of the war zone to even involve themselves and pay attention to the fact that Bremer was engaging in radical social and economic re-engineering. He was passing a radical new investment law that allowed foreign companies to own 100% of Iraqi assets and take 100% of their profits out; it was described by the *Economist* as the wish list for foreign investors. And in Sri Lanka, Klein learned that only four days after the tsunami hit – and that tsunami killed 40 000 people and displaced almost half a million people and the dead weren't even buried yet – in the capital, Colombo, a bill laying the groundwork for water privatisation was pushed forward. Obviously in this moment the entire attention of the country was focused elsewhere, and here is the most controversial plank of the privatisation agenda, water privatisation, being slipped through when no one is looking. That is a prime example of what Klein means by the 'shock doctrine' and 'disaster capitalism'.

Water privatisation is dealt with more fully as an integral part of neoliberal encroachment on human rights in Chapter 3. But the close link between increasing the scope of neoliberal financial control and a corresponding undermining of health rights is well documented by a report from the International Committee of the Red Cross (ICRC) showing how water privatisation can only threaten health in post-conflict Iraq. The report covered various regions throughout the country and noted the following:[8]

> In Al-Anbar province, west of Iraq, access to Ramadi is very restricted. As a result, food and medical supplies are running low, public services have almost ground to a halt and residents are reportedly trying to flee the area. Most of the city has been without power since 22 May and, owing to the shortage of fuel, back-up generators can only function for one or two hours a day. Consequently, water stations are unable to supply the city's 300,000 inhabitants or its medical facilities with clean water. The crisis is particularly acute owing to the current dry and hot weather.
>
> Through its network of local contractors, the ICRC has now begun delivering 30,000 litres of diesel to Ramadi's main water-treatment plant. This should make it possible to supply the city with water in sufficient quantity for the coming two weeks. On 18 June it also delivered 20,000 bags of drinking water to Ramadi's health authorities for distribution to various medical facilities in the area.
>
> The city of Fallujah, southeast of Ramadi, where access has been strictly controlled for months, is also experiencing acute fuel and power shortages. On 18 June the ICRC managed to deliver 15,000 litres of fuel to the city's two water-treatment plants and the same amount to its sewage-pumping stations.
>
> Sadr City, in Baghdad, has been suffering a chronic water shortage caused by the deficient water network and soaring temperatures. Over the past week, 30,000 litres of water have been dispatched daily by tanker trucks to Imam Ali Hospital, the main medical facility in the area. Moreover, the ICRC has installed four 10,000-litre water tanks to cater for the needs of 3,000 displaced families in sector 53 of Sadr City. These tanks are filled twice a day by tanker trucks.
>
> As a neutral, independent and humanitarian organisation, the ICRC endeavours to mitigate the impact of conflict on the daily life of civilians. In Iraq it is striving, within the limits imposed by security constraints, to respond to emergencies wherever they arise.

Their sombre report concludes that, despite their input – all of it from private contributions to the Red Cross and not from monies allocated through Paul Bremer or the corporate neoliberal resources to which he has access – health is severely undermined in Iraq through failure to get water supplies running.

Both the quantity and quality of drinking water in Iraq remain insufficient despite limited improvements in some areas, mainly in the south. Water is often contaminated owing to the poor repair of sewage and water-supply networks and the discharge of untreated sewage into rivers, which are the main source of drinking water. Electricity and fuel shortages and the poor maintenance of infrastructure mean that there is no regular and reliable supply of clean water and that sewage is often not properly disposed of.

In broader human rights terms then, the situation in Iraq meets all of the criteria of disaster capitalism, in this case based – not on the breakdown of society caused by flood, earthquake or other natural disasters – but on a carefully crafted war that could only strengthen the grip of neoliberalism on Iraq. Not only are its oil resources thus forfeit, but so is the health of its people and the strength of its civic institutions.

Klein's argument is that, in Iraq, we can easily see what the original plan was. It was to use the shock and awe of a sudden and catastrophically destructive invasion to create a corporate-controlled client state, a model free-market economy in the heart of the Middle East, and that obviously failed. But we can see that a new economy has emerged in Iraq, and it wasn't Plan A, but it was perhaps a Plan B, in the sense that the economic project of the war was rigged so that the US couldn't lose. Even if Wal-Mart and McDonald's were not arriving in downtown Baghdad to open up outlets and stores, the worse things are and continue to get in Iraq the more the economy of privatised occupation expands. From the beginning, the invasion and occupation of Iraq was another kind of shock therapy that actually began in the US under Donald Rumsfeld and radical measures to privatise the US military. So as things worsen in Iraq, the more functions private contractors take over and the larger the rôle they perform in the war zone.

NEOLIBERALISM AS A CAUSE OF COMMUNITY FRAGMENTATION

It is very strongly in the Iraqi context that we note another distinguishing feature of neoliberalism – namely its ability to create splits in the community, giving rise to pockets of mutual alienation and thus rendering it less likely and more difficult for people to act collectively to improve their condition. Loss of neighbourly trust decreases the likelihood of collective action. It is all an example of the author's previously enunciated argument that neoliberalism cannot logically represent a solution to increasing global inequity when it – by definition – requires competition to sustain itself.[9]

As we have noticed in Iraq and in many other trouble spots, neoliberalism creates surges of very rapid profits for a few, degradation and despair for many. It is quickly characterised by massive disparities. In fact, this is such a prominent feature of the process that it leads to the creation of the 'gated communities' one sees appearing all over the USA and beginning to appear in the UK, due to the fact that the few privileged beneficiaries of neoliberalism have to physically protect themselves from the large body of deprived 'neighbours' created by the very same neoliberalism. It is not realised, though, by many people that, in fact, the phenomenon of gated communities first appeared in the 1950s and 1960s in such less-developed countries as Jamaica, where the obscenely rich live almost cheek-by-jowl with the desperately deprived – from which the former employ their maids, gardeners, etc.

While working with UNESCO in such nations, the author and his family typically were housed in virtual stone fortresses with barred windows and immense grounds – maintained by houseboys and gardeners – surrounded by tall metal fences. Typically, if someone from the surrounding deprived sector needed to communicate with me, they had to hammer with a stone on the metal gate. One of the housemaids would run out, ascertain what they wanted and then return to the house to convey the message to myself. Only if I agreed would the maid unlock the gate and let the person in. I was constantly being warned against going to the gate myself in case I was assaulted – or worse!

Thus it also is in India, South Africa, etc., that one can still find magnificent modern factories surrounded by wretched hovels, open sewers and unpaved roads simply because the 'development' infrastructure always takes prior account of the profit-generating part of the community, depriving the rest. It is that sort of scene that is an identifying feature of neoliberalism – massive poverty interspersed with fortified 'safe zones'. In Iraq, as we know, this is a perfect reductio ad absurdum of the exercise of neoliberalism.

One recognises the same phenomena in special economic zones in Malaysia, Borneo, etc., and export processing zones in South Africa and Vietnam. We have many socially acceptable euphemisms for what is indeed nothing more than divisive, exploitative and totally inhuman conduct. In Naomi Klein's book, she refers to her experiences in the Philippines, where she lived temporarily in the famous Cavite Export Processing Zone. It derived its name from the town of Cavite outside of which the factory zone had been established as part of a World Bank-funded 'development project'. People from the town of Cavite could only enter the export zone if they were workers there, but could not live therein.

Inside the zone were 200 modern factories generating handsome profits, but somehow none of the 'development' money found its way into the garbage-strewn streets and disease-ridden households of the town. Medical facilities existed in the zone but there was even less access to healthcare in the town itself than had existed before the development loan had been negotiated by the Philippines with the World Bank.

VARIATIONS IN THE NEOLIBERAL ECONOMIC MODEL

While the reader will encounter in subsequent chapters considerable variations in the way that neoliberalism is implemented in different parts of the world, closer analysis shows that it is never a 'solution' to inequity but always a generator of it. In fact, it itself is the ultimate obstacle to global equity; the direct cause and sustainer of all of the individual obstacles – such as water privatisation, transnational production of pharmaceuticals, etc. – which we shall encounter. But this author will argue that, although neoliberalism itself is, if you like, the 'Mother of all Obstacles', we would get nowhere trying to attack neoliberalism directly and first. It is far too subtle and flexible. The recommended strategy will be to take on each of the main obstacles one by one. Having said that, let us consider some of the many ways neoliberalism expresses itself worldwide.

The most widely appreciated attribute of neoliberalism is that it both promotes and depends on 'free trade' – that is, on decreasing whenever possible the amount of local government interference, whilst encouraging unregulated markets. Long-established First World governments generally apply free trade neoliberal solutions to their corporate holdings in the Third World, but they are less able to do so at home because, since the industrial revolution, societies there have established a modus vivendi between trade union movements, reasonably democratic forms of government and state support of various social services such as schooling, health, etc. People are by and large aware of their 'rights' and an independent judiciary is at hand to defend them.

For that reason, some developed countries may have had short dalliances with foreign corporate and banking interests controlling their finances, but have – once a particular domestic financial crisis has been solved – managed to break away from World Bank SAPs and the like and re-erect protective tariffs, etc., so that they can protect their people to some extent from that neoliberal net. New Zealand is a relevant instance. That country did allow itself in the 1970s to undergo an IMF/World Bank-based 'shock therapy' programme because it had become mired in a series of balance of payments problems. But certainly by 1990 it had broken free of these and was holding the neoliberal whip hand in controlling the economics of a number of small South Pacific countries. Like many such newer industrialised members of the First World, it established its own 'special relationship' with the US. It has developed a much better level of social protections than the US has and such a strong welfare state that it has its own internal protection against the excesses of neoliberalism.

A lively democratic tradition often acts, at best temporarily, as a protection against domestic neoliberal machination. Where a democratic tradition has not been established, things are different. Take Singapore, for instance. It is a one-party state with an exploited ethnic underclass and a dominant state religion (Islam). The society is divided by a hugely different capacity for access to social significance and recognition of human rights. As Klein points out, it is those primed for emergence of the sort of social or economic shocks that would provide the perfect opportunity for the emergence of disaster capitalism. She argues that shocks and crises are a necessary prelude to the advance of neoliberalism. And it is considerations like this that expose the myth (so assiduously promoted by the international media and even by large state-run educational systems in designing their history and social studies examinations syllabi) that neoliberalism is the wave of the future, the solution to all of our previous problems and the only 'realistic' way forward. These same agencies would have us believe that free markets and free people are synonymous, when it will become obvious in succeeding chapters that the direct opposite is true. In other words, democratic traditions usually have to be beset by severe crisis before neoliberalism can get the upper hand over their finances. And, at the same time, crisis often circumvents democratic institutions.

KLEIN'S MODELS OF NEOLIBERALISM

It would seem from Klein's book, as well as from this author's field experience, that in such places as Hong Kong, China, Singapore, Malaysia, etc., we encounter a cruder and – in some ways – a more transparent view of neoliberalism than prevails in most First World countries. This backs up the author's view that the neoliberal system works most effectively without the checks of a free press and other democratic traditions. For instance, at the moment China seems to be the most thrusting economy in the world. Moreover, it has achieved this legacy by removing many previously existing democratic structures and expressly forbidding and suppressing new ones.

In many ways, China can be seen as a laboratory – rather like Chile was in the 1970s – for testing out those raw aspects of neoliberalism unhindered by the remnants of democratic traditions. There are several differences, of course. Chile had had a more prolonged experience of at least a quasi-democratic tradition – e.g. an opposition press, relatively unregulated levels of cultural expression, an unhindered church itself experimenting with a social gospel, etc. All of this constituted too formidable a barrier to wholesale imposition of free trade and anti-unionism from within the Chilean right wing itself. It depended instead on huge outside resources (largely US corporate and banking agencies) that could be involved over and above Chilean agencies.

China, on the other hand, has not been hindered to the same extent by internal

democratic traditions. Mao effectively eliminated all of that. But even more importantly, China's switch to neoliberalism largely came from within. After the bloody
repression of the populist opposition movement in Tiananmen Square in Beijing
in 1989, the Chinese leadership successfully managed to attract outside business
interests to China, whilst calling itself 'communist' and resolutely controlling all
business transactions. They set up their own indigenous business agencies, which
only 'welcomed' foreign input which it could oversee by offering as bait the
opportunity to exploit further a heretofore untouched mass market (the largest
in human history). Corporations cheerfully queued up for a piece of the action.
And the local workforce was effectively docile and non-unionised. China in effect
is running its own internal monetarist free market experiment with no coherent
opposition at all.

It is now a cutting-edge world economy with the potential to flood markets
and manipulate currencies almost at will. It has moved almost effortlessly into the
high-tech computer market, even bringing proud and supposedly incorruptible
Google to heel by denying access unless the Chinese government could control
access to the net. No other dictatorship has succeeded in doing this so comprehensively. For instance, when Libya was effectively quarantined by the US and the
EU in the late 1980s and early 1990s, and mail and faxes were routinely censured
both coming and going, the government seemed to have no way of blocking or
censuring emails. At the time, one of this author's postgraduate students was a
senior figure in Libya's Ministry of Health. Letters, faxes and telephone calls were
routinely censured and often blocked. An inappropriate word or phrase could at
any time have landed the man in prison, but we kept up a lively and productive
communication by email.

But with China's official control over Google, there is no such safety there. In
China today, they are pioneering the economy of surveillance – using everything
from CCTV cameras to GPS and biometric ID cards. As well, the sale of these
technologies to other countries (e.g. Burma and Singapore) is one of the fastest-
growing businesses in the Chinese economy. This in itself says much about the
link between market forces and freedom. After all, as Klein points out, a major
plank of the 'neoliberalism is the way forward' rhetoric in the 1990s was that when
expensive corporate-owned computer technology penetrated a society, it soon
brought democracy with it. In fact, the opposite has happened. All of this trade
has increased China's control over its citizenry, and one of its fastest growing areas
of trade is in the technologies of repression and surveillance.[10]

Another feature of media presentation of neoliberalism is that it constantly
conveys the idea that it is only through unregulated free trade that we can
ultimately achieve world peace and national security. With respect to this claim,
Klein comments on her recent experiences in Italy, Spain and the USA. She

mentions that her book was published in several languages – in the USA, Spain and Italy – but reactions to it differed according to national prejudices and worries, rather than to the specific issues she raised. Thus, in the USA, her ideas were held to represent a warning about terrorism – not that terrorism (or fear of it) is a frequent precondition for disaster capitalism! And in Italy and Spain, it was held to be a warning about the dangers of immigration! Others have seen it as an attack on Islamic fundamentalism.

In the meantime, concepts like homeland security (USA) and Fortress Europe (EU) crystallise many of these fears (shock), making way for the smooth insertion of neoliberalism. And even the administration of homeland security and Fortress Europe are themselves privatised and their funding swells the coffers of share-holders. This is sustained by our international news outlets constantly generating a growing fear of terrorism, immigrants and even climate change, etc., which in turn calls out for security fences, security passes, etc. and – above all – the voluntary relinquishing of hard-won democratic rights and mutual trust. All of this makes it possible to steadily transfer funds from the public sector to private security firms, etc., and hence to boardroom profiteers. What a scam, but very cleverly done!

EXCHANGING COMMUNITY FOR SECURITY

Neoliberalism, then, makes it more difficult for community trust to develop, because we are unaware whether our next-door neighbour is a terrorist or not. Since we must each face this inchoate and constant threat of terrorism alone – depending on strong but remote security forces rather than on one another – we have to realise that 'human rights' naturally make us less secure. Thus, there can be no overriding social or civic values. We cannot say that we are morally opposed to torture (whether water-boarding or anything else) if we cannot trust the community – e.g. the person beside us in the bus queue – to do the expected and decent thing. Frightened enough, it is easy to believe that if he or she is tortured perhaps we can be warned of imminent danger and our security can be assured.

One can only be amazed at how quickly people have got used to the extraor-dinary idea that a 'little bit' of torture should be allowed. It is a measure of the degree to which neoliberalism – with its capacity to commodify everything – has given us the idea that if we sacrifice our freedoms, such as human rights, including doing away with 'wasting money' on community welfare, we can 'buy' personal security.

This allows us to sell off our community responsibilities (would you help your assassin?) to 'the Empire' in one way or another and to concentrate on personal survival rather than on social interaction. The 'gated communities' discussed earlier fit so well with the scenario. As the profits of societies are increasingly concentrated by these attitudes into the hands of the few – who we look to to protect us – actions that only a few years ago would have been regarded as unthinkable became regarded as necessary for security. Now, in 2008, we can live with torture, extraordinary rendition and long-term imprisonment of people far away from their homes and language communities – for years on end and without charging them with anything.

That removal of 'assumed decency' is, of course, an essential part of the shock that creates the conditions, as described above, for imposition of neoliberalism. We can see it all more clearly if we look back at Chile and other parts of Latin America in the 1970s. In those first 'laboratories for testing neoliberalism' we can recognise that a 'triple shock' formula played the key rôle. Each of these shocks reinforced the preceding ones. There was the shock of the coup itself, the shock of the economic crisis, the shock therapy following it to restart the economy and then, finally, the shock of torture.

The latter is really the shock of 'enforcement', a mechanism by which society is warned not to question the necessity of the original economic shocks. If they were *not* unwanted, then military coups would be uncalled for. But, although discouraged from overt action on our own account, we are made aware of the fact that there is a constant (and unspecified) threat of rebellion and resistance. It is in *that* context that torture finds its true place in the neoliberal enterprise and as an astonishingly effective measure of social control.

This point is important because we have been conditioned to believe that the purpose of torture – in fact, its only moral justification, is to gain information in time to rescue ourselves from some planned disaster. But a moment's reflection will show that it is a most unreliable method of extracting information. The terror induced by even the anticipation of torture is so great that the victim will usually say anything to stop it – confessing to things of which he/she is accused, even listing the names of colleagues in often non-existent conspiracies. It is clear that our collective understanding of the rôle torture has played in repressive regimes is as a form of social control. It's not just an interrogation technique; it is a technique of state terror.

Commentators speak of torture in the United States as a question of whether or not it extracts useful information or reliable information. That whole debate overlooks the fact that torture is about communicating information, and it is communicating information to the broader society. While we're having debates about whether 'waterboarding' is torture or not, for the rest of the world and anybody who considers themselves potentially compromised by the US 'war on terror', the message is very clear: the US does torture. And that is a technique of state terror; that is a terrorist technique. People receive that message, and fear is spread – which is to say that torture works. It may not work to get effective information, but its primary rôle has never been just to get information. The primary rôle of torture is to communicate the message of obedience and the danger of resistance. We may even conclude that torture is working.

LATIN AMERICA AND THE WAY OUT

As we have seen then, neoliberalism did not just 'happen', but was the result of careful planning to prevent any chance of closing the equity gap and to sustain the 'ethics' of competition rather than a global survival tactic of cooperation. Is this, then, a counsel of despair? Have we gone too far? In this author's view we have not and for several reasons. As Klein points out, 'shock' provides the *vade mecum* for a panicked voluntary sacrifice of human rights in return for the promise of 'total security'. But people eventually became immune to shock. The crisis needs to be ever more threatening to bring about the melting away of community structure. That even began to happen in Chile during Pinochet's term in office.

And it is to Latin America – that first laboratory for testing Milton Friedman's theories – that we now turn for reassurance, because the siren call of neoliberalism there, so powerful in the 1980s and early 1990s, has become increasingly ineffective.

We will, in the next chapter, discuss the degree to which Latin America has successfully resisted the privatisation of water supplies. But at the more general level we have seen one country after another shift to the 'left' by adopting policies of national economic autonomy based on exploiting their own resources rather than letting transnational corporations buy them out.

The first to go in recent years was Venezuela, under Hugo Chávez, followed by Ecuador and Bolivia. Less spectacularly, Brazil and Chile have fallen prey to populist movements within their own countries. Generally, USA corporations are finding it more difficult to assert financial and trade compliance as the US dollar itself shifts from crisis to crisis. More detailed analyses of these specific cases are discussed in later chapters, but let us take a brief look at some examples.

STIRRINGS IN ECUADOR

Until 2006, Ecuador seemed to be rock-solidly safely ensconced in the US orbit. None of its recent leaders had been particularly 'revolutionary'. Its people were desperately poor – especially its indigenous people – but they had few resources of great significance, other than an extremely good potential for hydro-electric power, and its only systematic and regular contact with the USA centred on that country's largest military base in Latin America. But as a new leader (Rafael Correa) came to power, things began to shift. Or, as an Ecuadorian mathematics teacher put it to me when I was there in 2006, 'Suddenly the ground shook and we woke up!'

The military base in question is Manta, an accident of geography situating it in a key strategic position in terms of US military needs. No one would expect any drastic change. There was no real popular animus to US troops. They did not leave the base very often and many Ecuadorians were barely aware of their presence. But Correa, relatively new to politics himself and assumed to be an agreeable and easy sort of person for the US to push around, has turned out to be a frothing nationalist with a strong resentment at the US marginalisation of his country and its people.

The fact is that at the end of 2008, the peppercorn rental lease that the US has on Manta runs out. Correa pronounced on Ecuadorian TV that he would renew the US lease, but only on condition that they allow Ecuador to have a military base in Miami, Florida! Obviously he knew that the US could not agree to such an outrageously humiliating deal so, in effect, he has served them notice to leave.

But, as suggested earlier, this is not so much a reflection of one jumped-up politician's anti-Americanism, as it is a tendency that has already been growing in Latin America since 2002. In terms of disaster capitalism, this is an important event because, since 1970, such diplomatic shocks have tended to create conditions favourable to the imposition of US corporate control. But that did not happen this time!

Ecuador in the first decade of the second millennium was not the Chile of the 1970s. Things had changed – or as Klein might have said, people were becoming 'shock resistant'. If we look carefully at events in Latin America following Pinochet's dictatorship, we see that the change has been gradual, but consistently in one political direction. As Klein observed, during the 1980s and '90s, even though there was a gradual shift to more traditionally democratic forms, this did not prevent the shock strategy from going into operation.

In the 1980s and '90s, as dictatorships gave way to fragile democracies, Latin America did not escape shock doctrine. Instead, new shocks prepared the ground for another round of shock therapy – the 'debt shock' of the early '80s, followed by a wave of hyperinflation accompanied by sudden drops in prices of commodities on which economies depended. In Latin America today, however, new crises are being repelled and old shocks are wearing off – a combination of trends that is making the continent not only more resilient in the face of change but also a model for a future far more resistant to the shock doctrine.

When Milton Friedman died in 1995, the global quest for unfettered capitalism he helped launch in Chile three decades earlier found itself in disarray. The obituaries heaped praise on him, but many were imbued with a sense of fear that Friedman's death marked the end of an era. In Canada's *National Post*, Terence Corcoran, one of Friedman's most devoted disciples, wondered whether the global movement the economist had inspired could carry on. 'As the last great lion of free market economics, Friedman leaves a void . . . There is no one alive today of equal stature. Will the principles Friedman fought for and articulated survive over the long term without a new generation of solid, charismatic and able intellectual leadership? Hard to say.'[11]

It certainly seemed unlikely that he would be replaced! Friedman's intellectual heirs in the United States – the think tank neocons who used the crisis of September 11 to launch a booming economy in privatised warfare and 'homeland security' – were at the lowest point in their history. The movement's political pinnacle had been the Republicans' takeover of the US Congress in 1994, just nine days before Friedman's death – they lost it again to a Democratic majority in October 2006. The three key issues that contributed to the Republican defeat in the 2006 midterm elections were political corruption, the mismanagement of the Iraq War and the perception – best articulated by Jim Webb, a winning Democratic candidate for the US Senate – that the country had drifted 'toward a class-based system, the likes of which we have not seen since the nineteenth century.'

Nowhere, however, was the economic project in deeper crisis than where it had started: Latin America. Washington has always regarded democratic socialism as a greater challenge than totalitarian communism, which was easy to vilify and proved a handy enemy. In the 1960s and '70s, the favoured tactic for dealing with the inconvenient popularity of economic nationalism and democratic socialism was to try to equate them with Stalinism, deliberately blurring the clear differences between the world views. A stark example of this strategy comes from the early days of the Chicago crusade, deep inside declassified Chile documents. Despite the CIA-funded propaganda campaign painting Allende as a Soviet-style dictator, Washington's real concerns about the Allende victory were relayed by Henry Kissinger in a 1970 memo to Nixon: 'The example of a successful elected Marxist government in Chile would surely have an impact on – and even precedent value for – other parts of the world, especially in Italy; the imitative spread of similar phenomena elsewhere would in turn significantly affect the world balance and our own position in it.'[12] In other words, Allende needed to be taken out before his democratic third-way spread.

But the dream Allende represented was never defeated. It was merely temporarily silenced, pushed under the surface by fear. Which is why, as Latin America now emerges from its decades of shock, old ideas are resurfacing, along with the 'imitative spread' Kissinger so feared.

By 2001 the shift had become impossible to ignore. In the mid-'70s, Argentina's legendary investigative journalist Rodolfo Walsh had regarded the ascendancy of Chicago School economics under junta rule as a setback, not a lasting defeat, for the left. The violent terror tactics used by the military had put his country into a state of shock, but Walsh knew that shock, by its very nature, is a temporary state. Before he was gunned down by Argentine security agents on the streets of

Buenos Aires in 1977, Walsh estimated that it would take 20 to 30 years until the effects of the terror receded and Argentineans regained their footing, courage and confidence, ready once again to fight for economic and social equality. It was in 2001, 24 years later, that Argentina erupted in protest against IMF-prescribed austerity measures and then proceeded to oust five presidents in only three weeks.

In the years since, that renewed courage has spread to other former shock laboratories in the region. And as people shed the collective fear that was first instilled with tanks and cattle prods, with sudden flights of capital and brutal cutbacks, many are now demanding more democracy and more control over their markets. These demands represent the greatest threat to Friedman's legacy because they challenge his central claim: that capitalism and freedom are part of the same indivisible project.

The staunchest opponents of neoliberal economics in Latin America have been winning election after election. Venezuelan president Hugo Chávez, running on a platform of '21st century socialism', was re-elected in 2006 for a third term, winning 63% of the vote. Despite attempts by the Bush Administration to paint Venezuela as a pseudo-democracy, a poll conducted that year found 57% of Venezuelans happy with the state of their democracy, an approval rating on the continent second only to Uruguay's, where the left-wing coalition party Frente Amplio had been elected to government and where a series of referendums had blocked major privatisations. In other words, in the two Latin American states where voting had resulted in real challenges to the Washington Consensus, citizens had renewed their faith in the power of democracy to improve their lives.

Ever since the collapse of Argentina's government in 2001, opposition to privatisation has become the defining issue of the continent, able to make governments and break them. By late 2006, it was practically creating a domino effect. Luiz Inácio Lula da Silva was re-elected as president of Brazil largely because he turned the vote into a referendum on privatisation. His opponent, from the party responsible for Brazil's major sell-offs in the '90s, resorted to dressing up like a socialist NASCAR driver, wearing a jacket and baseball hat covered in logos from the as yet unsold public companies. Voters, in fact, were not persuaded, and Lula received 61% of the vote. Shortly afterward in Nicaragua, Daniel Ortega, former head of the Sandinistas, made the country's frequent blackouts the centre of his winning campaign; the sale of the national electricity company to the Spanish firm Unión Fenosa after Hurricane Mitch, he asserted, was the source of the problem. 'Who brought Unión Fenosa to this country?' he bellowed. 'The government of the rich did, those who are in the service of barbarian capitalism.'

In November 2006, Ecuador's presidential elections turned into a similar ideological battleground. Rafael Correa, a 43-year-old left-wing economist, won the vote against Álvaro Noboa, a banana tycoon and one of the richest men in the country. With Twisted Sister's 'We're Not Gonna Take It' as his official campaign song, Correa called for the country 'to overcome all the fallacies of neoliberalism'. When he won, the new president of Ecuador declared himself 'no fan of Milton Friedman'. By then, Bolivian President Evo Morales was already approaching the end of his first year in office. After sending in the army to take back the gas fields from 'plunder' by multinationals, he moved on to nationalise parts of the mining sector. That year in Chile, under the leadership of President Michelle Bachelet – who had been a prisoner under Pinochet – high school students staged a wave of militant protests against the two-tiered educational system introduced by the Chicago Boys. The country's copper miners soon followed with strikes of their own.

In December 2006, a month after Friedman's death, Latin America's leaders gathered for a historic summit in Bolivia, held in the city of Cochabamba, where a popular uprising against water privatisation had forced Bechtel out of the country several years earlier. Morales began the proceedings with a vow to close 'the open veins of Latin America'. It was a reference to Eduardo Galeano's book *Open Veins of Latin America: five centuries of the pillage of a continent*, a lyrical accounting of the violent plunder that had turned a rich continent into a poor one. The book was published in 1971, two years before Allende was overthrown for daring to try to close those open veins by nationalising his country's copper mines. That event ushered in a new era of furious pillage, during which the structures built by the continent's developmentalist movements were sacked, stripped and sold off.

Today Latin Americans are picking up the project that was so brutally interrupted all those years ago. Many of the policies cropping up are familiar: nationalisation of key sectors of the economy, land reform and major investments in education, literacy and healthcare. These are not revolutionary ideas, but in their vision of a government that would aim for equality, they stood as a rebuke to Friedman's remark in a 1975 letter to Pinochet: 'The major error, in my opinion, was . . . to believe that one can do good with other people's money!'

Whatever mistakes left-wing movements in Latin America may have made in the past, they have clearly learned to protect themselves more vigorously from neoliberal contoured financial shocks. For instance, the new crop of left-leaning Latin America leaders now anticipate US-backed counter-revolutionary tricks to destabilise their economies. Venezuela's new government under Hugo Chávez has offered both Bolivia and Ecuador military aid should Colombia violate their borders.

Hugo Chávez is probably the most 'classically socialist' of these leaders and he has made a priority of turning the vast oil profits, which previously had left Venezuela in the pockets of foreign (usually US) corporations, over to the construction of clinics and schools for the poorer Venezuelans who had never before had such luxuries. He has also been a strong and insistent influence in pushing for closer economic integration among the region's governments to help forestall US corporate control.

This has resulted in such powerful financial agreements as the Bolivarian Alternative for the Americas (ALBA in the Spanish acronym) and it represents a robust answer to the US-based multilateral Free Trade Area of the Americas (No trade barriers from Alaska to Tierra del Fuego!). It has been described as an ideal example of a system of fair trade. Each country provides what it can produce most efficiently and cheaply in return for what it cannot produce economically – totally independent of global market prices or of WTO manipulation. Under that enlightened system, Bolivia provides gas at low and stable prices, Venezuela offers heavily subsidised oil to poor neighbours and also provides engineering expertise in exploiting mineral resources, while Cuba not only offers doctors and complete medical teams to provide free healthcare whenever it is required, but also trains medical students from countries that either do not have medical schools or only provide them for wealthy students.

All of this means, of course, that none of those countries now need to fall into the snares of the IMF or the World Bank for financial assistance. The tyranny of Structural Adjustment Policies need no longer trouble them and their financial resources stay in their own countries.

HOW WILL THE EMPIRE RESPOND?

It would appear that in thus managing their own financial and trade needs locally, those countries had acted just in time. The IMF had been preparing to toughen further its loan conditionalities. At the 2006 meeting of the US Security Council, a strategy was adopted which included the phrase 'If financial crisis occur in a country, the IMF's response must reinforce that country's own private responses to financing the nation out of its problems.' A refocused IMF will strengthen market institutions (not government-run ones) and impose market forces discipline on them.

In this chapter, then, we have identified not one obstacle to be addressed before global equity in health can be realised, but several. As already indicated, though, short of a violent and worldwide revolution (which would be immensely destructive, compromise the environment catastrophically and lead to untold suffering, without necessarily succeeding), there is no practical way of trying to reverse the neoliberal agenda. What will be advocated in this book, though, is a system of picking off individual obstacles (each dependent on neoliberalism) one by one and in localised and specific campaigns.

This will, for one thing, have an impact on WTO trading controls and may even change present trade regulations based on the US dollar. This will provide an opportunity for the international community to consider alternative, more stable mechanisms, based – for instance – on fair trade zones rather than unregulated free trade. These issues will be considered in the final chapter.

The next chapter will address the first of several of the presently prevailing individual obstacles to global health equity – namely water privatisation.

REFERENCES

1 CNN. *Milosevic: architect of Balkans carnage.* Available at: http://edition.cnn.com/2006/WORLD/europe/03/11/milosovic.obit/ (accessed 28 Apr 2008).

2 Klein N. *The Shock Doctrine: the rise of disaster capitalism.* Tucker, GA: Metropolitan Books; 2007.

3 Tiwari P. A people's history of shock and awe. *Upping the Anti: a journal of theory and action.* 2007: 1–3. Available at: http://auto_sol.tao.ca/node/2877 (accessed 28 Apr 2008).

4 Wikipedia. *Monetarism.* www.en.wikipedia.org/wiki/monetarism (accessed 28 Apr 2008).

5 MacDonald T. *Health, Human Rights and the United Nations: inconsistent aims and inherent contradictions.* Oxford & New York: Radcliffe Publishing; 2007.

6 MacDonald T. *Sacrificing the WHO to the Highest Bidder.* Oxford & New York: Radcliffe Publishing; 2008.

7 McElroy D. *Paul Bremer Blamed for Iraq Mistakes.* 18 Mar 2008. Available at: www.telegraph.co.uk/news/worldnews/1582100/Paul-Bremer-blamed-for-Iraq-mistakes.html (accessed 30 Apr 2008).

8 ICRC. *Dirty and Scarce: the water crisis in post conflict Iraq.* 2008. Available at: www.icrc/org/web/Eng.siteeng0.nsf/html/Iraq–update–311207 (accessed 30 Apr 2008).

9 *Sacrificing the WHO to the Highest Bidder,* op. cit.

10 *The Shock Doctrine: the rise of disaster capitalism,* op. cit. p. 66

11 Klein N. *Development of Citizen Advice: Latin America's shock resistance.* 11 Nov 2007. Available at: www.venezuelanalysis.com/analysis/2822 (accessed 30 Apr 2008).

12 *The Shock Doctrine: the rise of disaster capitalism,* op. cit. p. 8.

Chapter 3

Inequity in access to water

ADAM WOULD BE CHARGED TODAY

When this author was a youngster in Canada, an expression commonly directed at school children was 'Travel on Shank's Pony and drink Adam's Ale, all for free!' 'Shank's Pony', of course, referred to walking to one's destination, rather than taking a tram or a bus, while 'Adam's Ale' was a glass of water. Now, many once walker-friendly roadways are so packed with fast-moving vehicles that poor old Shank's Pony doesn't get much of a chance, and as for Adam's Ale, well today he would probably have to pay for it.

We hear so much detail about the plight of many Third World communities with inadequate access to potable water, but comparatively few of us realise that even in the First World, easy-access free-of-charge drinking water is becoming problematical. Before dealing with the manifest iniquities in this regard, which lead to millions of unnecessary deaths in the Third World as water supplies in many communities become privatised, let us briefly consider the situation in many parts of the First World.

THE WATER BUSINESS IN BRITAIN

One could select virtually any First World country as an example of the way in which inroads over the control of privatised water supplies have become a major corporate preoccupation. Britain and France are the home bases for the most aggressive of these water-privatisation corporations, but the impacts of these firms are felt more keenly in other First World (and Third World) countries than in their own.

Most developed nations have government agencies which, nationally, provide some sort of brake, some sort of control, over large privatised agencies which dominate in the supply of such utilities as gas, water, electricity and telephone services. In the UK, the government agency responsible for overseeing water supply is the Water Services Regulation Authority (OFWAT).

OFWAT, like other similar agencies, has recently greatly angered ordinary British citizens by its recent requests to government to be allowed to increase the charges made to customers. Naturally this will hit pensioners (usually on fixed incomes) the hardest, also affecting single parents trying to meet the water needs entailed in raising children and keeping both them and their clothing clean. The average price increases mooted are about 5.8% or just over £300 a year. Perversely, too, the proposed price increases vary from one locality to another, but not according to local water table levels and rainfall. North Wales, for instance, is by no means an arid region in Britain, yet it is anticipated to experience cost increases considerably in excess of the aforementioned figures.

As already suggested, though, this is not a uniquely British phenomenon – and certainly not a uniquely First World phenomenon, as we shall see. As Steve McGriffen pointed out in a recent issue of the *Morning Star*, this is but part of a worldwide grab of water supplies being coordinated (often under UN mandates) by huge multinational corporations.[1] In fact, the IMF, along with various agencies in the EU, work together, using IMF SAPs as their weapon, quite commonly imposing water privatisation on any poor country desperate enough to approach the UN for a development loan. The EU connection with the IMF works through a series of contracts called 'Economic Partnership Agreements' (EPAs), with the aim being to force developing countries to open their service markets (including health and education!) to European corporate investments. The profits, of course, do not go to the Third World country involved, but to those European corporate agencies and their stockholders.

This is all part of the phenomenon of 'unrestricted free trade' (strongly endorsed by the World Trade Organisation (WTO)), analysed by the author in a previous volume.[2] 'Free trade' is, as shown in that publication, the major mechanism governing financial globalisation under neoliberalism. And, as we have seen in that account, a country relying on free trade (as opposed to some form of 'fair' or 'reciprocal' trade) quickly finds it impossible to develop except as a vassal of First World corporate interests. The health of its people is one of the first aspects of its supposed autonomy under the UN Universal Declaration of Human Rights (UDHR) to be sacrificed.

The overall strategy is simple. Just as in the EU itself, publicly owned service providers will be simply categorised as monopolies. In that way, any attempt to defend such sources or to improve their access to the population violates WTO regulations by 'supporting a restrictive monopoly practice'. As we shall see subsequently, this alone constitutes an enormous obstacle to global health equity. Others will emerge, and strategies will be required to eliminate them.

THE US'S CONTINUED RÔLE IN PRIVATISATION

Since the late 1980s, the European Commission has turned a jaundiced eye on publicly owned companies of all kinds. In its ultra-liberalising view, a public service which is owned by the people is no different to any other monopoly. The fact that Belgium, for example, has a legal ban on privatising water is, in this way of seeing things, merely a 'restraint on trade', as it prevents private companies from competing for contracts within the sector. Belgium can no longer claim (under WTO rulings) that this is Belgium's business and if any other country doesn't like it, they can lump it.

As a result of EU rules implicit in the 1957 Treaty of Rome, which were first made explicit 30 years later in the Single European Act and intensified with every new European treaty since, a foreign water privateer such as the French Vivendi has the right to muscle in on the Belgian 'market' for water. It is only a matter of time before someone insists on exercising that right. The fact that privatisation of water often does not deliver what it claims to and that the Belgian people might like the current arrangements or want to decide for themselves how they might be improved is, in the European Union's view, irrelevant.

Fortunately, reality is having its say. In France, the paramount lair of the water privateers, around 40 local authorities, including Paris, have taken water back into public ownership in the last decade. A rash of privatisations had followed the introduction of a new law passed in 1992. A few years of experience of rising prices and deteriorating levels of service were enough for most French people, however, and while French corporations scour the world looking for water to grab, France itself is turning away from this costly and inefficient 'solution'.

As well as trade negotiations, the EU organises the theft of people's property outside Europe through the European Union Water Initiative (EUWI). This makes it clear that the EU sees its prime responsibility as being to EU-based corporations, rather than to people in developing countries lacking access to clean, usable water. In the Commission's world view, the fact that water is a necessity makes it a great business opportunity, rather than a human right. The 1.4 billion people in the world who are without clean water, along with the 2.5 billion without even basic sanitation, are potential sources of profit. The Millennium Development Goal of halving these numbers by 2015 becomes simply a commitment to line the pockets of corporate shareholders.

The fact is that, in rich countries or poor, there is no way to make a service provider committed to delivering wholesome water and effective sanitation to every home into a profitable business. This is why, in common with other vital services such as public transport and postal delivery, it was in public ownership in the first place.

Privatisation is simply another way of transferring public wealth into private pockets. This is as true in Africa as it is in Accrington. Where a population is relatively wealthy, as in Britain, the money will come direct from people's pockets, in the form not only of raised prices but also in the taxes needed to cover subsidies which are, in reality, the only source of 'profit' for privateers.

Where the people are too poor to pay up, one of two things will happen. Services will improve, if at all, only for the rich. Or exceptions may be found in urban areas, but only if development money which originates with those same taxpayers in Europe and other wealthier parts of the world covers the costs, and then some. The market can deliver only to those who can pay. The poor will not get water, being unable to pay for it, unless someone else meets the expense.

Twenty-five million people a year die as a result of water-related diseases. Most readers would, I hope, be only too happy to see some of their taxes go to addressing the stark inequalities which lie behind these shortened lives. Lining the pockets of Vivendi's shareholders, however, is surely likely to be less popular. The real solution is, of course, to use our development money, our power as a trading bloc and our long experience and accumulated expertise to work with those communities and public utilities in developing countries which are really trying to solve this most fundamental of problems.

Partnerships between public utilities in Europe and developing countries, known as public-private partnerships (PUPs), to share expertise and improve service, innovative thinking such as the small solidarity levy paid by customers of Milan's publicly owned water company, together with a concerted effort to achieve and go beyond the UN Millennium Development Goal are what will help to end the thirst, hunger and disease which are the results of inadequate water supply and sanitation.

But, of course, the water issue is neither a discrete and separate 'issue' nor one confined to Europe. It is a global issue, very much more viciously crucial in the marginal economies of poorer countries, and it has far less to do with actual availability of water resources – an environmental and geographic phenomenon – than with control from abroad by people not directly dependent on those same sources of water for their own survival. While children in their millions die through use of polluted water or through lack of water altogether, corporate owners of the water companies responsible for supplying those people sit in boardroom meetings where clean bottled water is routinely available in abundance to slake the thirst of the very people profiting from the deaths of those children.

In August 2007, the former director-general of the UN, Boutros Boutros Galli, was quoted as saying on BBC Radio, 'Water will be more important to world peace in this century than even oil will be.'[3]

ESTABLISHMENT OF THE PEOPLES' WATER FORUM

As we know, the rôle of access to oil supplies has been recognised as an obstacle to world peace for much longer – at the very least since the 1960s – but the growing environmental crisis has been highlighting the pivotal importance of water. In fact, in 2004, the World Social Forum – an international human rights NGO – called for the establishment of a 'People's World Water Forum'.

Their statement read:[4]

> Water is life, and access to it is a fundamental birthright of all living beings.
>
> At the core of our concerns is the increasing control that global powers such as multi-national corporations, international financial institutions (including the World Bank and International Monetary Fund) exercise, and even in many cases, national governments are usurping water. Water is not a commodity to be controlled, bought and sold. Water cannot be owned. Water is a 'global common' to be accessible for the needs of all people. Our rivers cannot be diverted by major river-linking schemes, nor destroyed by large dams which displace millions of people. Our water cannot be privatised and sold for profit. We are the protectors and sustainable users of water, not the privateers. Water is a public good and must remain in public hands.
>
> Our collective concerns must lead us to collective action. Therefore people from all over the world met in Delhi January 11 to 14, 2004, for the People's World Water Forum in order to further build a common vision for action and to strategize how best to counter the global forces of destruction and privatisation.

The World Water Forum actually held an initial meeting in Kyoto, Japan, during the previous year – 2003. But at this preliminary meeting, they failed to address the needs of developing countries, which either lacked safe water altogether or were trying to survive on a very restricted access to safe water. They convened another meeting in Delhi in January 2004 and the group now considers this as their first meeting with a complete agenda.

Since then, they have established 22 March as 'World Water Day' and around that they are striving to focus worldwide attention on what they recognise as a major and growing obstacle to achieving even a basis for global equity in access to healthcare. But their annual meetings have signally failed to make a sustained impact on any major country's policy with respect to privatised water corporations or even to agree on a coherent policy. Typical was the meeting held on 24 March 2006 in Mexico City. The event attracted considerable media interest, but most of the reporters and commentators were very much under-whelmed by the whole thing and were critical of the way it had (or had not) been organised.

By the end of that World Water Forum (WWF) – World Water Day, 22 March – many of the Mexican newspapers had published articles recognising that it was, overall, a top-heavy event where a lot of money had been spent and little was achieved. And many participants seemed to agree. Meanwhile, behind closed doors, ministers of water, energy and environment from 78 countries, and 68 other ministerial delegations, negotiated the final Ministerial Declaration of the Forum. Rather than achieving consensus on the declaration, however, several Ministers – most notably Abel Mamani, water minister of Bolivia – demanded changes or additions to the document. By the closing ceremony of the WWF no agreement had been reached, though a bland and noncommittal document was agreed upon soon after.

The final declaration committed governments to prioritise water and sanitation as aspects of sustainable development and to continue efforts to reach the Millennium Development Goals of halving the number of people without water and sanitation services by 2015. It also committed funds to reducing risks from water-related natural disasters, among other commitments that do little, if anything, to recognise a need for a totally different approach to the water issue. Recognising the bland nature of the document, the ministries of Bolivia and Venezuela lobbied hard to add an addendum – in the Venezuelan minister's words, 'to add a little salt to a tasteless soup'. Several other governments – Cuba, Uruguay, Brazil, Angola and Argentina – have agreed, or nearly agreed, with the contents of the addendum – and at the end of the forum, the sense behind the scenes was that the discussion had only been of limited use.

When asked why they perceived a need for this addendum, Ernesto Paeva, the head of the Venezuelan delegation, said, 'It was not possible to have an open discussion about the issues that we see as important, and for this reason we have drafted a complementary document that we believe reflects the true interests of the people of the world.'

Asked if many governments disagreed with the addendum, and if their intervention had caused a severe disruption of the declaration process, Abel Mamani said 'Unfortunately in these processes, protocol often comes before real discussion of the issues. It is not that other governments do not agree with our point of view – it is that they believe in the importance of protocol. As you know, I do not come from the political class, but from the social movements – therefore I have little regard for protocol.' He continued, 'Our intention has not been to sabotage consensus. But consensus in our understanding is the complete agreement between 140 countries involved in the process – and we are not in complete agreement.'

The addendum was as follows:[5]

The Ministers or their representatives herein signing at the Fourth World

Water Forum, declare before the participants of this Forum, the international community and the people of the world, the following:

Access to water with quality, quantity and equity, constitutes a fundamental human right. The States, with the participation of the communities, shall make efforts at all levels to guarantee this right to their citizens, within their respective countries. Thus, we agree to continue making all efforts within the Commission on Sustainable Development of the United Nations and other international fora according to their mandates, to recognize and make this right effective.

We declare our profound concern regarding the possible negative impacts that international instruments – such as the free trade and investment agreements – can have on water resources, and reaffirm the sovereign right of every country to regulate water and all its uses and services.

We exhort the international community and multilateral entities to comply with the commitments repeatedly made to support efforts of countries to guarantee access to water and sewage treatment. We call on all States to develop the World Water Forum as a framework for an international multilateral system, based on the principles of full participation and inclusion.

How effective is all of this in confronting this one clear obstacle to global equity in health? As will become evident in succeeding chapters, idealistic talk is cheap. The above is the official statement, one that very few corporate leaders in the industry would lose much sleep over. Of course, as is almost always the case in these things, an alternative forum (drawn often from the idealistic fringe and sometimes singularly lacking in practical input) had been organised to run parallel sessions with the official one and their statement was much more explicit in stated objectives – always easy when one lacks real powers of implementation! In this case, though, it was the alternative group that zeroed in on the real solutions.

AN INTERNATIONAL PERSPECTIVE IN DEFENCE OF WATER EQUITY

The alternative statement emphasised two particular points at which practical action could be mounted, firstly that water has to be officially (and internationally) recognised as a fundamental human right (and hence enforceable under the UDHR) and not a merchandisable commodity and secondly, that commercial controls cannot be allowed to supervene this basic right. In other words: 'The WTO (and the IMF) has to get out of water supply decision-making.' As indicated in the author's book *Health, Human Rights and the United Nations*, it is this link with the UN's first mandate – to promote and defend human rights – that is the *only* way of overcoming the obstacle of corporate control over water supply.[6] This will, of course, be a recurrent theme throughout the book.

But it is at the international level, and through close and unconcealed cooperation between the IMF (a bona fide UN agency) and the WTO (not a UN agency) that the international protection theoretically offered by the UDHR is fatally compromised. We get nowhere unless and until we resolve that contradiction. It is at this level that the People's Health Movement (PHM) can play such an important rôle, as discussed in detail in the book cited above.

In addition to the basics, a number of subtle points were raised at public meetings that many feel have helped to sharpen the analysis of the water movement. For example, in the last few years the alternative to water privatisation has been made out to be 'public management of water services'. But several participants, most notably the Uruguayan delegation, who were, in their own words, 'the spinal column of Uruguay's movement to build a constitutional approach to water as a human right', insisted that the term 'public control' leaves too much up to states that may be corporate, corrupt and anti-democratic. The emphasis, agreed on the final declaration, is now on water management that is 'public, social, community controlled and participatory.'

The overall experience of the alternative forum was empowering and forward looking, especially in the fact that the forum was very much led by social movements and the NGOs that work with them. (This is very much like a People's Health Movement agenda, where activists from all levels of civil society manage to participate equally.) If there is one criticism of the alternative events, it would be the lack of practical, hands-on skills-building. There was much radical talk of participatory management, clear analysis of the problems and sharing of information between movements in many countries. But insisting on community-controlled water management means building both technical and social skills, and I would hope that future discussions would make room for workshops on home water treatment, ecological sanitation, grey water management, water conserving agriculture and other small-scale, community-controlled methods. These issues will be addressed in detail in the final chapter.

In the official forum, there were exactly two (amongst 2000) stands promoting these kinds of technologies.[7] One was an ecological sanitation stand, supported by the Swedish government and Mexican NGOs, and the other was a display, sponsored by the Dutch government, of simple ceramic water filters, low-tech rope pumps, hand-operated well-drilling equipment and that sort of thing. (All of these technologies are described in the Hesperian Foundation publications *Water for Life* and *Sanitation and Cleanliness for a Healthy Environment*.)[8]

APPROPRIATE TECHNOLOGY AND ACCESS TO WATER

The PHM is made up of people who are not merely academic commentators and observers, but who are very much concerned in providing access to health for communities of people in the Third World. As such, they confront the water/ health nexus daily and have elaborated a broad range of responses to it. The key phrase in much of this is 'appropriate technology' (AT) and that adjective 'appropriate' means, among other things, that it is so low-tech as to be of scant interest to commercial water providers.

In *The Watering Hole*, cited above, are a number of comments from people affected by AT. AT is, politically speaking, an important lever in removing the obstacles to health equity posed by corporate water providers. Consider the following four comments:

> One of the great debates in the forum is that some think the millennium development goals (MDGs) are very ambitious, while others say they are insufficient. To those pessimists who say that the goals are too ambitious, those of us working in AT say that it is not that the MDGs are too ambitious but that there is a lack of political will. If there were political will of all governments to improve health and services, it could be done. And if we were to be less ambitious, and choose simply one of the MDGs – the one for water, for instance – this would help us to achieve all the others.

> Another problem is that of administration. If we had good administration, we would give more emphasis to appropriate, small-scale solutions promoted by communities, and this would in turn create more democracy.

> The problem is political, because it has to do with power. Because people have no power, they have no water.

> Appropriate technology has a democratic affect, because it empowers people, and when the people are empowered, they resolve their own problems. Take for example, rainwater harvesting. Rainwater cannot be collected in one central place and then distributed to people. It is decentralized by its nature. Also there is the Nicaraguan rope pump, a simple pump made of rope, rubber gaskets, and PVC pipe that can be used to raise water in nearly any setting, and which is in wide use in Central America. If we have millions of people using rope pumps, we have millions of people protecting the aquifers – which means reforesting, protecting water catchments and ensuring that water goes back into the ground. In taking water, by hand, from the insides of the earth, the people are personally taking something from the earth, and this gives them the consciousness to also give back to the earth. In contrast to large systems of pipes and water storage, this gives people a direct relation with the water and with the earth. This doesn't mean we are against large systems in cities and elsewhere where they

are necessary, just to say they should be augmented by small scale systems that work towards developing democracy and ecological consciousness.

Finally, consider some of the views about the 'official' forum and its PHM-style 'alternative', in 'The Watering Hole' as cited above.

Clear ideological differences between the two fora emerged subsequently. The 'official' forum is supposed to be a place where stakeholders, technocrats and policy-makers address different problems together. But it is the PHM's view that this objective has been defeated. The PHM would like to see a platform where community people are brought together with academics and governments. But no such platform has emerged. As stated in 'The Watering Hole' account: 'The academics are locked in their rooms, the governments are locked in their rooms, and the community people are not invited.'

Most of the World Water Forum has been about things – what we have invented, what we can sell – rather than about actions – what we can do together. This is not right. It is a marketplace not for ideas, but for products. One delegate commented that everything he heard in the debates was no different from what goes on at a trade fair.

The PHM's comment went on to assert that if this is compared to the alternative forum, it is obvious that every single continent, indeed, every single sub-region, are linking together and resolving issues. 'It is not three people talking here and five people talking there, but everybody talking together. And they are talking about substantive issues – very big issues. This is how the official forum should be, but it is not. It would not be surprising if, in some years, the official forum becomes obsolete and everyone is coming to the alternative forum.'

All of the above comments constitute indicators of what will have to be done before all obstacles to equity of global access to healthcare can be overcome and real and lasting solutions can be found. It is an easy lesson to cite and to be aware of but a difficult one to implement. It confronts much that most of us have come to regard as 'legitimate authority' (governments, CEOs and experts of all kinds) with needs first felt and articulated at or near the bottom of the social order but which – under neoliberalism – are usually addressed and 'solved' at or near the top of social organisations – and their 'solutions' tend to be validated by the extent to which they enhance and secure the prevailing top-down authority structure.

It is the growing water crisis that has really brought this to the fore. People – all people of all races and social classes – have had a dependency relationship with water since (and before) civilisation and recorded history began. It long antedates, for instance, our relationship with oil. Water privatisation has only in the last few years, though, become widely appreciated as the dark side of global corporate control.

THE INTERNATIONAL WATER PRIVATISERS

As late as the 1970s, the idea of actually privatising a commodity which had from time immemorial been regarded as a universal human need and hence a basic 'right' had not been a serious prospect. In developed countries, water was regarded as something like air – so necessary to life that supply was not a problem.

But, as the author details in his 2005 book, a number of factors have suddenly rendered the easy availability of water far more problematical.[9] Climate change and associated levels of desertification and sudden increase in our commercial exploitation of aquifers, as well as the industrial-scale elaboration of golf courses and swimming pools, all have created a problem which we have never before faced – a global shortage of water.

Under those circumstances, privatisation of water supply as a purchasable commodity has become a reality. The idea of actually making people pay for what has universally been regarded as a basic right, of course, strikes many as so horrifyingly tactless that the issue doesn't perhaps attract the media attention it deserves, but let us acquaint ourselves with some of the facts.

We are told by the industry's yearbook, in 2004/05, that about 9% of the world's population (545 million people) were being served by private water providers. The three largest water corporations, and their approximate outreach, are:
- Suez (a French company) serves 117.4 million people
- Veolia Environmental (French) serves 108.2 million people
- RWE (German) – before it sold its subsidiary, Thames Water to Kemble Water, served 69.5 million people.[10]

The next largest corporations are: Aguas de Barcelona (35.2 million people), Saur (33.5 million people) and United Utilities (22.1 million people). It may strike the reader as odd, but none of these are US corporations. Water privatisation started mainly in certain sub-Saharan countries (often under IMF/WTO requirements), but increasingly private providers are supplying markets in such middle-income countries as Brazil, Malaysia and China. In addition, public utilities are increasingly going overseas and entering into contracts that do not require investment (such as management contracts). This will be explained below, but suffice to say, Rand Water (a South African firm) and Vitens (from the Netherlands) are the dominant players in Africa, especially Ghana. The use of the term 'public utilities' tends to blur the level of actual private corporate control, but this is only a smokescreen.

It goes without saying that privatisation of water, and of other key public services, is routinely strongly opposed and, in the Third World, such schemes often have to be enforced as part of IMF loan SAPs before local politicians and governments will accept them. There is, of course, little opposition from the stockholders of the First World corporation involved, as their dividends accumulate! The opposition viewpoint often focuses on worries that privatisation (from abroad) will lead to local monopoly formation and that profits will take precedence over service. All of this has been well borne out everywhere that such privatisation of water has been set up. Sometimes the opposition has led to direct violence, as happened in Bolivia and is detailed below.

Moral opposition to privatisation of water among First World populations has also sometimes been effective. For instance, in September 2004, the Netherlands government banned the practice. In another of his books the author dealt with the details of opposition to water privatisation in Ghana, Zambia and even in the US.[11] Those accounts showed how varied local oppositional response can be, both in the way it is organised by the people most directly affected and in the ways it can try to impact – largely through litigation – on official authority structures.

The important point for the reader to keep in mind is that reforms have rarely come from above. It only seems to be effective if it develops from the grassroots – bottom up. Therefore, when in the final chapter we address the issue of developing strategies for removing existing obstacles to global health equity, we will draw on these varied grassroots approaches. To make the point, we will now recount three different Latin American opposition campaigns to water privatisation. Let us begin with the events of 2000 in Bolivia.

COCHABAMBA PROTESTS OF 2000

These protests will, I predict, go down in socialist history as landmarks for action and they have become known as 'The Cochabamba Water Wars'. They arose during the four-month interval of January through April 2000 in street protests and more violent acts in opposition to legislation privatising the municipal water supply and sewage services.

The content was itself a blood-drenched one. Up until 1982, Bolivia had been a classical Latin American banana republic, with a military junta and a hugely disenfranchised and landless peasantry. In all, it was a far cry from Simón Bolívar's (1783–1830) intention to establish a 'liberated and democratic republic'. Although civilian rule replaced the military in 1982, this did not usher in economic stability. There were huge IMF loans – and an accumulated level of compound interest – yet to be paid off. By 1985, hyperinflation was at an annual rate of 2500% (!), and this insured that few foreign investors were ready to invest in Bolivia. The rest of the story is sickeningly familiar. The desperate Bolivian government turned to the World Bank to re-negotiate their deficits and, in order to qualify for such support, new SAPs were imposed – affecting various public services such as railways, the telephone system, national airlines and fuels. But worse was to come.

THE IMPOSITION OF WATER PRIVATISATION

As described in an article by Schultz, in 2000, the World Bank, under the belief that 'poor governments are often too plagued by local corruption and too ill-equipped to run public water systems efficiently (and that the use of private corporations) opens the door to needed investment and skilled management', declared it would not renew a $25 million loan to Bolivia unless it privatised its water services.[12] Believing that charging for resources encourages conservation and avoids shortages and environmental damage, the World Bank, with the goal of countering inefficiencies and waste, said that 'no subsidies should be given to ameliorate the increase in water tariffs in Cochabamba.'[13] The *New Yorker* reported on the World Bank's motives, 'Most of the poorest neighbourhoods were not hooked up to the network, so state subsidies to the water utility went mainly to industries and middle-class neighbourhoods; the poor paid far more for water of dubious purity from trucks and handcarts.' In the World Bank's view, it was a city that was crying out for water privatisation.

> Prior to privatization the water works of Cochabamba were controlled by the state agency SEMAPA. The Bolivian government put SEMAPA up for auction for privatization but not capitalization. Only one party was willing to bid on the project. This was Aguas de Tunari, a consortium led by International Water Limited (England), the utility Edison (Italy), Bechtel Enterprise Holdings (USA), the engineering and construction company Abengoa (Spain) and two companies from Bolivia, ICE Ingenieros and the cement maker SOBOCE. The water network that they envisioned was projected to provide drinking water to all of the people of Cochabamba. This was set to double the existing coverage area and also to introduce electrical production to more of the region.
>
> Without regard for its weak bargaining position, the Bolivian government under President Hugo Banzer agreed to the terms of its sole bidder Aguas de Tunari and signed a $2.5 billion, 40-year concession 'to provide water and sanitation services to the residents of Cochabamba, as well as generate electricity and irrigation for agriculture.' Within the terms of the contract the consortium was guaranteed a minimum fifteen per-cent annual return on its investment, which was to be annually adjusted to the United States' consumer price index. The implementation of Aguas de Tunari's program was set to correlate with a government plan to present a $63 million rural development package to peasants with funds for crop diversification, and extending electric and telephone services to remote areas.[14]

PRIVATE WATER ENSHRINED IN LAW

To ensure the legality of the privatization the Bolivian government passed law 2029, which verified the contract with Aguas de Tunari. To many the law appeared to give a monopoly to Aguas de Tunari over all water resources. Many feared that this included water used for irrigation by peasant campesino farmers, and community-based resources that had previously been independent of regulation. The law was seen as 'enabling the sale of water resources that had never really been a part of SEMAPA in the first place.' It was worried that independent communal water systems which had yet to be connected with SEMAPA would be 'summarily appropriated by the new concession.' By Law 2029, if Aguas de Tunari had wanted to, not only could it have installed meters and begun charging at independently built communal water systems, but it could have also charged residents for the installation of those meters. The broad nature of Law 2029 led many to claim that the government would require a license be obtained for people to collect rainwater from their roofs, an unenforceable policy. The first to raise concerns over the scope of the law was the new Feracion Departamental Cochabambina de Regantes (FEDECOR) under its leader Omar Fernandez. FEDECOR was made up of local professionals, including engineers and environmentalists. They were joined by a federation of peasant farmers who relied on irrigation, and a confederation of factory workers' unions lead by Oscar Olivera. Together these groups formed Coördinator for the Defense of Water and Life, or La Coordinadora which became the core of the opposition to the policy.[15]

WATER RATES JUMP

As a condition of the contract Aguas de Tunari had agreed to clear the $30 million debt accumulated by SEMAPA. They also agreed to finance an expansion of the water system, and begin a much needed maintenance program on the existing deteriorating water system. Dider Quint, a managing director for the consortium said 'We were confident that we could implement this program in a shorter period of time than the one required by the contract. [To accomplish this] We had to reflect in the tariff increase all the increases that had never been implemented before.'

On top of this, in order to secure the contract, Aguas de Tunari had to promise the Bolivian government to fund the completion of the stalled Misicuni dam project. The dam was purportedly designed to pipe water through the mountains, but the World Bank had deemed it uneconomic. While the consortium had no interest in building the dam, as it was backed by an influential member of Banzer's megacoalition, the mayor of Cochabamba, Manfred Reyes Villa, it was a condition of their contract. An attempt to privatize the water system had been made without the condition of building the dam in 1997, but Reyes Villa had used his influence to squash the deal. Critics of Reyes Villa held that the dam was a 'vanity project' which would profit 'some of his main financial backers'.

The officials in Bolivia for Aguas de Tunari were mostly engineers lacking marketing training. They were also foreigners unaware of the intricacies of Bolivian society and economics. Upon taking control the company raised water rates by an average of 35% to about $20 a month. While this seemed minuscule in the developed nations that the Aguas de Tunari staff had come from, many of their new clients only earned about $100 a month and $20 was more than they spent on food. In complete ignorance of the reality of his situation, a manager for the consortium, Geoffrey Thorpe, simply stated 'if people didn't pay their water bills their water would be turned off'. The poor were joined in their protest by January 2000, when middle-class homeowners and large business owners stripped of their subsidies saw their own water bills increase. As anger over the rates mounted, Reyes Villa was quick to distance himself from Aguas de Tunari.[16]

POPULAR RESISTANCE AND GOVERNMENT REACTION

There were many accounts in the media of these events, probably those on CNN being the most persuasive.[17] The following summarises those broadcasts. The use by grassroots organisations of existing state-supported human rights and media agencies and of legally recognised trade union organisation is significant.

Demonstrations erupted when Aguas de Tunari imposed a large rate increase, reportedly to finance the Misicuni Dam project, a week after taking control of the Cochabamba water supply system. In a country where the minimum wage was less than US$70 per month, many dwellers were hit with monthly water bills of $20 or more.

Starting in early January 2000, massive protests in Cochabamba began with Oscar Olivera among the most outspoken leaders against the rate hikes and subsequent water cut-offs. The demonstrators consisted of regantes (peasant irrigators) who entered the city either under village banners, or carrying the wiphala; they were joined by jubilados (retired unionized factory workers) under the direction of Olivera and cholitas. Young men began to try and take over the plaza and a barricade across incoming roadways was set up. Soon they were joined by pieceworkers, sweatshop employees, and street vendors (a large segment of the economy since the closure of the state owned tin mines). Self-styled anarchists from the middle-classes came from the University of Cochabamba to denounce the World Bank International Monetary Fund and neoliberalism. The strongest supporters of the demonstration were drawn from the city's growing population of homeless street children.

Protesters were able to halt Cochabamba's economy by holding a general strike that shut down the city for four straight days. A ministerial delegation went to Cochabamba and agreed to roll back the water rates, still the demonstration continued. On 4 February 2000 thousands marching in protest were met by troops and law enforcement agents from Oruro and La Paz. Two days of clashes occurred with the police using teargas. Almost 200 demonstrators were arrested, 70 protesters and 51 policemen were injured.

Throughout March 2000 the Bolivian hierarchy of the Roman Catholic Church tried to mediate between the government and the demonstrators. In the meantime, the Coordinadora made their own referendum and declared that out of fifty thousand votes 96% demanded the contract with Aguas del Tunari be cancelled. The Government's reply was, 'There is nothing to negotiate.'

In April 2000, demonstrators again took over Cochabamba's central plaza. When the leaders of the Coordinadora (including Óscar Olivera) went to a meeting with the governor at his office they were arrested. Though they were released the following day, some, fearing further government action, fled into hiding. More demonstration leaders were arrested, with some being transferred to a jungle prison in San Joaquin, a remote town in the Amazon rainforest on the border with Brazil. The demonstrations spread quickly to other areas including La Paz, Oruro, and Potosí, as well as to rural areas. The protesters also expanded their demands calling on the government to resolve unemployment and other economic problems. Soon demonstrators had most of the major highways in Bolivia barricaded. The protest even inspired officers in four La Paz police units to refuse to leave their barracks or even to obey superiors until a wage dispute was settled.[18]

OPPOSITION STRENGTHENS AND ORGANISES

The Bolivian Constitution allows the President (with the support of his Cabinet) to declare a 90 day state of siege in one or more districts of the nation as an emergency measure to maintain public order in 'cases of serious danger resulting from an internal civil disturbance'. Any extension beyond 90 days must be approved of by the Congress. Anyone arrested at this time must be released after 90 days unless criminal charges are brought against them before a court. With the roads cut off and fearing a repeat of the 1781 Tupac Katari Amero-Indian uprising that trapped white Spaniards in the city of La Paz for 109 days (forcing them to eat rats and shoe leather to survive), President Banzer on 8 April 2000 declared a 'state of siege'.

Banzer said, 'We see it as our obligation, in the common best interest, to decree a state of emergency to protect law and order.' Information Minister Ronald McLean described the rationale for the decree, saying 'We find ourselves with a country with access roads to the cities blocked, with food shortages, passengers stranded and chaos beginning to take hold in other cities.' The decree suspended 'some constitutional guarantees, allowing police to detain protest leaders without a warrant, restrict travel and political activity and establish a curfew.' Meetings of over four people were outlawed, and the freedom of the press was curtailed with radio stations being taken over by the military and some newspaper reporters being arrested. The police moved in to enforce the policy with nighttime raids and mass arrests. At one point 20 labor union and civic leaders were arrested. The police's tear gas and rubber bullets were met by protesters' rocks and Molotov cocktails. Continuing violent clashes between the demonstrators and law enforcement led to internal exile, 40 injuries, and 5 deaths. International human rights organizations decried the 'state of siege' declaration. This was the seventh time since Bolivia returned to democracy in 1982 that the 'state of siege' decree had been employed.

On 9 April 2000, near the city of Achacachi, soldiers met resistance to removing a roadblock and opened fire killing two people (including a teen-age boy) and wounding several others. Angry residents overpowered soldiers and used their weapons against military leaders. They wounded Battalion Commander Armando Carrasco Nava and army captain Omar Jesus Tellez Arancibia. The demonstrators then found Tellez in hospital, dragged him from his bed, beat him to death and dismembered his body.[19]

The AI report cited above went on to report subsequent events. On 9 April 2000, nearly a thousand striking police officers actually fired tear gas at government soldiers. The soldiers, astonishingly disciplined in their response, only fired their weapons into the air. At this point, the government weakened noticeably, giving a 50% increase in wages to the La Paz police to end the strike. The effect of this was that the police in other cities, such as Santa Cruz, went on strike in demand for equal treatment!

THE GOVERNMENT RESPONSE

The government gradually became less able to oppose the resistance, as little by little, some of its strongest supporters joined forces with the rebels. The last straw occurred when the ordinarily reactionary coca producers (led by Evo Morales, who himself was elected on a reform government ticket to the presidency in December 2005), also became involved. The ranks clearly were splitting. The coca farmers demanded an end to US attacks on their coca plantations. The government tried to deflect this level of opposition by saying that the coca producers were really working hand in glove with terrorists financed by the illegal narcotics trade. They even tried to claim that all of the anti-government resistance had been directed by international terrorism!

But such official responses and overt attempts to secure the sympathies of US corporate interests began to appear increasingly suspect as important branches of the public services began to rally behind the protests. Teachers at state schools went on strike and students battled the police in the streets.

THE PROTESTS GAIN THE MORAL HIGH GROUND

After a televised recording of the Bolivian Army captain, Robinson Iriarte de la Fuente, firing a rifle into a crowd of demonstrators wounding many and hitting high school student Víctor Hugo Daza in the face, killing him, intense anger erupted. The police told the executives of the consortium that their safety could no longer be guaranteed. The executives then fled from Cochabamba to Santa Cruz. After coming out of four days of hiding, Oscar Olivera signed a concord with the government guaranteeing the removal of Aguas del Tunari and turning Cochabamba's water works over to La Coordinadora. Detained demonstrators were to be released and Law 2029 repealed. The Banzer government then told Aguas del Tunari that by leaving Cochabamba they had 'abandoned' the concession and declared the $200 million contract revoked. The company, insisting that it had not left voluntarily but been forced out, filed a $40 million lawsuit in the International Centre for Settlement of Investment Disputes, an appellate body of the World Bank against the Bolivian government, 'claiming compensation for lost profits under a bilateral investment treaty.'

On the day following Víctor Hugo Daza's funeral, Óscar Olivera climbed to his union office's balcony and proclaimed victory to the exhausted crowd. The demonstrators declared that they would not relent until Law 2029 was changed. To get a quorum to amend the law the government even rented planes to fly legislators back to the capital. In a special session on 11 April 2000 the law was changed.[20]

But this was by no means the end of the matter, for as is customary in these situations of grassroots-organised resistance, the Empire soon struck back – this time invoking the authority of the World Bank. At that time, the World Bank was under the presidency of James Wolfensohn, famous for his attacks on UN human rights activities and for his undiminished support of free trade under global neoliberal control.

On 12 April 2000 when asked about the outcome in Bolivia, World Bank President James Wolfensohn maintained that free or subsidized delivery of a public service like water leads to abuse of the resource; he said, 'The biggest problem with water is the waste of water through lack of charging.'

In Washington, D.C. at the 16 April 2000 IMF and World Bank meetings protesters attempted to blockade the streets to stop the meeting. They cited the Water Wars in Bolivia as an example of corporate greed and a reason to resist globalisation. Oscar Olivera attended the protests, saying, 'The people have recaptured their dignity, their capacity to organise themselves – and most important of all, the people are no longer scared.'

On 23 April 2002 Oscar Olivera led 125 protesters to the San Francisco headquarters of Bechtel, the only member of Aguas del Tunari located in the Americas. Olivera says, 'With the $25 million they are seeking, 125,000 people could have access to water.' Bechtel officials agreed to meet him.

The victory gained the cocalero and campesino groups international support from anti-globalisation groups. Oscar Olivera and Omar Fernandez have become sought-after speakers at venues discussing how to resist resource privatization and venues critical of the World Bank. His actions in the Water Wars raised the profile of Congressman Evo Morales and he became President of Bolivia in 2005. Omar Fernandez joined Morales' socialist party Movimiento al Socialismo and became a Bolivian senator.[21]

RESOLUTION

The people did succeed to some degree in thwarting the international power of corporate finance and – as we shall see – provided valuable organisational and tactical lessons. But neoliberalism is not that easily halted in its tracks and that particular obstacle to equity of access to health has not yet been overcome. On 19 January 2006, a settlement was reached between government (with Evo Morales now President) and the people, but the statement absolved the government of blame by stating that an agreement was reached only under pressure of civil unrest, not because of any interference by outside corporate interests!

In the meantime, the people (except for the very wealthy) had been left with many unresolved water supply problems.

On 19 January 2006 a settlement was reached between the Government of Bolivia (then under the Presidency of Evo Morales) and Aguas del Tunari, in which it was agreed that 'the concession was terminated only because of the civil unrest and the state of emergency in Cochabamba and not because of any act done or not done by the international shareholders of Aguas del Tunari'. With this statement both parties agreed to drop any financial claims against the other.

[. . .]

In the end water prices in Cochabamba returned to their pre-2000 levels with a group of community leaders running the restored state utility company SEMAPA. As late as 2005, half of the 600,000 people of Cochabamba remained without water and those with it only received intermittent service (some as little as three hours a day). Oscar Olivera the leading figure in the protests admitted, 'I would have to say we were not ready to build new alternatives.' SEMAPA managers say they are still forced to deal with graft and inefficiencies, but that its biggest problem is a lack of money (it can not raise rates and no international company will give them a loan). Luis Camargo, SEMAPA's operations manager, in an interview with the New York Times said they were forced to continue using a water-filtration system that is split between 'an obsolete series of 80-year-old tanks and a 29-year-old section that uses gravity to move mountain water from one tank to another.' He stated that the system was built for a far smaller city and worried about shrinking aquifers.

A system to bring water down from the mountains would cost $300 million and SEMAPA's budget is only about $5 million a year. The *New Yorker* reports 'in Cochabamba, those who are not on the network and who had no well, pay ten times as much for their water as the relatively wealthy residents who are hooked up and with no new capital the situation cannot be improved. A local resident complained that water truck operators 'drill polluted water and sell it. They [also] waste a lot of water.' According to author Frederik Segerfeldt, 'the poor of Cochabamba are still paying 10 times as much for their water as the rich, connected households, and continue to indirectly subsidize water consumption of more well-to-do sectors of the community. Water nowadays is available only four hours a day and no new households have been connected to the supply network.' Franz Taquichiri, a veteran of the Water War and an SEMAPA director elected by the community, said, 'I don't think you'll find people in Cochabamba who will say they're happy with the service. No one will be happy unless they get service 24 hours a day.' Another Cochabamba resident and activist during the unrest summed up her opinion of the situation by saying, 'afterwards, what had we gained? We were still hungry and poor.'[22]

From the foregoing account, a number of patterns emerge. Most conspicuously, strong movements originating from the grassroots tend to lose their focus as they impact further up the power hierarchy. They can become deflected by having to make compromises. In Cochabamba's case, much of the finance and administrative structure has remained in the same hands. Does the situation in Uruguay and elsewhere in the Americas offer useful alternatives?

FREE TRADE AND EXPENSIVE WATER

As we have seen, globalisation of financial control by neoliberalist corporate interests has widely impacted negatively on the health rights of us all, but particularly of the already disadvantaged. The author has argued in a previous publication that neoliberalism, by definition, relies on unfettered competition and hence can only widen the health inequity gap globally.[23]

We see this illustrated most effectively in multilateral or bilateral agreements based on 'free trade'. The gap between the initially powerful and the underdog partners widens. A good example is provided by the FTAA (Free Trade Area of the Americas), which has not only had adverse impacts on Canadian and Mexican workers, but has rendered many US workers much less secure in their employment than before. The main beneficiaries have been the corporate CEOs in US boardrooms. With respect to water privatisation, Carmelo Ruiz Merrero has given an excellently comprehensive account.[24]

As he points out, control over water is the main threat in the proposals put forward by FTAA. They seek to use neoliberal mechanisms (such as the WTO and IMF SAPs) to privatise water resources, and ultimately they will not hesitate to use that authority to alter the flow of complete river systems to establish profitable megaprojects. As we have already seen, though, ordinary people in Latin America are beginning to learn how to organise and protect their access to water. In this respect, let us look first at Uruguay.

URUGUAYANS VOTE AGAINST WATER PRIVATISATION

Marrero (cited above) reminds us that:

> on 31 October, Uruguayans expressed their opposition to water privatization at the ballot box. In a plebiscite, the electorate approved a constitutional reform that defines water as a good belonging to the public trust and guarantees civil society's participation in the management of the country's hydrological resources.
>
> The resulting article in the Uruguayan constitution says that 'water is a natural resource essential to life,' adding that access to it and to sewage treatment services are 'fundamental human rights.'
>
> The plebiscite was promoted by the National Commission in Defense of Water and Life, made up of the state water company's labor union and various civil society groups. The proposal obtained the support of 60% of the electorate. Presidential candidate Tabaré Vázquez, winner of the election that took place the same day, also supported the water plebiscite.
>
> Subsequently, 127 organisations from 36 countries endorsed an open letter in support of the Uruguayan people's decision. According to the document, the vote set 'a historic precedent in defence of water, through its inclusion in a country's Magna Carta by means of direct democracy.' They also pointed out that the approved constitutional reform 'ensures the defence of sovereignty over a natural resource from the onslaught of transnational corporations.'

One of the enterprises most affected is the Spanish-based Aguas de Costa. After it took charge of services in the Uruguayan department of Maldonado in 1992, water tariffs rose seven times higher than in the rest of the country.

'The people have voted confirming that water, a scarce and perishable natural resource, must be a right of all and not a privilege of those who can pay for it,' said Uruguayan author Eduardo Galeano, commenting on the plebiscite. 'The people have confirmed also that they're not ignorant, and they know that sooner than later in a thirsty world water reserves will be as coveted as petroleum reserves, or more. We in countries that are poor but water-rich, must learn to defend ourselves. More than five centuries have passed since Columbus. How long will we keep trading gold for mirrors?'

'Wouldn't it be worthwhile for other countries to submit the subject of water to popular vote?' Galeano suggested. 'In a democracy, when it is real, who should decide? The World Bank or the citizens of each country? Do democratic rights really exist or are they just little fruits that decorate a poisoned cake?'

In fact, as Cochabamba made clear, privatisation of water in Latin America has not been a resounding success. Similar schemes have run amok in Puerto Rico, Argentina, Brazil, Columbia and Chile, as well as elsewhere in Bolivia than in Cochabamba itself.

Advocates of neoliberalism are anxious to gain the impression that the only alternative to neoliberalism is constricting public ownership of utilities, monopoly control of various types, totalitarianism and loss of involvement. Considering the record of neoliberalism thus far, one is rather reminded of pots calling kettles 'black'! Marrero (cited above) draws our attention to some instructive examples in Brazil and Bolivia.

PUERTO ALEGRE IN BRAZIL

The Brazilian city of Porto Alegre is famous for hosting the World Social Forums. The aqueducts of this city of 1.4 million people, capital of the southern state of Rio Grande do Sul, have been under the people's control ever since the Workers' Party (PT) won the municipal elections in the 1990s. The entity that manages them, the Departamento Municipal do Agua e Esgoto (DMAE), belongs to the public sector but is financially independent from the state government and is funded by ratepayers. It is a non-profit enterprise that reinvests its income in infrastructure improvements.

DMAE's workings stand out because of the advanced level of public participation and democratic control over its operations and investments. It is governed by a council of local civil society representatives; operational and investment decisions must go through a participatory budgetary review. It's part of a system also applied to many other areas of public life in Porto Alegre, as well as in Rio Grande do Sul, in which the citizens directly decide budget priorities.

The results of this participation policy are concrete. In Porto Alegre, a full 99.5% of the population has access to clean drinking water, a rate higher than any location in Brazil. The sense of belonging and responsibility that residents feel toward DMAE translates to a high level of consciousness among the population regarding water conservation. People also willingly accept occasional rate hikes because they believe the money they pay is used prudently and responsibly. In any case, the DMAE's rates are among the lowest in the country. At the same time water consumption in Porto Alegre is low because of educational campaigns and a progressive rate scale that favours the poor.[25]

AN ALTERNATIVE APPROACH IN BOLIVIA

Ratepayer co-ops are another alternative to privatization. Since 1979 the company that provides water to the Bolivian city of Santa Cruz has been run by the Cooperativa de Servicios Publicos Santa Cruz (SAGUAPAC) and is today one of the best-managed water companies in all of Latin America. All ratepayers are members of the co-op and have the right to vote in the general assembly of delegates, which in turn elects part of the administrative and supervisory boards of the water company. SAGUAPAC is financially independent and has a rate scale that favors those who use less water. Between 1988 and 1999 it was able to increase its service coverage from 70% of the population to 94%.

After studying the Santa Cruz model even the World Bank admitted 'that cooperative solutions can be superior to either public or private approaches to utility management.' In one study, the bank praises Santa Cruz for its 'efficient and transparent administration that appears to have virtually eliminated corruption.' It also states that 'the Bolivia experience confirms that privatisation is not a panacea.'[26]

NEOLIBERALISM'S SURVIVAL RESTS ON PRIVATISATION

Any socially acceptable alternative to neoliberalism, any political or social system that emphasises international cooperation and a rational sharing of the world's resources, has to be anathema to neoliberalism and other competition-based doctrines. Therefore, First World governments and their large network of banking and transnational corporate interests are gradually being morally isolated, so to speak, as the negative and divisive consequences of privatisation become more evident to more people.

In its advocacy of privatisation, the US is at present the hegemonic influence, but one wonders for how long. A hungry China and a hungry India are waiting! Labels such as 'communist' for China mean little when it comes to the mad rush for profits first. One can wonder 'What for?' If we have to mortgage the environment, world peace and civilisation itself to keep the game going, it is a pointless exercise. But those who would privatise the air we breathe seem oblivious to all of this.

In spite of these cases of positive engagement, the U.S. government and transnational corporations insist on privatization and neoliberal orthodoxy in the management of water. The main tool to push the privatization agenda is the Free Trade Area of the Americas (FTAA). Under the FTAA's terms, foreign investors will be able to sue and demand compensation from governments for any law or rule that affects their profits. This could mean costly economic sanctions to the country that revokes privatizations of aqueducts or tries to limit or prevent the international trade in water, even if such attempts are motivated by environmental or public health reasons.

Such investor protections already exist in the North American Free Trade Agreement (NAFTA), which covers Canada, the United States, and Mexico. The treaty defines water as a tradable good, obligating all levels of governments – from Puerto Rico to Hawaii and from Chiapas to Alaska – to sell their water resources to the highest bidder under threat of being sued by private companies.

The ill effects of this approach can be seen in the 1998 case in which the U.S. company Sun Belt sued the Canadian government for $10 billion for violating NAFTA. The grievance was that the government of British Columbia prohibited the mass export of its potable water when Sun Belt wanted to import it to thirsty California. In another case, the U.S. company Metalclad Corp. successfully sued the Mexican government for $17 million after Mexican authorities barred the operation of the company's hazardous waste treatment and disposal facility in San Luis Potosí state, and the company claimed that was an unjust expropriation. These and many other NAFTA cases are omens of what Central and South America can expect from the FTAA.

The investor protections provided by NAFTA and the proposed FTAA do not even exist in the World Trade Organization (WTO). At this time only states can present grievances to the WTO, but this will change if the Multilateral Agreement on Investment (MAI) is approved. With the MAI, transnational corporations will be able to use the WTO to sue any member country that limits their activities and profits in any way.

With neoliberal globalization a massive increase is expected in activities that consume fresh water, such as manufacture, monoculture-based agribusinesses, and urban concentration. According to the World Bank the next world war will not be over oil but over water. The U.S. Central Intelligence Agency claims that by 2015 water will be one of the major causes of international conflict. And the

United Nations forecasts that the demand for the liquid will exceed the supply by 56% in 2025, should current trends continue.[27]

TRANSLOCATING RIVERS

Of course, privatisation of domestic water supplies, profitable as it is, represents not a patch on the profits to be made from damming rivers for hydroelectric power, flooding out entire communities and compromising the environment irretrievably. But it creates splendid dividends for people living in First World urban opulence, who will never experience its adverse effects. As Marrero's paper points out, in this we are speaking of very long-term damage for every short-term advantage. It is a process which is continuing without effective social control, and we have to find elaborate mechanisms for reasserting global control before it is too late.

The effects of large-scale water privatisation are immense and even the FTAA's activities in the field rapidly transcend the Americas in their negative impacts on global health.

> The FTAA's neoliberal regime comes with a series of megaprojects of unprecedented proportions, which aim to detour water flows throughout the hemisphere. These projects are charted in three infrastructure plans: the North American Water and Power Alliance (NAWAPA), the Plan Puebla Panama (PPP), and the Initiative for the Integration of the Regional Infrastructure of South America (IIRSA).
>
> NAWAPA includes designs to build aqueducts, tunnels, and pumping stations to divert fresh water from Canada's mountainous west and Alaska, where this resource is abundant, toward the United States' arid west. This water would be stored – among other places – in a reservoir some 308 kilometres long planned for the Rocky Mountains.
>
> The PPP has as one of its key elements the establishment of industrial corridors with transportation and communications infrastructure from Mexico to Panama, and several inter-oceanic roads. Its objective is not only to facilitate the movement of commodities between the Pacific and Atlantic oceans, but also to take maximum advantage of the region's cheap labour and natural resources in export agribusiness, maquiladoras, and tourist resorts. All of this will require considerable quantities of electricity and fresh water, which will come from large reservoirs and hydro projects, especially in Guatemala's Petén and Mexico's Chiapas state. Part of this water would be pumped north to facilitate the growth of maquilas and agribusiness in northern Mexico, where rain is scarce.
>
> IIRSA includes plans for industrial corridors, water canals, and super highways that will connect the most remote corners of South America to the global economy. Some of these would cross the Andes mountain range to link the

Amazon Basin, which contains 20% of the world's drinkable water, to megaports to be built on the Pacific Coast.

One of IIRSA's projects is the construction of a Grand Canal that will connect the Plata, Amazon, and Orinoco rivers. This hydro pathway must be visualized as a direct exit to the Caribbean and a route toward the Mississippi River in the United States, says Mexican economist Giancarlo Delgado Ramos, a researcher with the Latin American Social Sciences Council. 'Here is where the scenario of super giant bags full of South American water being dragged toward the northern power (Florida) could unfold.'

Other ambitious IIRSA hydro projects are planned for the Plata River, whose basin (3.1 million square kilometres) is the nodal axis of Mercosur's productive zone. The US National Science Foundation has set up a multidisciplinary project to study the basin and its resources. It is also being surveyed by the American Association for the Advancement of Science as part of its Science for Sustainable Development project, with financing from the Ford and Rockefeller foundations, as well as corporations including Coca Cola, Nestle, Kellogg, IBM, and Kodak. Grassroots and progressive sectors in South America hold that all this scientific research is being carried out in the service of the transnational corporations' agenda.[28]

ACTUALLY RUNNING OUT OF WATER

The reader will recall the author's reference to recent exploitation of precious aquifers in our headlong rush into establishing golf courses for the ultra-privileged classes. In Latin America, much of the supply of clean and safe water depends on the huge Guarani Aquifer, which snakes its way underground from Argentina up to Brazil, embracing an area of 1.2 million km^2 and producing about 60 km^3 of water annually.

Another closely watched resource is the Guarani Aquifer, located between Argentina and Brazil, with a dimension of 1.2 million square kilometres and a production of 40 to 80 cubic kilometres of water a year.

The Global Environmental Facility, the environmental arm of the World Bank, is financing the Environmental Protection and Sustainable Development Project of the Guarani Aquifer. This project, based in Montevideo, has the support of the Organization of American States, the International Atomic Energy Agency, and the governments of the Netherlands and Germany. Its alleged end is the protection of the aquifer by insuring its rational use, but popular organizations and progressive sectors suspect that its real motivations are different.

The Brazilian movement Grito Das Aguas notes with concern that the project will consolidate the knowledge accumulated during years of research in different Latin American universities to put it at the disposal of corporate interests. With this information, the great economic groups will be able to steer their investments toward their primary objective: the creation of a water market. This de facto implementation of a new hydro-geopolitic of domination would jeopardise Latin American sovereignty.

Rich countries need the developing world's natural resources to continue to make the profits that are necessary to the neoliberal capitalist model, warns Grito Das Aguas. The group adds that since in the past their wealth was generated through super-exploitation of their own reserves, developed countries today face serious problems in increasing their productive capacity.

Hydroelectric projects and the looting of Latin America's blue gold and other natural strategic resources, such as biodiversity and oil, will run into difficulties if the opposition manages to coordinate its efforts, notes Delgado Ramos. The possibility of reversing the march toward mayhem depends on how solid the social wall is that is built to detain the different projects. But it also depends on how active a role the Latin American elites take in promoting and implementing them.

For its part, the Corporate Europe Observatory affirms the need to support popular initiatives like those in Porto Alegre, Cochabamba, and Santa Cruz, but at the same time to question the policies of institutions such as the Inter-American Development Bank and the World Bank, which favour privatization at the expense of any other option. The pivotal but sensitive issue of foreign debt must also be dealt with since the debt burden undermines the sovereignty of countries and causes a disastrous flow of capital from the poor South to the rich North.

Ultimately, the future of water access and use will depend in large part on the success of resistance to free trade regimes such as those of the WTO and the FTAA. These agreements force member countries to sell their water resources to the highest bidder, at the expense of any social or environmental consideration.[29]

As the author has indicated, it would appear that our only realistic hope is to make ourselves thoroughly aware of how these various resistance movements have developed and mobilised, the strategies they have adopted socially, legislatively and politically, and above all, how to counter the present obstacles to global equity in health.

We will close this chapter on the obstacle of water privatisation by briefly considering what strategic lessons we can learn from the situation in Ecuador.

ECUADOR

Ecuador is a country with not a great deal to offer in terms of precious minerals or oil but much to offer as a possible site for US military bases and, of course, a likely target for water privatisation. Until November 2006, Ecuador's rôle as a US ally and economic pawn was more or less taken for granted. It had rarely been the arena for violent revolutionary activity, and on the whole it acquiesced with the preferred right-wing approach of US business interests.

But the Ecuadorian people suddenly awoke – in September 2000 – to find that their government had 'dollarised the Ecuadorian currency'. Financiers and bankers, both Ecuadorian and American, could of course advance various arguments for the tactic, but its negative impacts on the poorest Ecuadorians (especially its ethnic minority American Indian communities) quickly became obvious. This author was in Ecuador at the time, and while in government offices or speaking to people in positions of authority, one only heard upbeat comments about dollarisation. But out in the streets and in the rural areas, I met little but hopeless despair. Rarely have I experienced at first hand such a divide between government and governed anywhere.

Therefore, the water privatisation scandal was really all it took to push out that compliant government and to bring in a more hard-nosed leftist government under Rafael Correa. But this author argues that the water privatisation scandal would not have been enough by itself. It was dollarisation that set the Ecuadorians for a fall. Thus some space must be devoted to summarising the events of that disaster.

IMPACTS OF DOLLARISING ECUADOR'S CURRENCY

Of course, there appeared to be good arguments for dollarisation. Some economists, for instance, argued convincingly that it allowed more financial flexibility at the local and community level, for the very cheapest commodities were still bought and sold with the old currency. In fact, dollarisation, by 2000, was regarded as a firm trend in Latin America. First Ecuador and then a month later El Salvador followed suit. But as well, dollarisation was even being considered by the wealthier English-speaking Latin American/Caribbean nations.

The 'flexibility' argument is based on the fact that:

> Third World economies have traditionally operated 'soft peg' exchange rate policies, whereby central banks determine the exchange rate they want to achieve between their currency and a stronger one, usually the US dollar, and then buy and (very occasionally) sell their own currency in international markets in order to keep it at that 'pegged' level.
>
> Such a policy makes a currency vulnerable to attack by foreign speculators,

however. If speculators are able to generate a panicked sell-off of the local currency by other foreign investors, they can force the central bank to sell them its foreign reserves on the cheap, in a vain attempt to keep the currency at the level of the peg.

This is exactly what happened to the Mexican peso in 1994 and to the East-Asian, Russian and Brazilian currencies during the world financial crisis of 1997–98 – all came under sustained and successful attack by speculators. Defending its soft peg drained Brazil's central bank of US$56 billion in reserves within a year, according to IMF figures.

Since the crisis and the desperate failure of the 'soft peg', the conventional wisdom among neoliberal economists has reduced Third World governments' exchange rate options to two polar opposites: either a freely floating currency, in which the central bank makes little or no attempt to keep it at a set level, or a 'hard peg', an irrevocable linking of the local monetary unit with a stronger one, either by law or through adopting the stronger currency outright, as in dollarisation.

But neither policy course offers much chance of improving the people's welfare. Both policy courses only further Third World countries' dependence on First World central banks and financial markets.

The perils of a freely floating currency are obvious: it offers no protection whatsoever from increasing volatility of international currency markets. Countries which choose a free float, as Brazil and Mexico now have, thus become painfully dependent on their own 'credibility', a financial press euphemism for the good will of the major foreign investors. Any false move and instantly the currency is sold down, inflation kicks in and capital flees.[30]

INFLEXIBILITY AND STABILITY

The appeal of a 'hard peg' is that it promises to do away with this instability, most especially the threat of the hyperinflation which has long plagued Latin America. Third World governments trade in their currencies for the unassailable 'credibility' of the greenback and the US Federal Reserve.

The ability of the 'hard peg' to deliver stability and economic growth is questionable, however, as delivery is highly dependent on local elites' disavowal of profiteering, something which very rarely happens. Even more importantly, the 'hard peg' severely restricts anti-recessionary policy options. Monetary policy – such as currency devaluations, drops in its official interest rates and expansions of the money supply – is completely closed off and handed over to the US Federal Reserve. Fiscal policy – such as running government deficits to stimulate demand – is severely restricted, both by the necessity to keep large foreign currency reserves in order to cover demand for US dollars and by countries' massive debt repayment commitments.

The price, then, of dollarised 'stability' is that any economic shocks can only be dealt with by deflation – more specifically, by a sharp reduction in workers' living standards. Austerity becomes the only policy option.

Since then-President Jamil Mahuad announced Ecuador's dollarisation plan on 9 January 2000, for example, the impoverished Andean nation has experienced its worst-ever inflation rate – 91% – largely due to the local elite running up a 50% US dollar loan default rate and stripping domestic banks of assets.

The shift to the dollar has been universally condemned by Ecuador's popular sectors. Within three months of announcing the plan, Mahuad was forced to resign by a near-insurrection in April, led by the country's indigenous communities. Protests have continued since, albeit on a lesser scale, against his successor, Gustavo Noboa.

The social impact has even been recognised by officials of the World Bank, which backed dollarisation. According to the bank's Ecuador chief, Augusto de la Torre, since the adoption of the dollar, 'the economic system has become more corrupt, more politicised and therefore there is more room for the traditional oligarchy to come back, with force'.

Western bankers, such as Federico Kaune, vice-president for 'emerging markets' at the US investment bank Goldman Sachs, now advise Ecuador that dollarisation will only work if a 'fiscal adjustment' is carried out, including a hike in the rate of value-added tax and the privatisation of state assets.[31]

It was dollarisation, this author argues, that finally woke the Ecuadorians up and gave the lower social classes, including the largely neglected ethnic minorities, the impetus to oppose authority. The débâcle of water privatisation only confirmed the rectitude of that quasi-revolutionary point of view.

DOING THE WORLD BANK'S BIDDING – PRIVATISING WATER AT GUAYAQUIL

The actual transnational water privatisation firm which gave rise to the corruption and ineptitude that set off the Bolivian resistance in the Bolivia city of Cochabamba was Bechtel, and, as the fates would have it, Ecuador – as part of an Inter-American Loan (under World Bank auspices) – was required to privatise its water supply via Bechtel. The plot unfolds almost as ineluctably as a Greek tragedy!

As Sara Grusky reported in October 2007, it was only a few months after the resolution of the Cochabamba fiasco that Bechtel found itself engaged to service the water and sewage needs of yet another Latin American city, this time Guayaquil, the largest city in Ecuador.[32] Details of the agreement were not widely proclaimed over the government-controlled media because of the disgrace at Cochabamba. However, the truth soon enough leaked out, even though the deal was signed with another company, Interagua, a subsidiary of Bechtel. The government signed – under the duress of Structural Adjustment Policies – a 30-year concession contract to run all water and sanitation services in Guayaquil.

The privatization process was promoted by loans from the Inter-American Development Bank and a guarantee from the Multilateral Investment Guarantee Agency (MIGA), a World Bank agency. Now, more than six years later, the residents of Guayaquil are demanding damages from the company for water contamination, an end to water cut-offs, and a return to local, public control.

On Sept. 28 residents in Guayaquil gathered in front of the offices of the undersecretary of the economy to protest the contract. On Oct. 18 thousands gathered to proclaim that water is a human right, demanding that their 'water debts' are forgiven and that their water services are reconnected. A local advocacy organization, the Observatorio Cuidadano de Servicios Publicos (Citizen's Observatory of Public Services), is seeking to stop the water cut-offs through legal action.

One in six people in the world lack access to clean and affordable water and thousands of children die of water-borne diseases every day. Corporations like Bechtel seek to profit from providing water, often elevating the narrow interests of their companies and its shareholders above social and environmental goals. Around the world, privatization has led to large rate hikes and poor service, while failing to solve the problem of lack of access, leaving the poorest communities with no water services at all. This is now the situation in Guayaquil, where there are hundreds of documented complaints due to the appalling service of Bechtel's subsidiary, Interagua. The citizens of Guayaquil are demanding accountability from the company. The Ecuadorian regulatory agency ECAPAG recently fined Interagua $1.5 million for contractual violations. Some of the problems that face the residents of Guayaquil include:

- Repeated residential water cut-offs for up to 12, 24, 36, or more hours at a time;
- Residential water cut-offs of senior citizens and other low-income residents due to inability to pay;
- Failure to extend services to specific neighbourhoods, especially to low-income residents;
- Failure to meet contractual obligations for rehabilitation and expansion of services;
- Public health problems such as respiratory problems, skin rashes, asthma, and diarrhoea due to lack of wastewater treatment;
- Environmental contamination due to lack of wastewater treatment;
- Hepatitis A outbreaks, such as one in June 2005, investigated by local

authorities (Commission for Civic Control and the Public Defender's office) who concluded that the water was 'not apt for human consumption.'[33]

THE DEAL COLLAPSES

In 2006, Bechtel's total revenue amounted to $20.5 billion and Interagua's operations in Guayaquil earned $300 million in revenue. Despite these profits, Interagua did not initiate the rehabilitation programs it had promised. Concerns and complaints mounted over broken pipelines, floods due to malfunctioning sewage systems, exorbitant water rates, poor water quality, and environmental damage due to the lack of wastewater treatment during this first five-year period. Lack of investment in storm drainage forced many residents to suffer the health effects of constant flooding. In 2002 the company was treating only 5% of the sewage and releasing the rest, including fecal material, and domestic and industrial waste directly into the local river, Guayas. The health department began to issue reports documenting health problems that children were experiencing in communities located north of the city, such as Acuarelas del Río and Guayacanes, where the sewage was being released. The health problems included skin rashes, asthma, and gastric problems such as diarrhoea.

Along with overflowing sewage and illegal dumping, unsafe tap water has also contributed to the serious health crisis. Residents complain about the 'nauseating' and 'unbearable' odor coming from the tap water. Interagua has refused to make public information regarding water quality. In June 2005 over 150 children were infected with Hepatitis A from drinking dirty tap water. The outbreak was concentrated around the western suburbs of Guayaquil, where 76% of residents described their water as cloudy and foul-smelling. Interagua denied responsibility for the outbreak but studies have shown that it was a combination of the nonfunctional sewage system and poor water quality that contributed ultimately to the outbreak of Hepatitis A. The Commission for Civic Control and the Public Defender's office declared that Interagua held some responsibility for the Hepatitis A outbreak and concluded that the water was 'not fit for human consumption.' But problems persist including repeated cut-offs of water service that last for more than 24 hours, which is illegal unless the company provides alternative sources of water for the residents. In some areas Interagua cut the water for 23 hours a day in order to evade the responsibility of providing an alternative water source. In addition, the company continues to cut off water services when consumers accumulate too much debt.[34]

PEOPLE'S POWER ASSERTS ITSELF

Of course, by the time all of this was happening, the Ecuadorian government was no longer the compliant and long-suffering vassal of US corporate interests that it had been – and President Correa, who had already established good relations with both Fidel Castro in Cuba and Hugo Chávez in Venezuela – had a politically energised people behind him.

> Guarantees and loans provided by the World Bank and the Inter-American Development Bank have ensured a profitable investment for one of the world's most influential corporations, Bechtel. But, similar to the experience of many other cities across the world, water privatization has not solved water problems in Guayaquil. Instead, Bechtel has delivered water not suitable for drinking, refused to expand access to services, cut off water to those unable to pay, and neglected responsibilities to provide wastewater treatment compromising the local environment and public health.
>
> The Observatorio Cuidadano de Servicios Públicos is working tirelessly to document Bechtel's contract violations. The group – which brings together numerous civil society organizations in Guayaquil to monitor and help improve public services – has exposed the constitutional, legal, and contractual violations of Interagua and is working to ensure that action is taken. They will continue to organize and demand that water and other public services be locally and publicly owned, controlled, and managed with active citizen oversight and participation.
>
> The recognition of water as a human right and the push for citizen oversight and participation in public services is also being acknowledged and supported on an international scale. The United Nations Committee on Economic, Social, and Cultural Rights adopted the human right to water on Nov. 26 2002 and the United Nations Development Program's Human Development Report of 2006 calls on all governments to enshrine the right to water in enabling legislation. The human right to water is indispensable for leading a life of human dignity. Everyone should have secure access to sufficient safe water and sanitation to meet their basic human needs. To ensure that safe and affordable water is available to the 1.2 billion people across the globe that currently do not have proper access, international financial institutions and aid agencies need to abandon failed policies and stop pushing countries to privatize water services. Governments need to involve residents in solutions and recognize the human right to clean and affordable water.[35]

Thus the Ecuadorian experience has provided yet another model of how to organise resistance and of the social and political contexts which render success more likely. It provides us with further insight into overcoming one particular obstacle to global health equity.

REFERENCES

1 McGriffin S. The water robbers. *Morning Star.* 19 Mar 2008. p. 8.

2 MacDonald T. *Health, Trade and Human Rights.* Oxford & New York: Radcliffe Publishing; 2006. p. 47.

3 Galli, B. Quoted on the *BBC World Service.* 15 Aug 2007.

4 World Social Forum. *Addressing Global Water Access Inequities.* Available at: www.ukabc.org/wsf2003.htm (accessed 27 Apr 2008).

5 World Water Forum. Last days of the Water Water Forum. *The Watering Hole.* 24 Mar 2006. Available at: www.lipmagazine.org/conant/archives/2006/03/last_days_of_th_1.html (accessed 27 Apr 2008).

6 MacDonald T. *Health, Human Rights and the United Nations: inconsistent aims and inherent contradictions.* Oxford & New York: Radcliffe Publishing; 2007. p. 9.

7 Last days of the Water Water Forum, op. cit. p. 3

8 Hesperian Foundation/UNDP. *Water for Life: community water security.* Available at: www.energyandenviroment.undp.org/undp/index.cfm?DocumentID=5637&module=Library&page=Document (accessed 27 Apr 2008).

9 MacDonald T. *Third World Health: hostage to First World wealth.* Oxford & New York: Radcliffe Publishing; 2005.

10 Wikipedia. *Water Privatization – Multinationals.* http://en.wikipedia.org/wiki/water_privatisation (accessed 27 Apr 2008).

11 MacDonald T. *The Global Right to Health: dream or possibility.* Oxford & New York: Radcliffe Publishing; 2007. pp. 24–8.

12 Schultz J. The politics of water in Bolivia. *The Nation.* 28 Jan 2005. pp. 4–7.

13 Finnegan W. Leasing the rain. *The New Yorker.* 8 Apr 2002. p. 2.

14 The politics of water in Bolivia, op. cit.

15 *Water Privatization – Multinationals,* op. cit.

16 *Water Privatization – Multinationals,* op. cit.

17 CNN: Broadcast under World News, 10 Apr 2000.

18 *Water Privatization – Multinationals,* op. cit.

19 *Water Privatization – Multinationals,* op. cit.

20 *Water Privatization – Multinationals,* op. cit.

21 *Water Privatization – Multinationals,* op. cit.

22 *Water Privatization – Multinationals,* op. cit.

23 MacDonald T. *Sacrificing the WHO to the Highest Bidder.* Oxford & New York: Radcliffe Publishing; 2008. pp. 180–2.

24 Marrero C. *Free Trade and Water Privatization: the wet side of the FTAA.* 2 Dec 2004. Available at: www.americaspolicy.org/articles/2004/0412water.html (accessed 29 Apr 2008).

25 *Free Trade and Water Privatization: the wet side of the FTAA,* op. cit.

26 *Free Trade and Water Privatization: the wet side of the FTAA,* op. cit.

27 *Free Trade and Water Privatization: the wet side of the FTAA,* op. cit.

28 *Free Trade and Water Privatization: the wet side of the FTAA*, op. cit.

29 *Free Trade and Water Privatization: the wet side of the FTAA*, op. cit.

30 Healy S. *Latin America: trend toward dollarisation accelerates.* 24 Jan 2001. Available at: www.greenleft.org.au/2001/433/26904.

31 *Latin America: trend toward dollarisation accelerates*, op. cit.

32 Grusky S. WHO controls Ecuador's water. *Food and Water Watch.* 30 Oct 2007. Available at: http://Americas.irc-online.org/am/4686 (accessed 30 Mar 2008).

33 WHO controls Ecuador's water, op. cit.

34 WHO controls Ecuador's water, op. cit.

35 WHO controls Ecuador's water, op. cit.

Chapter 4

Neoliberalist approaches to healthcare and the transnational pharmaceutical corporations

PHARMACEUTICAL CORPORATIONS AND MEDICAL PROGRESS

In the past five or six decades the progress made in humankind's ongoing war against disease has been nothing short of remarkable. Illnesses which only 20 years ago were regarded as death sentences can often now be cured by swallowing a pill three times a day for a week or so and never missing a day of work while doing so. Our astonishing medical victories have occurred right across the healthcare spectrum, from heroic advances in surgery to modern insights into nutrition and huge technical advances in diagnosis, but it is broadly agreed that pharmaceutical corporations have played an enormous rôle in the ongoing war against disease. Indeed, this is so much the case that the names of some of the more famous pharmaceutical corporations, and of many of the remedies they have produced, have become household words worldwide.

Of course, such activity is hugely expensive to carry out, and as a consequence, the remedies themselves are expensive. It is not difficult to understand why this is so. Behind the emergence of every new wonder drug is an army of expensively-trained medical researchers, some of them in international demand as leaders in their field. Typically, a new medication has involved years of laboratory research and carefully monitored drug trials, so that by the time a remedy has been proven safe and effective and is ready for distribution, it has involved millions of pounds in accumulated costs. In order to stay in business – and we would all quickly suffer if those pharmaceutical firms did not – they have to continuously recoup the expenses they have generated.

In some First World countries the citizens are lucky enough to have a universal health service, like the NHS in the UK, and thus each patient only pays a fixed contribution to the cost of any prescription required. But the cost is not trivial and it is said that the NHS spends more on pharmaceuticals from multinational pharmaceutical corporations than any other bulk customer. In the USA, by contrast, each patient pays for their own prescriptions and consequently many do not bother having them filled. This, of course, condemns many US citizens to levels of ill-health and/or suffering that a British person can hardly imagine.

But it is in Third World countries that the neoliberal financial rules by which corporations live condemn many – especially among children or the elderly – to unnecessary death. There are two broad reasons for this, which serve to help maintain the widening gap of global health inequity.

1   Many tropical diseases – most Third World countries have tropical climates – can now be cured quite easily by recently developed pharmaceuticals, but these cost too much for all but a small and privileged portion of a Third World country's population to access.

2   A large number of common and distressing tropical illnesses have not attracted the interest of the major pharmaceutical corporations and consequently no remedies have yet been developed. The reason for this is plain – the corporations have to realise a profit from the massive investment in preliminary biochemical research required to elaborate a remedy. But if the disease concerned mainly attacks people too poor to pay for the prescriptions, the profit incentive is gone and the necessary research never undertaken.

The following two quotes state the issues rather well:

> Millions of people, most of them in tropical countries of the Third World, die of preventable, curable diseases. . . . Malaria, tuberculosis, acute lower-respiratory infections – in 1998, these claimed 6.1 million lives. People died because the drugs to treat those illnesses are nonexistent or are no longer effective. They died because it doesn't pay to keep them alive.[1]

> The establishment of the World Trade Organization . . . imposed US style intellectual property rights around the world. These rights were intended to reduce access to generic medicines and they succeeded. Developing countries

paid a high price for this agreement. But what have they received in return? Drug companies spend more on advertising and marketing than on research, more on research on lifestyle drugs than on life-saving drugs, and almost nothing on diseases that affect developing countries only. This is not surprising. Poor people cannot afford drugs, and drug companies make investments that yield the highest returns. The chief executive of Novartis, a drug company with a history of social responsibility, said 'We have no model which would [meet] the need for new drugs in a sustainable way . . . You can't expect for-profit organizations to do this on a large scale.[2]

That, of course, is why treatments are available for a host of less serious diseases – but ones which afflict wealthy people in First World countries, while diseases such as malaria, which wipe out millions a year, remain far down the research list of problems to address.

HIV/AIDS, for instance, was merrily wiping out millions of economically deprived people for two or three decades before it began to attack and kill people in the First World in the 1980s.[3] At that point, serious money was put into the necessary research, and a sequence of drugs, of which various antiretrovirals (ARVs) are the latest, were developed.

But, as we shall see, the problems do not stop there, because, although most sub-Saharan African victims of HIV/AIDS cannot afford the ARVs (the wealthier First World victims keep the companies in business), some countries (such as India and Brazil) set about producing generic copies of these expensive ARVs. Generic copies, of course, cost far less to produce than the originals because no money has had to be spent on the research and development phases. As the author has pointed out in previous books, the pharmaceutical corporations – and the forces of neoliberalism behind them – have not reacted kindly to such developments and have used all sorts of strategies to prevent Brazil and India from making generic copies available (at greatly reduced prices) to the masses of people who would otherwise not be able to access effective treatment.[4]

THE TRANSNATIONAL PHARMACEUTICAL INDUSTRY AS A BARRIER

It is issues like that – issues which impose restrictions on access to healthcare in the name of enhanced profits for unaffected shareholders living thousands of miles away – which render the transnational pharmaceutical corporations themselves obstacles to global health equity. They are also aided in this policy of generating financial profit by effectively preventing poorer people from accessing needed health by the IMF, the World Bank and the WTO.

Poor countries driven to approach the IMF and the World Bank for development loans often find that, as a result of imposed Structural Adjustment Policies (SAPs), their own existing government-financed public health programmes become restricted in favour of engaging private contractors. If they try to solve the problems by using generic copies of ARVs from Brazil or India, they often find themselves in violation of Trade-Related Aspects of International Property Rights (TRIPS) regulations under patent legislation, as explained by the author in a previous book.[5]

As Marwaan Macan-Marker of the Third World Network (TWN) reported as far back as 2001 the patterns of the emerging conflict were already becoming clear.[6]

> The battle lines between the Western-based transnational pharmaceutical industry and companies in the developing world that produce generic drugs have grown sharper this month, with anti-AIDS drugs being at the heart of this dispute.
>
> Among the catalysts in such a turn of events include Cipla, an Indian pharmaceutical company, and the government of Brazil, both of which are adamant on challenging the stance of the pharmaceutical industry that it decides who should produce anti-AIDS drugs and at what price they should be sold.
>
> Significant in the Cipla challenge, which came to light on 6 February, is the price at which it is prepared to sell large quantities of the triple-therapy cocktail of anti-AIDS generic drugs to African countries. The amount ranges from $350 per year if the drug combination is sold to patients to $600 per year if the same combination is sold to African governments.
>
> By contrast, the same combination of drugs sold in the United States by the pharmaceutical companies that hold the patents costs between $10 000–15 000 per year.
>
> On 15 February furthermore, the Cipla offer is due to evolve from an announcement to action, when company representatives meet the Paris-based medical aid agency Doctors Without Borders (known by its French acronym MSF, for Médecins Sans Frontières) to work out plans to distribute its generic drugs.
>
> The Cipla offer has received a nod of approval from the World Health Organization (WHO). In a statement issued on 9 February, the leading UN health agency declared that it 'welcomes recent reports' of the combined triple-therapy medication of anti-AIDS drugs being made available cheaply in Africa for those afflicted with HIV and AIDS.
>
> 'The cost of medication is one of several factors limiting access to life-extending care for people living with HIV/AIDS,' the Geneva-based health body states. 'The reduction in the cost of anti-retroviral medicines and other drugs

combating opportunistic infections is one of the key objectives of accelerating access to effective care for people living with HIV.'

The dispute between Brazil and the pharmaceutical industry centres on the right to produce generic anti-AIDS drugs. At the beginning of this month, the South American nation made its intentions clear, when it threatened to back local production of generic versions of two anti-AIDS drugs if the pharmaceutical companies making those drugs refused to lower their prices by June.

Such defiance came after the US government filed a complaint with the World Trade Organization's (WTO) Dispute Settlement Body over Brazil's intention to 'violate' patent rights, consequently defending a US pharmaceutical company involved in this discord.

'The US complaint threatens the Brazilian AIDS policy, which includes providing free drugs to HIV-infected people. The lives of hundreds of thousands of patients depend on this system,' declared Bernard Pecoul, director of MSF's Access to Essential Medicines campaign.

'The Brazilian government is currently treating over 90 000 patients afflicted with the human immunodeficiency virus (HIV) that causes the acquired immune deficiency syndrome (AIDS) through the generic anti-AIDS drugs produced domestically. Since such efforts began, moreover, it has resulted in a decrease of AIDS deaths by 50 percent.'[7] And since then, as cited above, the neoliberal interests have succeeded in stifling the export of generic copies to the Third World countries.

> Such determination, in fact, is amplified in a court case due to commence in South Africa early March. . . . In this legal dispute, 40 pharmaceutical companies will be suing the South African government for enabling the import of generic anti-AIDS drugs into South Africa under the country's Medicines Amendment Act of 1997.
>
> For Richard Jeffreys, project director at the New York-based AIDS Treatment Data Network, such a court case is 'morally repugnant'. In Ghana, he adds, patients with HIV who were taking the generic version of Combivir, an anti-AIDS drug, 'have literally had their drug supply cut off' following a lawsuit by Glaxo Smithkline, a leading pharmaceutical company. 'They are already the most profitable industry in the world, and lives surely do not have to be sacrificed to keep their stockholders happy,' he asserts.
>
> Moreover, there are other factors that explain why such challenges are being mounted against the drug industry. According to MSF, for instance, even when pharmaceutical companies have demonstrated a will to cut the prices of anti-AIDS drugs, they have been slow to deliver on their commitments or the

cheaper drugs were still prohibitively priced for the developing world.

By last December MSF points out, there had been 'little progress' on a promised discount on anti-AIDS drugs made last year by five pharmaceutical companies to nations in Africa, where close to 25 million people are infected with HIV out of the 36 million people infected worldwide.

To date, only agreements with three African countries have been reached under that initiative, 'Accelerating Access', which is backed by the Joint United Nations Programme on HIV/AIDS (UNAIDS). The three countries are Senegal, Uganda and Rwanda.

And for MSF, not only is the amount that Senegalese pay under this initiative too high – between $1000–1800 per patient for annual treatment – but the number of patients who would benefit under such effort would only be around 900.

For James Love, director of the Consumer Project on Technology, a Washington DC-based consumer rights group, the attitude of the pharmaceutical companies has left governments in the Third World with little alternative but to turn to generic anti-AIDS drugs as a remedy against the killer disease.

'Governments have a responsibility to protect their people and they should draw the line when the price for medicines is too high,' he argues. 'You have to look at the reality, since drug companies are determined to control prices at the expense of the sick.' The pharmaceutical industry will have more challenges to contend with in the future, given the emergence of generic-drug manufacturers in Thailand, Pakistan, the Philippines and China.

Adds MSF: 'Developing countries should take full advantage of their rights to produce or import generic drugs under the WTO's TRIPS (Trade-Related Aspects of Intellectual Property Rights) Agreement.' Such a view by MSF stems from the conditions spelled out under the TRIPS Agreement, which allows for a special provision, called 'compulsory licensing', that permits countries to produce drugs which are under patents in cases of public health emergencies or where there is unfair pricing. If heeded, it could propel the animosity between the patent-holding drug companies and advocates of generic alternatives to a more intense level in the future.

But the United States is trying to use its power of bilateral threats, (. . .) bilateral and regional agreements, as well as the negotiations for the Free Trade Area for Americas, to tighten up investment and intellectual property rules – to take away even the limited leeway now available under the WTO accords.[8]

NEOLIBERALISM AND HIV/AIDS IN SOUTH AFRICA

The profit motive produces two noticeable effects – it widens any inequity gaps which already exist and, as indicated in Chapter One, it establishes a basis for allowing neoliberalism to assume hegemony over human rights. One sees this illustrated with respect to, say, the rôle that HIV/AIDS in any Third World country can effectively have in dividing societies. South Africa provided an excellent example when, in 1999, the South African government was moved – by the South African Communist Party – to condemn the US government for backing the WTO in trying to prevent the Republic from gaining access to generic copies of RARVs. Key Martin reported the event in the *Workers World* newspaper, published in Durban.[9]

He argued that the world is faced with a struggle between Third World countries like South Africa and the neoliberal forces (especially transnational pharmaceutical corporations) to secure equity of access to effective HIV/AIDS remedies. The South African Communist Party saw it in ideological terms, asserting that problem was that the US government had backed a legal action by the Pharmaceuticals Manufacturing Association and 41 drug companies in the South African Constitutional Court.

> The suit aims to block implementation of the Medicines and Related Substances Act.
>
> This Medicine Act uses provisions of World Trade Organization procedures to license domestic generic production of medicines. It also allows purchasers to import medicines from third countries rather than buy from the patent holders when discounts are available.
>
> Pharmaceutical companies were given a lot of benefits by the old apartheid regime to attract them to the country during the years of the economic boycotts. They have a stranglehold on the industry.
>
> If this law helps South Africa to meet the HIV/AIDS crisis, it will open up a strategy for all of southern Africa. Already, in Zimbabwe, the morgues are open 24 hours a day because of the dramatic death toll from diseases brought on by AIDS.
>
> The US trade representative, however, has placed South Africa on a 'watchlist' and withheld trade benefits for some South African products, charging 'piracy' of 'intellectual property rights', a process that could lead to an even bigger economic blockade.
>
> Years have already been lost to corporate greed in the fight against AIDS in Africa and thousands have died. According to Umsebenzi, a publication of the South African Communist Party, last year 3.5 million South Africans had HIV and 100 000 were estimated to be dying each year.[10]

Protests coincided with health campaigns involving a variety of groups in the USA during October of 2001.

A COMMUNIST VIEW

The general secretary of the South African Communist Party made a statement on the situation which was relayed and read out to the US protestors. In it he stated:[11]

> One of the biggest threats that we face as a country, as a region, as a continent, is the scourge of HIV/AIDS. One should not be surprised at this because poor countries are unable to provide some of the necessary tools to fight HIV, like education, literacy and so on. What this also illustrates is the extent to which the Western world seems to be turning a blind eye, particularly to sub-Saharan Africa.
>
> The pharmaceutical companies are just not interested in providing even some drugs that could assist in trying to contain or prevent some aspects of the epidemic, like the passing of HIV/AIDS from mother to child. The United States government's behaviour in this regard is shocking because it has backed these pharmaceutical companies to the hilt, which prevents us from finding mechanisms to deal with this and many other problems and diseases because of the high costs of medications.
>
> We are really pleased and appreciate the fact that our comrades and other people have waged these high-profile protests. I think they are beginning to make it felt because we hear now that even Vice President Al Gore is trying quietly to plead with the ANC and the South African government to assist in containing some of these protests.

The protests in the US energised AIDS activists, including ACT-UP (AIDS Coalition To Unleash Power) and other American groups, to actually intrude in late October on the Presidential campaign of Al Gore, President Bill Clinton's vice-president. They did this by handing out leaflets exposing Gore's links to the large pharmaceutical companies and demanding that they stop using the WTO and various patent law legal actions against generic copy producers.

Although that particular statement had been a policy statement of the South Africa Communist Party, the sentiments it expressed were also warmly endorsed by the African National Congress (ANC). In fact, the ANC General Secretary, Kgalema Mortlante, stated:[12]

> Today it's the pharmaceuticals, tomorrow it's something else. The issue is really about how transnationals operate in essentially Third World countries.
>
> The 'pharmaceuticals' issue now is typical of the manner of operation of most transnational [corporations]. They tend to dictate, use their power, to give prices, to determine and load terms of trade in their favour regardless of the consequences to those they are doing trade with.

And in the case of these pharmaceuticals, the South African approach, the ANC's approach to issues of health, is to have a national primary health system, where you lay emphasis on prevention. This requires lots of education, lots of generic medicine, which can be affordable and therefore accessible to poor communities.

In this respect he seemed far more realistically aware of how transnational corporations operate – responsible only to their First World stockholders and not to the people who suffer their policies – than do our First World politicians. He went on to observe that the pharmaceutical corporations are energised only to generate higher dividends for their First World stockholders and nothing else, and that for this reason they seek only to maximise profits and thus be in a position to exercise complete control over the logistics so that they can fetch higher prices. 'From an affordability point of view, this control would actually exclude the majority of people who need such medicines. When they deal with Third World countries, even given what they normally describe as "market forces" doesn't apply. They set prices because they determine the terms of trade.'

In that long and diluted speech, Kgelama Mortlante kept emphasising the link with US banking and business interests by pointing out that in this sort of action they did not represent what he termed 'ordinary working Americans'. He emphasised the fact that it was 'ordinary American wage earners' who were so stalwartly protesting against the pharmaceutical industry, and that South Africans should regard them as being allies as they engage in the struggle to save humanity. He also reflected the belief that such protests would ultimately cause the corporations to retract, as happened in the US in response to anti-Vietnam war protests. In this, of course, he was clearly wrong, but he insisted that struggle must not be allowed to be sequestered in different campaigns in different countries, but must be coordinated transnationally. This will be dealt with in the final chapter.

In closing, Mortlante reminded his audience that if they were to read through any of the corporate policy statements, they would easily ascertain their purpose in using US influence and cash to derail South Africa's attempts to establish a domestic health policy based on people's needs. They could only come to one conclusion – and that is that neoliberalism is guided only by a business philosophy. The corporations have not the slightest concern for the health of South Africa's people, especially the most deprived. Their primary goal is to make profits, even out of people who are dying and who will have no share in those profits.

THE POWER AND INFLUENCE OF THE PHARMACEUTICAL INDUSTRY

From the above, it should be clear that equity of access to primary healthcare will have to involve considerable action on a number of fronts. But one of the fundamental ones has to address the issue of making pharmaceuticals available where the medically determined need is, and not primarily where the greatest profits are to be made. Despite all that has been said (and will be said) about the intimacy of the relationship between US government interests and corporate power in sustaining a neoliberal agenda, some of the best resistance to this relationship comes from within the USA itself. An example, however, of just how well 'plugged in' the pharmaceutical industry is to the levers of corporate power is exemplified by a group calling itself the Pharmaceutical Research and Manufacturers of America (PhRMA). In the USA, groups opposed to its activities refer to it as 'Big Pharma', and that ironic term, along with references to 'the Empire', now has considerable currency globally.

Various analyses have suggested that links between European and, later, American imperialist expansion and the phenomenal growth of capitalism are reflected in the current activities and attitudes of Big Pharma. In other words, it was the need to protect colonial interests, and especially the health of settlers and soldiers, that drove early and prolonged medical research into such tropical diseases as malaria and yellow fever.

According to the Wikipedia entry, PhRMA represents the pharmaceutical research and biotechnology companies in the United States. It is one of the largest and most influential lobbying organisations in Washington, DC.

On its website, PhRMA states its 'mission is winning advocacy for public policies that encourage the discovery of life-saving and life-enhancing new medicines for patients by pharmaceutical/biotechnology research companies.' It goes on to say, 'To accomplish this mission, PhRMA is dedicated to achieving in Washington, DC, the United States and in the entire world the following:

❐ Broad patient access to safe and effective medicines through a free market, without price controls
❐ Strong intellectual property incentives, and
❐ Transparent, efficient regulation and a free flow of information to patients.'[13]

PhRMA tries to present an image of caring concern and devotion to helping the sick, but its neoliberal intentions and fixation on its wealthy shareholders is never far from the surface.

In keeping with its transnational representation of corporate interests, PhRMA's lobbying activities have extended outside the United States. 'America's big drug companies are intensifying their lobbying efforts to change the Canadian healthcare system and to eliminate subsidised prescription drug prices enjoyed by Canadians,' Canwest News Service reported on 9 June 2003.[14] 'A prescription drug industry spokesman in Washington confirmed to Canwest News Service that information contained in confidential industry documents is accurate and that $1 million US is being added to the already heavily funded drug lobby against the Canadian system.' PhRMA was the leading drug industry trade group behind the increased lobbying and PR campaign. PhRMA was also independently spending $450 000 to target the booming Canadian internet pharmacy industry, which has been providing Americans with prescription drugs at lower prices than they can obtain in the United States.

It is the hostility which PhRMA exhibits toward generic copies that gives us a true picture of its intentions. As Robert Weissman says, 'Whenever developing countries seek to improve access to essential medicines by hastening the introduction of generic competition and reducing prices, they invariably must confront a single overriding claim: their actions will undermine incentives for research and development (R&D) of important new drugs.'

Weissman goes on to observe:[15]

> PhRMA is deeply troubled by the recent trend toward the issuance of compulsory licenses for pharmaceutical products,' said Billy Tauzin, President and CEO of PhRMA, the U.S. pharmaceutical companies' trade association, in 2007. Tauzin's statement followed Thailand's decision to import significantly cheaper generic versions of three life-saving drugs and Brazil's decision to use the generic version of a key treatment for HIV/AIDS. 'This misguided focus on short-term "budget fixes" could come at a far greater long-term cost, potentially limiting important incentives for research and development that are necessary to positively impact the lives of millions of patients worldwide.'
>
> It is expensive to develop new drugs, but not nearly as costly as the pharmaceutical industry suggests.

TRUTH ABOUT R&D COSTS

Numerous independent studies and investigations show that the world's largest drug companies' R&D spending claims are misleading and overblown, and that they spend much more on marketing than on R&D for new products. These findings undermine the pharmaceutical industry's repeated assertion that high drug prices are justified by the cost of research, and that generic competition in the developing world will undermine the industry's ability to develop new treatments.

Although PhRMA asserts that U.S. brand-name pharmaceutical companies invest more in R&D than marketing, independent investigators reach different conclusions. A January 2008 article, published in the peer-reviewed journal *PLoS*, concluded that U.S. drug companies spent almost twice as much on marketing as on R&D. Researchers Marc-Andre Gagnon and Joel Lexchin of York University in Toronto found that U.S. companies spent 24.4% of their U.S. sales on marketing and 13.4% on R&D in 2004. U.S. sales that year totalled US$235.4 billion. Gagnon and Lexchin based their findings on data and estimates drawn from industry sources.

'These numbers clearly show how much promotion predominates over R&D in the pharmaceutical industry, contrary to the industry's claim,' wrote Gagnon and Lexchin. '[This] confirms the public image of a marketing-driven industry and provides an important argument to petition in favour of transforming the workings of the industry in the direction of more research and less promotion.'

And while companies argue that high drug prices are necessary to cover the cost of R&D – implying that companies make only modest profits after the cost of R&D is paid for – pharmaceuticals remain one of the world's most profitable industries. The industry's 2006 return on investment was 19.6%, according to *Fortune*, second only to the oil and mining industry. Pharmaceuticals almost always rank in the top three industry sectors by this measure.

Current R&D incentives often result in limited health benefits as well as high prices. The investments that Big Pharma does make into R&D are driven by market demand, not public health need. One result is a surplus of 'me-too' drugs, treatments that are similar to existing products and offer limited therapeutic benefits over existing medicines.

When new drugs are submitted to the US Food and Drug Administration (FDA) for marketing approval, the agency classifies them as meriting either 'priority review' (conferred for drugs that offer 'major advances in treatment, or provide a treatment where no adequate therapy exists') or 'standard review' (applied to a drug that offers 'at most, only minor improvement over existing marketed therapies'). Only about one third of FDA approvals reach 'priority.'

Other reviews find that only about one in ten new drugs offer substantial therapeutic gains:

- Between 1999 and 2004, 122 new active substances were introduced into Canada. Only 10 percent were designated as major therapeutic advances or breakthrough products, according to a report by the Patented Medicine Prices Review Board of Canada.
- Since 1981, Prescrire, a leading review offering independent comparative information on drugs and other therapeutic interventions, has been evaluating new drugs and new indications for older drugs. By 2003, it had completed almost 2900 such assessments and found that only 11 percent of medications constituted substantial advances.

Big Pharma is very concerned about developing country markets, where drug sales are growing at a faster rate than in rich countries. However, it remains the case that developing countries represent only a small fraction of Big Pharma's revenues. Developing country markets account for less than 13 percent of global pharmaceutical sales, according to IMS Health. Slightly more than 1 percent of sales are attributed to sub-Saharan Africa, the world's poorest region.

Any lost revenue from developing countries therefore and by definition can only have a limited impact on Big Pharma's capacity to undertake R&D.

The limited contribution that developing countries are now making to Pharma's R&D budget opens the possibility of exploring new methods of funding R&D. Developing countries should be able to pay a fair share of drug development costs through means other than high drug prices unaffordable to most people in those countries.[16]

If, as suggested above, the real cost of research and development has been cancelled from close media analysis, we can see why shares in pharmaceutical corporations remain so attractive to investors. Anup Shah, in an essay for an online journal, has produced an exceedingly comprehensive account of how research in and by pharmaceutical corporations really operates.[17]

STRUCTURE AND ORGANISATION OF BIG PHARMA

Modern science has been able to research and develop cures for most illnesses and diseases, yet, politics and corporate greed affect who can benefit from this, resulting in what a French newspaper, *Le Monde*, describes as an apartheid of pharmacology.

In addition, as observed by the British newspaper, the *Guardian*, more emphasis is placed on profitable research and cures for problems such as impotence and 'diseases of affluence and longevity', while many tropical diseases are given far less attention.

'Multinational pharmaceutical companies neglect the diseases of the tropics, not because the science is impossible but because there is, in the cold economics of the drugs companies, no market. There is, of course, a market in the sense that there is a need: millions of people die from preventable or curable diseases every week. But there is no market in the sense that, unlike Viagra, medicines for leishmaniasis are needed by poor people in poor countries. Pharmaceutical companies judge that they would not get sufficient return on research investment, so why, they ask, should we bother? Their obligation to shareholders, they say, demands that they put the effort into trying to find cures for the diseases of affluence and longevity – heart disease, cancer, Alzheimer's. Of the thousands of new compounds drug companies have brought to the market in recent years, fewer than 1% are for tropical diseases.

In the corporate headquarters of major drug companies, public relations posters display the image they like to present; of caring companies that bring benefit to humanity, relieving the suffering of the sick. What they don't say, is that, so far, their humanity has not extended beyond the limits of the pockets of the sick.' – Isabel Hilton, A Bitter Pill For The World's Poor, *The Guardian*, January 5, 2000.

Additionally, corporate priorities of profits can imply that the most appropriate treatments won't always apply (especially when they are cheap). 'There is a fundamental flaw [in corporate takeovers of medical complexes, hospitals etc, and the apparent efficiency gains that will come from it]; corporate owners of facilities, tools, and services must maximize their use and price to maximize their profits. There is a direct conflict between the pursuit of health and the pursuit of wealth. If they have their ways, the pharmaceuticals, surgical procedures, and hospital corporations they own or control will be used at a level way beyond true need.' – J.W. Smith, *The World's Wasted Wealth 2* (Institute for Economic Democracy, 1994), p. 82.

J.W. Smith's concerns do not seem too far-fetched given just a few examples: In May 2001 the *Guardian* newspaper reported that a pharmaceutical company, Aventis, used to produce the only safe medicine for the late, fatal, stage of sleeping sickness. However, they stopped making it in 1995 because they couldn't make any profit from it. In 2000, Bristol Myers Squibb used the drug for profitable purposes in the West – as an ingredient in hair-removing cream – under licence from Aventis. That, together with public outcry over the shortage of medicines in Africa at that time, and over the court case brought by 39 pharmaceutical companies against the South African government over access to cheap drugs, Aventis agreed to donate the drug to the World Health Organization and help fund research and treatment programs. While that was definitely welcome, it was criticized that it had only arrived after public outcries, given that sleeping sickness 'affects 500,000 people in 36 African countries, and 60m at risk of its spread.'[18]

CREATING A MARKET WHERE THERE IS PLENTY OF CASH

Anyone living in First World countries like the US, Canada or Australia is made very much aware of Big Pharma's capacity to generate a market for their products. That is, one does *not* have to be ill to be persuaded to purchase remedies for headaches and various other usually transitory discomforts. Of course such a market can only be created in communities where people have ready cash at hand to cope with such discomforts. Headache tablets are probably the most common of these 'pharmaceutical marvels', closely followed by indigestion remedies of various sorts. But a quick walk through any high street pharmacy, or 'drug store', as they are called in North America, will reveal dozens and dozens of over-the-counter (no prescription required) remedies for itchy skin, watery eyes and bad breath.

It is advertising, of course, which increases demand for these pills and potions, tonics and liniments, ointments and powders, off the druggist's shelves and into people – or often enough onto the back of bathroom shelves from which they eventually get thrown away without being used. The corporations do not mind *what* has happened to products once they have generated a profit. But where there is shortage of disposable cash, there is no point in producing or advertising such usually unimportant and rarely urgently required remedies.

And it is not simply a case of people being able to treat themselves when they want to or need to. The high-powered advertising has to *stimulate* a felt need for treatment! It cannot simply be left to chance!

This author recalls a concentrated advertising campaign taking place in a small Ontario town near where he was working. The remedy being promoted was Anicin, a well-known headache remedy produced by the German pharmaceutical corporation Bayer. It was so widely used in Canada that one saw packets of it in almost any house one visited, but the advertising campaign (in July and August 1958) was intended to double purchases of it over that time period. Accordingly the new advertisements made statements like:

> A good day ruined. I made a fool of myself at our sales meeting yesterday because I suddenly had a blinding headache – and no Anicin to hand! Don't let it happen to you. Have a packet in your pocket just in case; a packet in the glove compartment of your car and in your briefcase.

Another of the radio commercials went something like this:

> When you wake up, everything is fine. You don't have a headache – yet. But, you know the feeling. You can tell when one is coming on! The wise person stops it first by swallowing a couple of Anicin – and then you can face your day with confidence!

There are dozens of variations on this theme of deception. Get people to feel that the minor discomforts to which we are all prey require expensive medication. And why is it expensive? Not because of costly, scientifically driven research and experimentation. The R&D usually costs very little because most remedies are close variations of standard ones that have been around for years. No. It is the advertising which costs the money and that level of advertising would hardly be likely to pay for itself in, say, a Nigerian village in which most people are surviving on less than US$1 a day.

In New York in the 1960s, there was a radio/TV programme transmitted on a Public Service Licence.[17] On 19 January 2007 it broadcast a programme called 'Big Bucks, Big Pharma: Marketing Disease and Pushing Drugs'. The programme ran two pharmaceutical corporation advertisements, as follows, to illustrate the point. And the point they were trying thereby to make was that at almost any cost, pharmaceutical companies have gone to excessive lengths to portray common ailments and problems as diseases and have even highlighted obscure problems as common diseases. Through the use of uncertainty and fear in advertising campaigns, people are therefore encouraged to purchase drugs as solutions. As *Democracy Now!* found out when broadcasting the documentary. Many examples are given. Here are some advertisements from their transcript:

> It's frustrating. Just when you're ready to relax, that's when it happens: the urge to move, along with uncomfortable sensations in your legs. They're hard to describe, but they can even keep you from getting to sleep. You feel the urgent need to get up and move, just to get some relief. There's a name for it: restless leg syndrome. And if you have it, you're among the nearly one in ten US adults who do. Want to know more? Visit restlesslegs.com or talk to your doctor.

> I've got to remember that appointment tomorrow. Did I send the car payment? What made me volunteer for that assignment in the first place?' (In a high-strung male voice) Introducing Lunesta, a sleep aid that can give you and your restless mind the sleep you need. (In a soothing sweet female voice)

> At work, I'm tense about stuff at home. At home, I'm tense about stuff at work. If you're one of the millions of people who live with uncontrollable worry, anxiety and several of these symptoms for six months or more, you could be suffering from generalised anxiety disorder and a chemical imbalance.

The programme's host was Amy Goodman, and she then explained that:[19]

> Because patent life can be extended if new indications are approved, companies are constantly searching for new diseases to treat with old drugs. Antidepressants of the Prozac variety, or SSRIs, are a good example of this practice. Originally approved for major depressive disorder, these drugs are now prescribed for a variety of mood and anxiety disorders. Each new indication approved promises increased profits and must therefore be promoted heavily to the public. A striking example is how Paxil was revitalized as a treatment for Social Anxiety

Disorder. Its company hired a public relations company to frame this condition as a major and common medical problem, and the company launched a multifaceted campaign that moved beyond advertising to obtain stories about Social Anxiety Disorder placed in print media and on television.

The following provides an example of this advertising: the anchorman is speaking softly and says, 'This morning, we begin a special two-part series on social anxiety disorder. Many of us have suffered from shyness or fear of social situations at some point in our lives, but for millions of Americans, their anxiety could be debilitating.'

Paxil's award-winning product director was quoted as saying, 'Every marketer's dream is to find an unidentified or unknown market and develop it. That's what we were able to do with Social Anxiety Disorder.'

The prestigious *British Medical Journal* also asked, 'Who needs health care – the well or the sick?'[20] An interesting observation was noted whereby 'the rates of self-reported illness are paradoxical: low in Bihar [the poorest state in India], where low expectations of health are disturbing, and enormously high in the United States, which is equally disturbing but for different reasons.' In summary, it seemed that 'the more people are exposed to contemporary health care, the sicker they feel.' A key reason for this appears to be related to the industrialisation of health: 'more money can be made from selling healthcare interventions for the healthy majority than for the sick minority.'

The problem for pharmaceutical companies in wealthy countries (where most of their money can be made) is that the population is generally too healthy! They therefore have to be fed fear and anxiety so that they will buy more products.

The accepted approach to healthcare generally is to treat symptoms, of course, but also to address the causes, as preventative care will not only put less burden on health services, but also mean people are healthy and have the chance to live more meaningful lives. Yet the preventative medicine that pharmaceutical companies need in order to stay in business partly requires using fear and anxiety, thereby getting people to purchase preventative health rather than encouraging them to be healthy in the first place, so that they typically minimise the amount they need to spend.

IS GLOBAL HEALTH EQUITY A LEGITIMATE GOAL?

For some thousands of years, and definitely antedating systematic written recorded history, humankind has felt that various patterns of moral belief were of basic importance in establishing communities. Most of these were based on some sort of transcendental reference points and gave rise to religions. Such beliefs, and the forums of social organisation and values flowing from them, may in time be shown to (in the long run) contribute to the survival of the species. But we know that these same beliefs have often led to practices and actions that could be interpreted, at least in the short term, as threatening the survival of the species. For instance, it is often difficult to see how altruism can generally be of evolutionary value to the species. Sacrifice of one's life in defence of a weaker person or even an idea – to take an extreme example – would deprive the gene pool (if the martyr concerned died before reproducing) of a residue of altruism.

The question, therefore, must arise: 'Why should such moral concerns enter the equation? Why should pharmaceutical corporations put the welfare of poor and deprived communities ahead of making a profit?'

Among some business-friendly think-tanks in developed countries there are people who argue that criticising pharmaceutical companies for not spending as much on diseases of the poor is unfair, and that instead it should be up to those nations affected by such problems to invest in appropriate research; private corporations cannot be expected to solve all of the world's problems and they would also go bankrupt themselves if they tried. Furthermore, they provide jobs, which helps create wealth. However, a number of issues, rarely discussed in the mainstream, make this picture more complicated.

First World nations, in which the pharmaceutical corporations are typically based, have through colonialism and post-war global economics fostered an environment that has led to further poverty and dependency of the poorer nations on the First World countries. Post-war policies from the IMF and World Bank have forced most developing countries to cut back on such social expenditure as health and education, and many countries have faced downward spirals due to such policies.

Furthermore, pharmaceutical companies often tout their strengths of having vast capital resources to fund research, bringing benefits to humanity the world over. Unfortunately though, the quest for ever more profits is a hindering factor in what they will research. Tropical disease cures are not profitable for them, because most people with such diseases are too poor to afford cures. Of course, as well as addressing the excessive quest for profits, poverty should be addressed too. Yet, poverty is also impacted severely when international trade rules and institutions are influenced by power politics as they so often are. As Julian Borger commented:[21]

> There was a time not long ago when the corporate giants that PhRMA represents were merely the size of nations. Now, after a frenzied two-year period of pharmaceutical mega-mergers, they are behemoths which outweigh entire continents. The combined worth of the world's top five drug companies is twice the combined GDP of all sub-Saharan Africa and their influence on the rules of

world trade is many times stronger because they can bring their wealth to bear directly on the levers of Western power.

Even more sharply to the point was a comment in the US weekly journal on international affairs *The Nation.* Ken Silverstein, cited previously in this chapter, writes:[22]

> A corporation with stockholders can't stoke up a laboratory that will focus on Third World diseases, because it will go broke,' says Roy Vagelos, the former head of Merck. 'That's a social problem, and industry shouldn't be expected to solve it.'
>
> Drug companies, however, are hardly struggling to beat back the wolves of bankruptcy. The pharmaceutical sector racks up the largest legal profits of any industry, and it is expected to grow by an average of 16 to 18% over the next four years, about three times more than the average for the Fortune 500 . . . Profits are especially high in the United States, which alone among First World nations does not control drug prices. As a result, prices there are about twice as high as they are in the European Union and nearly four times higher than in Japan.
>
> It's obvious that some of the industry's surplus profits could be going into research for tropical diseases,' says a retired drug company executive, who wishes to remain anonymous. 'Instead, it's going to stockholders.' Also to promotion: In 1998, the industry unbuckled $10.8 billion on advertising. And to politics: In 1997, American drug companies spent $74.8 million to lobby the federal government, more than any other industry; in 1998 they spent nearly $12 million on campaign contributions.

And, as already observed, the WTO over the past decade has devoted much of its time and energy to trying to prevent nations from trading in generic copies or otherwise trying to surmount the corporate obstacles to access to life-saving pharmaceuticals. I have already mentioned this with respect to HIV/AIDS, where the corporations affected put pressure on the US government to threaten South Africa with legal action.

Another recently employed strategy of Big Pharma has been to invoke TRIPS as a means of protecting patents of dubious legal standing. In fact, pharmaceutical companies often claim they need intellectual property enforcement to help recoup their investments. Many have argued that pharmaceutical companies owe a lot to the public education sector for providing the scientific basis. Pharmaceutical companies do note that their taxes on profits are ploughed back into government and contribute to the GDP, so that it can appear as a spiral of financial advantage to both the corporations concerned and to neoliberal bank stockholders generally.

It should come as no surprise that Noam Chomsky commented on the situation in a speech at University of Calgary in Canada, as follows:[23]

> Well, the pharmaceutical corporations and others claim they need this [protection via patents and intellectual property rights] so they can recoup the costs of research and development. But have a close look. A very substantial part of the research and development is paid for by the public anyway. In a narrow sense, it's on the order of 40–50%. But that's an underestimate, because it doesn't count the basic biology and the basic science, which is all publicly funded. So if you get a realistic amount, it's a very high percentage that's publicly paid anyway. Well, suppose that went to 100%. Then all the motivation for monopolistic pricing would be gone, and there'd be a huge welfare benefit to it. There's no justifiable economic motive for not doing this. There's some economic motive, profit, but it is an effort to impede growth and development.

As well, it can be argued that pharmaceutical corporations do not even really own the rights to such patents because many of the ARVs used to treat HIV/AIDS today are directly derived from US government-funded cancer research carried out 25 or more years ago. The intimate link between the US government and neoliberalism is again underlined by the fact that the US government sold its rights to government-created innovations to pharmaceutical corporations – and at knock-down prices at that! The legality of such extraordinary behaviour is currently being questioned by US legal authorities. But, in the meantime, it has had the outlandish effect of guaranteeing that such multinationals as Bristol-Myers Squibb can make enormous returns on a derisorily modest investment. The as yet undecided legal question is whether private corporations can have publicly funded research results sold to them. After all, despite the fact that the research was publicly funded by US taxpayers, the government has – in effect – handed the results over. That is, unelected agencies (the pharmaceutical companies) can decide who can have access to the remedies produced thereby.

It also needs to be borne in mind that much of what goes on operates under the assumption that laboratories (working for private financial gain) can be regarded as creating the discoveries that improve the quality of life. In fact, the truth is the direct opposite, as pointed out by Wayne M O'Leary in 2002. Data made available to the US Congress showed that the truth is mostly the reverse.

> Data submitted to the Joint Economic Committee of Congress by the National Bureau of Economic Research reveals that public research, not private, led to 15 of the 21 most therapeutically valuable drugs introduced between 1965 and 1992, and other studies made in the 1990s suggest that only a minority of

important drug discoveries in recent years – estimates range from 17% to 40% – were the result of commercial research. Those new cures were instead the product of the federal National Institutes of Health (NIH), either the 'intramural' (or in-house) research performed by NIH scientists, which accounts for 10% of the agency's $20 billion annual budget, or the 'extramural' research contracted out through NIH grants to universities, medical and pharmacy schools, non-profit foundations, and private laboratories, which accounts for most of the rest.[24]

The HIV/AIDS crisis is in some ways exceptional because it *also* affects people in First World countries and so attracts research by transnational pharmaceutical corporations. But speaking generally, TRIPS and WTO integration of patent laws further increase the healthcare access gap between the First and Third World, and these are three main reasons for this:[25]

1   Large corporations from developed countries are patenting so many resources from developing countries that it makes it difficult for those nations to be able to produce medicines for themselves.
2   The World Trade Organization's TRIPS agreement (Trade-Related Aspects of Intellectual Property Rights) makes it difficult for other countries to produce medicines if the product has already been patented.
3   There are some provisions in the TRIPS agreement, but that is only when there is an emergency and the products are not used for commercial use (and even this clause is under attack from the US and pharmaceutical companies).

The above, then, all makes it abundantly clear that if the moral perspective has any legitimacy at all in human affairs, the pharmaceutical corporations – on their present record – stand well beyond the pale. One can have no difficulty whatever in regarding them as a major obstacle to the moral and ethical desideratum of global equality of access to healthcare. In that case, then, can 'intellectual property rights to crucial health discoveries' really be on the same ethico-legal plane as, say, a weathervane that crows if a rainstorm approaches or bedroom slippers that light up when worn in the dark so that the wearer can find their way?

Joseph Stiglitz, in a 2006 editorial on the issue in the *British Medical Journal*, goes on to explain how so-called intellectual property rights differ from others, especially when applied to health:[26]

Intellectual property differs from other property – restricting its use is inefficient as it costs nothing for another person to use it . . . Using knowledge to help someone does not prevent that knowledge from helping others. Intellectual property rights, however, enable one person or company to have exclusive control over use of a particular piece of knowledge, thereby creating monopoly power. Monopolies distort the economy. Restricting the use of medical knowledge not only affects economic efficiency, but also life itself.

We tolerate such restrictions in the belief that they might spur innovation, balancing costs against benefits. But the costs of restrictions can outweigh the benefits. It is hard to see how the patent issued by the US government for the healing properties of turmeric, which had been known for hundreds of years, stimulated research. Had the patent been enforced in India, poor people who wanted to use this compound would have had to pay royalties to the United States.

[...]

The establishment of the World Trade Organization imposed US style intellectual property rights around the world. These rights were intended to reduce access to generic medicines and they succeeded. As generic medicines cost a fraction of their brand name counterparts, billions could no longer afford the drugs they needed.

[...]

Developing countries paid a high price for this agreement. But what have they received in return? Drug companies spend more on advertising and marketing than on research, more on research on lifestyle drugs than on life saving drugs, and almost nothing on diseases that affect developing countries only. This is not surprising. Poor people cannot afford drugs, and drug companies make investments that yield the highest returns.

As well, it is obvious that some pharmaceutical remedies cannot really be regarded as can other commodities, because they directly affect a person's basic right to life, something which a self-defrosting refrigerator cannot.

SHOULD PHARMACEUTICAL SUPPLY DEPEND ON NEOLIBERALISM?

The economic significance of our discussion so far confronts the social/moral perspective with official business practice, because if all pharmaceuticals were affordable by everybody, then no profit could accrue by their sale, and trade in them would fall outside the ordinary business model and even outside of the laws of supply and demand! This potentially paradoxical situation has been at the back of much of the recent human rights-driven campaigns to eradicate poverty – such as the Live 8 programmes and the 'Make Poverty History' campaign.

Even the WTO has had to back down somewhat with respect to using TRIPS as a basis of imposing punishment for breach of patent laws. In this context, for instance, arose the DOHA Agreement described by the author in a previous publication.[27] What this does basically is to suspend TRIPS-based patent rights if a member of state of the WTO is faced with a grave health problem against which it cannot finance a pharmaceutical response. This, in turn, has given rise to various provisions, as follows:[28]

- WTO patent rules allow 20 years of exclusive rights to make the drugs.
- Hence, the price is set by the company, leaving governments and patients little room to negotiate, unless a government threatens to overturn the patent with a 'compulsory license.'
- Such a mechanism authorizes a producer other than the patent holder to produce a generic version of the product though the patent-holder does get some royalty to recognize their contribution
- Parallel importing allows a nation to effectively shop around for the best price of the same drug which may be sold in many countries at different prices.

In moral terms this all sounds most commendable, a very 'let's care for the underdog' sentiment, but it cuts little ice in neoliberal circles. The main transnational pharmaceutical comparatives have remained stalwartly opposed to such considerations interfering with business. In fact, there has been constant threat by the large pharmaceutical industries in the US and Europe, for example, that feel threatened by these mechanisms; they have sought to pressure nations and international agreements in various ways to minimise the impact these would have on them. In this grey area, there have been accusations by the industry of piracy, for example, and groups have lobbied the US government to exert pressure on other countries about this (such as to threaten sanctions on South Africa for trying to develop cheaper and generic drugs, as mentioned earlier).

THE STATUS OF GENERIC COPIES

As we know, some countries that are classified as 'developing countries' and thus part of the Third World in fact occupy a middle economic position between the very poor and the industrial First World countries. Among these are countries like India, Brazil, Thailand and Egypt, which have tried to meet this real need. Brazil, for instance, has concentrated on producing cheaper generic copies themselves, while others (such as South Africa) have tried to act as entrepreneurs in buying up such drugs and selling them on at a slight profit.

The Brazilian ambassador to the WTO, Celso Amorim, points out that the United States provides vast amounts of aid and subsidies to its pharmaceutical corporations to research drugs and so forth, yet when other developing countries try this, the US often acts through the WTO to oppose it.

In fact, pharmaceutical corporations and the United States challenged Brazil, South Africa and others' attempts by claiming that they were breaching the above-mentioned TRIPS. The fear has been that if a few developing countries succeed in this sort of independent path, then other developing countries will follow suit, and this will threaten corporate markets.

India's successful pharmaceutical industry, built on its patent laws that allow the development of very cheap generic drugs, has been under threat from WTO property rights rules on patent protection and under pressure from large pharmaceutical companies.

The additional fear is also based on companies from developing countries making inroads on profits from marketing products that are not actually sold successfully by large multinational pharmaceuticals, instead of other products that generate more sales and profits; companies from developing countries could pose a real threat to their profit margins.

Furthermore, if other companies are able to offer similar drugs at much lower prices, it indicates potentially how much the public of the industrialised world are being overcharged. And, even if such production of generic copies can be made legal for Brazil, the WTO – with the backing of the US government itself – can require that corporate control is exercised over it. This is because, according to a 2001 amendment to the US patent laws, Brazil would be required to inform the US Department of Commerce at least 10 days in advance of any generic drugs being developed; this allows the US, in effect, to monitor Brazil's public health policies in these areas. Also, other countries might think twice about doing what Brazil and some others have tried – legally – to do here, as the fear of US pressure might be persuasive enough.

Just a couple of months later Brazil made a bold but important move to produce AIDS drugs themselves, but at the same time breaking the patent rights of the Swiss pharmaceutical company Roche. The Brazilian currency, the Real, has become weaker with its devaluation, which therefore makes the costs of imports even more expensive. This is important because it highlights the importance of self-dependency – especially in things like health. If such emergencies are left solely to the whims of the market, then there is no guarantee that real medical needs will always be met.

Furthermore, a subsequent global AIDS fund set up by the UN also led to warnings at concerns such as patents, pricing and so on, which is captured well by Philippe Riviére:[29]

The Indian firm Cipla's offer to MSF to provide a cocktail of antiretrovirals for less than $350 a year (compared to the big boys' $10,000) resounded like a thunderbolt. Suddenly, the emergence in the South of very low cost generics producers seems credible.

James Love, coordinator of the Consumer Project on Technology in Washington and kingpin of the Cipla offer, stresses: 'The success in the developing world of the southern producers is quite important. Otherwise there is no real leverage. It is important not to link use of the global fund to purchases from European and US producers, but rather, to permit competition and buy from the firms with the best price that have acceptable quality. Sachs has been terrible on this, urging purchases from big pharma exclusively.'

Is that why the Harvard mechanism found favour with the Bush administration, the European Commission, the WHO experts, UNAids, the Bill and Melinda Gates Foundation and the pharmaceutical industry? It offered an answer to 'medical apartheid' without dropping the guard on patents.

The reference in Riviére's statement to such large-scale private donations to world health carries important implications in its own right and is dealt with below. Suffice to say, though, that the Doha Agreement is not nearly the bulwark against the erosion of health rights in the Third World that people imagined it would be in 2001. In 2001, this author detailed various ways in which the promises for global justice inherent in the Doha Agreement were being whittled away to protect corporate interests.[30] Even within a year of that first Doha Agreement, it was being threatened with corporate subversion in the following ways:[31]

- All the other 140 countries of the WTO unsuccessfully opposed United States desire to block access for poor countries.
- This was due to pressure from the pharmaceutical industry. The Guardian newspaper reports, for example, that 'Dick Cheney, the US vice-president . . . blocked a global deal to provide cheap drugs to poor countries, following intense lobbying of the White House by America's pharmaceutical giants.'
- Since the Doha Agreement, 'America's drug industry has fought tooth and nail to impose the narrowest possible interpretation of the Doha declaration, and wants to restrict the deal to drugs to combat HIV/Aids, malaria, TB and a shortlist of other diseases unique to Africa' rather than all developing countries, as originally agreed. (The U.S. was part of that agreement process as well.)
- The repeated concern has been that copycat drugs will under price and override patents, and research will dry up.

Yet, as *The Guardian* article continues, 'cut-price drugs will only be sold in countries which cannot afford to buy them at first-world prices.' In addition, 'Aside from HIV/Aids, drug companies do almost no research into the diseases on the US shortlist. It excludes diseases like cancer, asthma and pneumonia which are killers in the developing as well as the developed world.'

In other words, dents on profits wouldn't be as big as feared.

The above adds further consideration to the actions of pharmaceutical companies in response to growing criticism of the way they are pricing drugs and the way they are researching.

❐ That is, in response to the criticism while it is good they have reduced prices, the dependency on them that still exists remains a problem.

❐ When fluctuations in currencies can be sharp, especially for poor countries, the effects can be enormous, as mentioned above with respect to Brazil's currency devaluation. This has a sharp impact on the affordability of external medicines from expensive multinational pharmaceuticals.

❐ More ideal would be for pharmaceutical companies to help with real technology transfer and sharing with others around the world. Currently, they are hiding behind their patents more to accumulate profit than to help others. Only when it is profitable or not harmful to them too much will they 'help', it seems.

❐ After all, the public 'shared' their wealth in the form of huge government funds, public research and subsidies etc. to help pharmaceutical companies. It is only fair that the corporations 'share' back!

IMPACT OF MULTINATIONAL PHARMACEUTICALS IN THE THIRD WORLD

Of course there is no question that the large pharmaceutical firms, often regarded as Big Friendly Giants in highly developed nations, have done much good in the Third World, too. However, this has been incidental to making a profit. While pharmaceutical companies have no doubt created drugs that have saved millions of lives, they have also participated in practices around the world that have come under a growing amount of criticism. For example, various NGOs have alleged that the Big Pharma and their agencies:

❐ sell products in developing countries that have been withdrawn in the West

❐ sell their products by persuasive and misleading advertising and promotion

❐ cause the poor to divert money away from essential items, such as foodstuffs, to paying for expensive, patented medicines, thereby adding to problems of malnutrition

❐ sell products such as appetite stimulants which are totally inappropriate

❐ promote antibiotics for relatively trivial illnesses

❐ charge more for products in developing countries than they do in the West
❐ fail to give instructions on packets in local languages
❐ resist measures that would help governments of developing countries to
    promote generic drugs at low cost
❐ use their influence to try to prevent national drug policies
❐ give donations of drugs in emergencies which benefit the company rather
    than the needy
❐ use their home government to support their operation with threats if
    necessary, such as withdrawing aid, if a host government does anything to
    threaten their interests.

As John Madeley put it:[32]

> The methods used by the corporations are highly controversial. Making use of
> advertising that is inexpensive in comparison to what they pay in industrialized
> countries, the big drug multinationals use the most persuasive, not to say unethi-
> cal, methods to persuade the poor to buy their wares. Extravagant claims are
> made that would be outlawed in the Western countries. A survey, in the Annals
> of Internal Medicine found that 62% of the pharmaceutical advertisements in
> medical journals 'were either grossly misleading or downright inaccurate.

Madeley goes on to provide an example (amongst many others) in which the US-
based drug company Eli Lilly made the largest single pharmaceutical donation at
that time, to provide an antibiotic to Rwanda during its refugee crisis in 1994. They
donated enough for 1.3 million people. However, the World Health Organization
didn't list this drug on their list of essential drugs for treating refugees. He also
pointed out that 'Médicins sans Frontiéres said it would never prescribe such
medicines in the camps.'

Many of the pills were past their expiry date, which added additional resource
burdens to a country already suffering from the aftermath of a civil conflict. Madeley
also shows some additional reasons to this apparent generosity as follows:[33]

> While Eli Lilly conceded that the tablets donated were excess stock nearing
> expiry date, they 'felt it was the right thing to do.' ... although drug donations
> may seem pure altruism, they can sometimes harm rather than help the victims
> of emergencies. However, they nearly always help a company's balance sheet.
> European and USA-based TNCs receive substantial tax benefits when they give
> donations. For gifts to the needy, US tax regulations allow a write-off for tax
> purposes of up to twice the production costs.

A question which must arise when discussing the response of Big Pharma to research and development of medications for people in less developed countries is how potentially useful remedies are trialled on people. In the First World countries, great care is ordinarily exercised in this regard – although even in that context, things sometimes go wrong. But in poor countries one often cannot fulfil such preconditions as 'informed' consent and lack of any confounding illness.

As noted above, though, the First World is not entirely immune to such ghastly accidents.[34] One has only to think back to an event on 24 March 2006, when a group of healthy volunteers were being used at the final stage of testing of a new monoclonal antibody. What was expected to be a dull routine went disastrously wrong and the volunteers who had taken the experimental dose suddenly underwent a series of grave, and in one case almost fatal, reactions. The causes are still, as I write, under intense investigation as to experimental protocol.

But when it comes to Third World countries, not only are such 'accidents' far more frequent, but the victims usually lack that matrix of human and legal rights, and other social securities, that they could rely on to represent their needs and prosecute their case. The situation was graphically brought to the attention of mass audiences in the developed world by the remarkable film *The Constant Gardener*, released in October 2005.

Only slightly deviating from the drama of the film, the script tells an essentially true and horrifying story of how large pharmaceutical corporations readily and routinely used Africans of all ages (but almost all unable to give anything like 'informed consent') to test out new pharmaceuticals. The consequences were often devastating.[35] Such crimes (no other word suffices) of pharmaceutical corporations are well documented and there are enormous sums involved with relatively little, and often nothing at all, going to the victims. Even worse, Sir David Weatherall, Regius Professor of Medicine at Oxford University, stated that the editors of such eminent medical journals as the *Lancet* (in the UK) and the *Journal of the American Medical Association* (in the US) had come under pressure not to publish data from such experiments, nor to edit or alter them.[36]

Without going into detail about the film itself, it is important to realise that it is based on a real case, and moreover, the attitude of the pharmaceutical giants, of Big Pharma, in other words – although it comes across stereotypically in the film – has been well documented in real life. It is a fact of commercial life that multinational drug companies collectively form the most profitable industry on the stock market. Dr Marcia Angell, former editor in chief of the prestigious New England *Journal of Medicine*, has stated, 'The combined profits for the ten drug companies in the Fortune 500 ($35.9 billion) were more than the profits for all the other 490 businesses put together ($33.7 billion).' What follows exposes a lack of concern by multinational drug companies about experimenting with the lives of

African children and how many who question these practices are silenced. The children become like guinea pigs used to qualify drugs worth many millions of dollars. Should the drugs eventually pass muster, very few in Africa could ever afford to use them. Readers of this book, for instance, can help to change this by sharing this information with friends and colleagues and the media might be persuaded to cover these important stories. Together, we can and will make a difference.

The 'real case' referred to is that of a little Nigerian boy named Anas, from the northern town of Kano. The film shows Anas, with a group of other children, playing in the dusty school playground with a football. But Anas cannot really play. He spends most of the time sitting on the sidelines because he has a pain in his knees that is exacerbated if he tries to run. The clinical truth (outside of the fiction story) is that no one can hazard a guess as to why Anas' knees hurt, but the local community pinpoints the blame on Big Pharma.

The fact is that six years previously, Anas had been put forward as a volunteer by his mother to participate, with other children, on tests of a new pharmaceutical. Usually such tests generated a small payment from the company. In this particular case, however, the drug being tested was Trovan. A known side effect of it was pain in the joints. But neither Anas, nor the other guinea pigs, their families or the community had been given this information.

Whatever the full truth in the Anas case, we definitely know of two other cases in which named pharmaceutical corporations had been accused of such slip-shod research protocols and such contempt for human rights, and it was those two cases that suggested the plot of *The Constant Gardener* to its author, John La Carré.

In real life, in 1996 the town of Kano became victim of a combined cholera and measles outbreak. This was followed up by a much more deadly outbreak of meningitis. Within a month thousands of children were seriously ill. Although the outbreak was obviously of concern to the local people affected, it did not feature in the reportage of the big corporate media owners. However, local agents from Pfizer, the US-based pharmaceutical firm later responsible for developing Trovan, were quickly informed and they equally quickly informed the parent company in Connecticut. Pfizer had been experimenting with Trovan as a cure for meningitis, but they had never been able to test it on children.

> The Infectious Diseases Hospital in Kano was under siege from desperate parents who brought their dying children begging for help. One of these was Anas, then aged six. His father, Mohammed, said his son was given a drug by 'a doctor from overseas' and put to bed. Mohammed assumed the doctors who treated his son were from Médecins Sans Frontières, an independent medical organisation, which had arrived several weeks before the Pfizer team. Only later when he examined a card he had been given did he realise that Anas had been

included in a trial of the new drug Trovan. The card was numbered 0001 – Anas was the first.

His story was told in the Channel 4 documentary *Dying for Drugs*, broadcast in 2003, which alleged that Pfizer had failed to obtain informed consent from the parents of the children tested, and had back-dated a letter granting ethical approval for the trial from the ethics committee of the Aminu Kano Teaching Hospital. Pfizer said it remained satisfied the Kano experiment was conducted properly.

Since the trial, Anas has had a pain in his knee which X-rays showed was inflamed and which prevents him from running. Trovan was not used in the US because it caused side effects including joint pain. It is impossible to tell whether Anas's knee problem was caused by the drug or was a consequence of meningitis. Trovan was later withdrawn from the market for unrelated reasons, after it was linked with a number of deaths of patients from liver damage.

But the case against Pfizer did not end there. Lawyers seeking damages for the children involved in the Trovan trial obtained a letter sent by Pfizer's childhood diseases specialist, Dr Juan Walterspiel, protesting strongly about it. Dr Walterspiel set out eight grounds for opposing the trial including the fact that Trovan had 'not been tested for its sensitivity before the first child was exposed to a live-or-die experiment.' His contract with the company was terminated soon after.

Brian Woods, who made *Dying for Drugs*, met Meirelles and Le Carré, during the development of *The Constant Gardener*. 'We had an entertaining lunch in which we were all frothing about the pharmaceutical industry,' said Woods, who last week won a commission from Channel 4 to make a follow-up film.[37]

The public significance of the film *The Constant Gardener* did not end, though, with the exposure of Pfizer. The film draws on another drug-testing scandal involving a different pharmaceutical giant.

A Canadian specialist in blood disorders, Dr Nancy Olivieri, was employed at the internationally famous Toronto Hospital for Sick Children. She was engaged in particular on the blood disease thalassaemia – a genetic disorder in many respects like sickle-cell anaemia. She was asked to participate in trials of a new drug called Deferiprone, produced by the US pharmaceutical firm Apotex.

Deferiprone helps clear iron from the blood which builds up in patients with thalassaemia and can prove fatal. At first the trial went well and Dr Olivieri published promising results in the *New England Journal of Medicine*. Then she noticed worrying liver changes in some of her patients. She raised her concerns with the company and tried to find a way of adapting the trial. But she was unprepared for the response of the company, whose potential million-dollar drug she was now questioning.

Mike Spino, the vice-president of Apotex, informed her that the trial had been terminated, and warned her that she would face legal action if she spoke about it to anybody, in breach of her duty of confidentiality. That triggered a dispute between Dr Olivieri and Apotex that has dragged on for more than five years, during which time she has not published new research. Sir David Weatherall, Regius Professor of Medicine at Oxford University and a supporter of Dr Olivieri, said the case raised a 'fundamental issue of academic freedom'. Nor was it an isolated case. Sir David added that editors of medical journals including the *Lancet* and the *Journal of the American Medical Association* had come under pressure not to publish data or to change it.

This story is also told in *Dying for Drugs*. Deferiprone is now licensed in more than 24 countries, including the UK, and Apotex insist it is safe and effective. The company also accused Dr Olivieri of making errors in the trial that made her results worthless.

Wherever he truth in the cases of Pfizer and Apotex, the behaviour of Big Pharma will come under renewed scrutiny thanks to *The Constant Gardener*. Even if its picture of multinational corporations engaged in global conspiracies with corrupt governments seems excessively paranoid, there are real issues to confront. The bigger scandal lies not in the forging of consent forms to clinical trials, nor even in the intimidation of recalcitrant researchers. It lies in the rapacious pricing policies of the pharmaceutical industry that puts life-saving drugs out of reach of individuals, hospitals and even nations. The words used to justify these prices are 'research and development'. But in truth, the industry's biggest cost is marketing. Extraordinary sums are spent persuading doctors to prescribe new drugs only fractionally different from older, cheaper ones, which ramp up prices.[38]

EXPERIMENTATION, EXPECTATION AND HUMAN RIGHTS

Of course, it is not difficult to cite many examples of experiments being carried out on Third World citizens without due regard to informed consent and other niceties of human rights. But almost routine are situations in which the protocols are relatively sound on paper, but in such a way that a casual sort of immoral behaviour is allowed to govern the process. In 1983, 1984 and 1985 – before more sophisticated remedies such as AZT (azidothymidine) was developed – some random field trialling took place. Cohorts of 30 were being tested in Ghana and in each group of 30, 15 were randomly assigned the AZT concerned, while the other 15 were given a placebo. These were double-blind trials, of course, in which neither the subjects nor even the nurses administering the materials were aware of which people were getting the AZT and which the placebo. But, although many of the subjects were aware that there was only a 50-50 chance that they were getting the real thing, they found it worthwhile to take part, just in case it worked.

What was required was that each subject sign up for two years of free treatment. The AZT worked extraordinarily well and – despite the fact that volunteers had to take 30 pills a day and to eat often – they generally found it all worthwhile. It soon became abundantly clear who were getting the real thing, because of their rapid health improvement and much higher energy levels. Of course, if they were to stop the AZT treatment, they would quickly revert to serious illness and ultimately death. After two years, the drug companies had established all they needed to know. The subjects who had been receiving the AZT were told that they were free to continue taking it, but that they would have to pay the full market price that the drug could command in First World countries. Almost none of them could do so, and they were simply dismissed and told that the trials were over.

There was nothing technically illegal about this. The subjects (one assumes) knew the conditions before they started and could give informed consent. But the moral deficit is obvious in several ways. The Ghanian subjects had, in effect, been used to test a drug which would largely benefit only wealthy people who had taken no risks in the trial stage. As well, the corporations were not really obliged to sell the drug at full price to subjects who wanted it. They could have even continued to provide it free of charge to them at only a minor loss compared to the millions they could make in the First World. Finally, surely those subjects who had taken the placebo had a moral right to the real thing once its effectiveness had been established.

This points to the fact that goals such as diminishing the global health inequity gap require that moral consideration be taken into account. If we are – as a global village – to tackle this particular obstacle to global health equity, we must inform our social choices with poorly defined, but easily recognised, moral imperatives. In drawing this long chapter to an end, therefore, we should be reminded of just how fickle and undesirable the neoliberal emphasis on profits really is in determining the priorities and goals of pharmaceutical corporations.

GENES, HEALTH AND PROFITS

Genetic research, and the insights derived from it, has been probably one of the most lively and exciting areas of science over the past three decades. We are constantly being made aware both of the increasing possibility that any distressing medical condition may have a provable genetic basis and the likelihood that it can be addressed by genetic engineering. When the author was doing medical studies only half a century ago, who would have thought of being able to slice bits off chromosomes and attach other bits; or of using genetic material from other sources to be injected into different tissues; or of isolating certain types of stem cells? Now all of that is almost a pedestrian routine.

That focus on the gene has, to a degree, distorted the allocation of funds and the focusing of specialist interest generally. The danger in this is that it can have the effect of causing the scientific/medical community to ignore stubborn diseases such as polio, cholera, TB and malaria that effect millions and instead focus our attention on such gold-plated areas as Parkinson's disease, Alzheimer's, motor neurone disease and so on. These are, of course, worthy and fascinating areas, but they are of less importance to most people than some of these older known enemies of the human race.

As we have seen, though, the pharmaceutical corporations are overwhelmingly attracted to wherever the money is. As Joe Cummins reminds us, the monies potentially available for research tend to be attracted to high-tech genetic research, wherein lies not only fortune but fame.[39]

It is clearly in the interests of the genomics industry to argue that genes are the most important cause of disease, given the commercial pressure to develop and retain investor confidence in a promise of drugs and treatments for the future. The multinational pharmaceutical companies Aventis and Novartis, in particular, have made large investments in this research field.

Against a backdrop of genetic 'hype', secrecy, the privatisation of basic knowledge and profit-driven motives, the benefits of gene therapy may not only be more elusive than predicted, they may also be restricted to the few who can afford them. In the meantime, corners are likely to be cut in safety testing. Evidence of such trends is already emerging.

The profit motive also means that the interests of the rich may drive the exploitation of technology. There are already fears that gene therapy may be misused in sport. Desirable 'improvements' to people's appearance, skills and personality could become the target of gene therapists and herald the prospect of designer babies.

Placing too much emphasis on gene therapy may also give rise to new insidious practices of genetic discrimination in areas such as employment, insurance and healthcare. Avoiding the pitfalls, whilst reaping the benefits of gene therapy, is a moral challenge for politicians and regulators. Crucially, society must not be overcome by 'genetic determinism' or 'genetic thinking' and the hype of the biotechnology companies if healthcare issues are to be addressed effectively.

The problems are many, but it is clear that it is not only strategy and tactics that are required to surmount them. An important front lies in the need to re-examine attitudes and then come to terms with the moral dimensions. This aspect will emerge with even greater force in the next chapter, in which we address the commerce of war.

REFERENCES

1 Silverstein K. Millions for Viagra – pennies for diseases of the poor. *The Nation*. 19 Jul 1999. pp. 10–13.

2 Stiglitz J. Scrooge and intellectual property rights. *BMJ*. 2006; **333**: 1279–80.

3 MacDonald T. *The Global Human Right to Health: dream or possibility*. Oxford & New York: Radcliffe Publishing; 2007. pp. 132–3.

4 *The Global Human Right to Health: dream or possibility*, op. cit.

5 *The Global Human Right to Health: dream or possibility*, op. cit.

6 TWN. *Generic Drug-makers Brace for Battle with Pharmaceuticals*. 11 Feb 2001. Available at: www.twnside.org.sg/title/brace.htm (accessed 15 Mar 2008).

7 *Generic Drug-makers Brace for Battle with Pharmaceuticals*, op. cit.

8 *Generic Drug-makers Brace for Battle with Pharmaceuticals*, op. cit.

9 Martin K. *Leaders Condemn US in HIV/AIDS Drug Policy*. Available at: www.workers. org/ww/1999/aids0902.php (accessed 15 Mar 2008).

10 *Leaders Condemn US in HIV/AIDS Policy*, op. cit.

11 *Generic Drug-makers Brace for Battle with Pharmaceuticals*, op. cit. p. 3.

12 *Generic Drug-makers Brace for Battle with Pharmaceuticals*, op. cit. p. 4.

13 Wikipedia. *Pharmaceutical and Research Manufacturers of America*. Available at: http:// en.wikipedia.org/wiki/pharmaceutical_research_and_Manufacturing (accessed 15 Mar 2008).

14 Weissman R. PhRMA and global access to medicines. *The Global Access to Medicines Bulletin*. Available at: http://salsa.democracyinaction.org/0/1678/t/5144/signup. jsp?key=2959 (accessed 15 Mar 2008).

15 Weissman R., Rimmington, S. High drug prices, access to medicines and the cost of R&D. *Essential Action's Global Access to Medicines Bulletin*. 14 Feb 2008. Available at: www.essentialaction.org/access/index.php?/archives/113-Gobal-Access-to-Medicines-Bulletin-High-Drug-Prices,-Access-to-Medicines-and-the-Cost-of-RD.html

16 High drug prices, access to medicines and the cost of R&D, op. cit.

17 Shah A. *Pharmaceutical Corporations and Medical Research – Global Issues*. pp. 1–29. Available at: www.globalissues.org/TradeRelated/Corporations/Medical.asp (accessed 15 Mar 2008).

18 Democracy Now. *Big Bucks, Big Pharma: marketing disease and pushing drugs*. 19 Jan 2007. Available at: www.democracynow.org/2007/1/19/big_bucks_big_pharma_marketing_disease (accessed 15 Mar 2008).

19 Who needs health care – the well or the sick? [editorial]. *BMJ*. 2005; **330**: 394.

20 Borger J. Industry that stalks the US corridors of power. *The Guardian*. 13 Feb 2001. p. 7.

21 Millions for Viagra – pennies for diseases of the poor, op. cit. p. 6.

22 Chomsky N. Whose World Order: conflicting visions. Speech given at the University of Calgary in Canada on 22 Sep 1998. Available at: http://legalminds.1p.findlaw.com/list/cyberjournal/msg00563.html (accessed 15 Mar 2008).

23 O'Leary W. *The Real Drug Lords*. 13 Aug 2002. Available at: www.alternet.org/story/13831 (accessed 15 Mar 2008).

24 *Pharmaceutical Corporations and Medical Research*, op. cit.

25 Scrooge and intellectual property rights, op. cit.

26 MacDonald T. *Health Human Rights and the United Nations*. Oxford & New York: Radcliffe Publishing; 2007. pp. 20–1.

27 *Pharmaceutical Corporations and Medical Research*, op. cit.

28 Rivere P. Southern sickness, northern medicine – patently wrong. *Le Monde Diplomatique*, 28 Jul 2001, p. 11.

29 *Health Human Rights and the United Nations*, op. cit.

30 *Pharmaceutical Corporations and Medical Research*, op. cit.

31 Madeley J. *Big Business Poor Peoples: the impact of transnational corporations on the world's poor*. London: Zed Books; 1999. pp. 145–6.

32 *Big Business Poor Peoples: the impact of transnational corporations on the world's poor*, op. cit.

33 American Academy of Science. *Drug Trials – Violent Reaction to Monoclonal Antibody Therapy Remains*. Available at: www.sciencemag.org/cgi/contents/full/311/5768/1688 (accessed 18 Mar 2008).

34 Mormon News. *Pharmaceutical Greed – Using African innocents for Illegal Testing: liver damage, deaths, horrible side effects ignored for big profits*. Available at: www.mormon.citymax.com/Drugmoney.html (accessed 18 Mar 2008).

35 *Pharmaceutical greed – using African innocents for illegal testing: liver damage, deaths, horrible side effects ignored for big profits*, op. cit. p. 1

36 Laurance J. The true story of how multinational drug companies took liberties with African lives. *The London Independent*. 26 Sep 2005. Available at: www.utexas.edu/conferences/africa/ads/1193.html

37 Ibid.

38 Cummins J. Safe gene therapy. *Journal of the Institute for Science in Society*. 22 Oct 2002.

Chapter 5

The obstacle of war

THE PROBLEM

Warfare is one of the most complex and puzzling aspects of human behaviour and seems to have been a part of the human condition from time immemorial. Some have even spoken of it as a basic human instinct and ineradicable. But even if early in our evolutionary history it provided a rather rough and ready way of promoting the survival of the gene pool of the most hardy and adroit – a good breeding stock, if you will – this certainly has not been so since the 15th century at least. As far as we know, it has not even served as an important natural selection mechanism for long, in terms of evolutionary history, for it does not seem to be a feature of primates other than humans and has not been a salient feature in the evolution of lower forms.

In terms of purpose, it has often been seen as resembling another uniquely human activity based on what amounts to violent assault – namely, surgery. Warfare is full of a phraseology parallel with medical operations – surgical strikes, quarantine, cordon sanitaire and so on; however, the ultimate rationale for heavily destructive surgery – amputations, transplants, and the like – is that in the long run it is designed to alleviate the patient's suffering, as indeed the guillotine certainly does! People who justify war – not often those actually engaged in it – have done so on the basis of two broad rationalisations, which this author refers to as the 'surgical' and the 'moral'.

The 'surgical' involves invasion and destruction of people and/or regions perceived as incompatible with the continued survival of some other people or regions that has been, is and no doubt will continue to be the basis of wars of competition for oil, water, and territory. The 'moral' rationalisation would presumably be completely beyond the mental or psychological capacities, of two coyotes fighting over possession of an injured rabbit. Moreover, this author would argue that it is our capacity to conceive of situations on some sort of moral plane that renders warfare, on the one hand so difficult to explain, and on the other so difficult to eliminate. For this state of affairs religion (of almost all brands) bears an enormous responsibility. It beyond the scope of this book to deal in any exhaustive way with such questions, but a basic idea of the dimensions of the moral arguments – and their compelling influence – is necessary if we are to seek ways of overcoming it. That we must regard the human proclivity for war as a barrier that has to be overcome if we are to close the global health equity gap hardly needs arguing.

This is more so today than at any other time in the desolate history of warfare. There was a time when wars were fought – often on a specific 'battlefield' – between two groups of protagonists. Sometimes the contest even attracted crowds of civilian spectators, ordinary folk who themselves were reasonably safe from being killed in the conflict. Some of the more recent wars (historically speaking) – such as the Thirty Years War(s) (1618–48) or, more recently, the First World War, involved the loss of prodigious numbers of civilian lives, and modern developments in military technology mean that in very recent wars, the number of civilian dead hugely exceed the number of soldiers killed on both sides.[1]

Moreover, over and above those killed or injured, are a much greater number who suffer and die from illnesses or levels of deprivation directly caused by the military destruction of hospitals or of means of access to them. Such sombre considerations, therefore, make it necessary to scrutinise the category of what might be called the 'moral' arguments in support of war as a means of settling disputes.

THE IDEA OF THE 'JUST WAR'

Since war has been such a steady companion of humankind, the idea of trying to find a 'moral' basis for large-scale armed conflict had certainly antedated the Christian tradition of the 'Just War'. For instance, the great Roman orator and politician Cicero (106–43 BCE) drew up what he regarded as two criteria which needed to be satisfied for a war to be 'just'. These were: to protect one's community from outside attack; and to defend the honour of one's community.

But it goes without saying that both the concept of 'honour' and the perception of 'danger' are highly subjective. Both criteria, indeed, could have been used to justify any war already fought and any future ones! They cannot realistically be invoked as a workable moral basis for either forestalling a war or for minimising its ferocity. Here the religio-philosophical grasp of what constitutes 'morality' comes to our rescue.

Almost all of the great religious leaders have declared the killing of people in any way as 'immoral' and/or 'sinful'. In the Judaeo-Christian tradition, for instance, murder is an extremely serious sin. Moses included the anti-murder commandment in the Decalogue and Jesus strenuously seconded the motion! And yet, almost without exception, every war of consequence since has gained the religious endorsement of religious leaders in the belligerent nations. This apparently yawning inconsistency gave one the Christian (primarily Roman Catholic) doctrine of the just war, coherently expressed by Thomas Aquinas (1225–74). Obviously it had been invoked in all but name throughout the intervening twelve centuries whenever it was needed but, although Aquinas formalised the arguments, in fact, even as early as the 4th century AD, Augustine of Hippo – a deeply revered father of the Church – made a statement of what criteria had to be met before fighting a war could be justified.

But Aquinas, committed logician that he was, tightened up the arguments and they appear in Vol II of his 4 volume treatise *Summa Theologica*.[2] In that work, only three criteria appear, as follows:

1   The war must be both started and controlled by the ruler or leading authority of the state prosecuting the war.
2   The war must be 'for good', or 'against evil' and after the actual fighting has finished, law and order must be restored.
3   The cause for the war must be a 'just' one.

Like almost any such exhortation, the principles may be easy to state, but difficult to apply. Take the first criterion. What it says is that for a war to be just, only the king or head of the nation has the right to initiate it. One of the clear implications of this is that it effectively rules out civil wars and revolutions, even if the ruler is such a tyrant that there appears to be no other way of getting him out. The French Revolution and the American Revolution, for instance, did not satisfy Aquinas' criteria for a 'just war'. More importantly, the 'enemy' has no say in the matter!

Consider the second criterion. It rules that no one prosecuting a war should ever find themselves supporting evil. It also implies that there is a duty to restore life back to normality after the war is finished. This criterion was not satisfied, for instance, in the Boer War, because the British immigrants had revolted against the Afrikaners only because the former wanted the Afrikaner territory to be part of the British Empire.

The third criterion is almost impossible to satisfy, because only the state starting the war determines whether or not it is 'just'. For instance, the most elementary meaning of 'just' is that any hardship incurred is a legitimate punishment. Thus, everyone in the enemy state who suffers as a result of the conflict had to have deserved it!

Things were not helped when the Roman Catholic Church, in an attempt to tighten things up, added two more criteria:

4   The war has to be a 'last resort'. This means that all other methods of reaching agreements have been tried and have failed.
5   The war must be fought proportionately – inflicting the minimum death and destruction required.

It is clear that these two additional criteria only muddy the waters further. What is meant by 'last resort'? Is the potential enemy consulted in determining what that is? And to discuss 'proportionality' is to rule out killing more people than necessary. Even in 'conventional' warfare entire families – including babies in arms – are wiped out. Nuclear war, as in the bombing of Nagasaki in 1945, falls completely outside this fifth criterion.

But, despite logical, philosophical and even religious arguments, wars continue to be fought – and to give an impression of 'high minded morality' – reasons as to how and why the rules can be broken are offered up without difficulty for John Q Public to swallow down with his evening meal. One of the most commonly used get-out clauses is that the particular enemy being fought is so *completely* unlike us that they cannot possibly share or even understand our moral distinctions. For this to work, the enemy has to have a sort of inhuman quality. It also helps if they are easily identified by skin colour or some other easy to assess difference.

In the Second World War, the Japanese fell into this category. *They* tortured people for fun and even committed hari-kari on themselves. *They* were fanatics and flew explosive-laden planes into Allied ships while singing the praises of the emperor! The distinctive Japanese facial characteristics became – in the allied countries – a symbol of all that was so essentially evil and atavistic that the Japanese simply fell out of the moral equation.

We still haven't learned, for now many people have invested 'Islam' with much of the same diabolism, even to the extent that we are told that we are justified in using torture, or in redefining that word so that it becomes not only 'legal' but morally acceptable to say that practices such as water-boarding are *not* torture – even though before September 11 they were regarded as torture.

The famous US popular writers on philosophy – a man and wife team – Will and Ariel Durant, in 1968 commented to the effect that in the last 3421 years of recorded history only 268 were not scarred by major wars.[3] Between 1968 and 2008, there has been at least one major war on the go in every year, so that – by comparison – the figure of only 268 war-free years was not too bad! This only represents 8%, if accurate, of the time of recorded human history. That being so, can we be surprised that humans have been so unsuccessful in controlling the phenomenon?

CIVILISATION AND WAR

Durant's statistics cited above give some indication of just how central a theme war has played in our various civilisations. Moreover, the theme of an enemy so atavistic as to fall below and outside any moral desiderata of the societies calling themselves 'civilised' keeps reoccurring. It is amazing just how persuasive this theme is. Read almost any of the Athenian plays of the 4th and 5th centuries BCE, for example, *Women of Troy* by Euripides[4] or even Thucydides' *Peloponnesian Wars*[5] and you run across this idea again and again, whether it is Athenians versus Trojans or Athenians versus Persians. Both Trojans and Persians are represented as having totally 'ungentlemanly' attitudes to the 'higher moral values' of the Athenians. The Persians, in particular, come across in many of the great plays as vain and effeminate, taken up with appearances and – of course – lacking in decency, courage, and manly virtues. Therefore, in dealing with such an enemy we can forsake such civilising virtues as restraint, respect for property, and respect for women and children.

In the ghastly Peloponnesian War (a totally unnecessary and prodigiously expensive war), we are told by Thucydides that when the Athenians, with their superior manpower, fell on their foe, the former made it clear that when the end came that the Athenians would insist that there would be no arguments about 'justice' or 'mercy', as the enemy were outside of that 'moral ambit'! Rather, the defeated enemy must accept that their position renders them undeserving. The victors would do as they wished and the losers would do as they were obliged to do.

IS PACIFISM AN ANSWER?

One obvious way out of the fact that no amount of religious or philosophical quibbling seems to prevent wars, suggests that the tendency for organised group conflict is a sort of 'relict psychological pattern', that once in the distant past it had served some evolutionary advantage, but has since become not only useless, but an actual threat. There are many physiological and anatomical parallels with this, such as the possession of a vermiform appendix, which no longer serves a useful purpose to omnivorous humans. Clearly, as we have evolved, we have become much more efficient and technologically efficient in fighting one another and, at some point, war became of negative evolutionary value. The tipping point might have been the invention of gunpowder, or maybe even the invention of the crossbow. Nuclear warfare has made feasible the idea of war vanishing altogether, as have other destructive refinements such as bacteriological warfare.

How do we stop it? How do we get off the merry-go-round?

One honourable tradition springs to mind, and that is Pacifism. In its most famous manifestations, it has been religiously affiliated. One thinks of George Fox (1624–91), Founder of the Society of Friends or 'Quakers', and of Mohandas Gandhi (1869–1948) of the Hindu tradition. But like all religion-linked ideas, pacifism is dependent on religious faith, and this in turn involves a larger agenda than simply avoiding military conflict, and is probably too easily equivocated or sidestepped in times of urgency.

Certainly, large numbers of people who have actually fought as soldiers now reject warfare as a reasonable solution. One of this author's colleagues, on his return from three years war service in Korea commented: 'I just had never before considered pacifism and have never really been able to understand it. An armed pacifist would presumably stand by and watch his mother get raped without shooting the attacker. But, I tell you, actual experience of warfare sure gives pacifism a good name!' It also seems evident that the most insistent proponents of war are either young idealists who have been influenced by accounts of the glorious traditions of dying bravely for one's country, or are people beyond call-up age who, a few even sitting complacently in board rooms, are safe from bullets as they make good dividends from a war killing off the young.

As will be seen in the final chapter, a secular basis for pacifism needs to be worked out and argued – not to *replace* religiously based pacifism, but to *extend* its social cogency. The 'winds of change' (to paraphrase a former British prime minister!) do seem to be blowing through the ranks of the youthful idealists, at last. Throughout his working life, this author has been privileged to have continuously been involved with adolescents, and the evocative power of 'guts, glory, bravery and sacrifice' of military service seems to be weakening by the day. Part of the reason for this change is due to recent media coverage of wars in such places as Liberia, Darfur, former Yugoslavia, the Palestinian Occupied Territories, and of course, Afghanistan and Iraq.

Space does not permit discussion of all of them, but Iraq serves as a particularly poignant example for a number of reasons. The 'just war' criterion of proportionality did not play a major part in either the planning or the execution of the original attack on Iraq by the Coalition Forces. The Ba'ath regime may have been comprehensively defeated on the battlefield and even Saddam himself captured and hanged. But the parallel disruption and even wholesale destruction of critical aspects of civic life has been indescribably immense.

COSTS OF THE WAR IN IRAQ

Before looking at Iraq specifically, we must appreciate that relative to any index of inflation or cost of living, warfare is becoming much more expensive by the day with the elaboration of more refined technologies. During the Korean War, Canadian servicemen were told (in one of the lectures given aboard ship on the way over) that every North Korean they shot cost about US$1.10. Each shot Iraqi today costs about US$895 minimum, according to this author's calculations from the figures available!

What this author quickly noticed, in his reading of any part of history from

the Greek and Roman empires until now, is that wars have been amazingly ineffective in meeting any long-term goal. What tends to happen is that subsequent
developments in agriculture, trade and technology, fairly quickly render previous
ideologies irrelevant and the immediate problems – which had ostensibly been
the 'cause' of the war in question – tended to re-assert themselves in different
state/national contexts. The actual detailed figures for the wars in classical times
are largely inaccessible, although some accounts of specific battles are horrifically
compelling as evidence. It is only when we get up to and beyond, say, medieval
Europe, that we begin to have access to much hard data.

Take the so-called Thirty Years War, for example. It forms a good parallel to the
sorts of modern wars fought since the First World War (1914–18) in the way it gradually sucked more and more nations into the vortex of conflict. It may have started
primarily as a 'religious' war, but – because its impacts on local trade and commerce
gradually widened – the doctrinal basis of its origins were often lost sight of. The
other feature which becomes obvious is the degree to which it grossly undermined
health and all other aspects of civil life over such an astonishingly wide area.

Wikipedia gives as good and compact an outline of the conflict as most
standard sources and from it we gather that, as indicated above, it was not fought
over an uninterrupted 30-year period in one place, or throughout, even between
two easily defined states or nations.[6]

In many ways, the war could be seen as a 'model' of all the European military
campaigns since then, including the conflict arising over the dismemberment of
Yugoslavia and the emergence of Kosovo. It started in the part of Europe presently comprising Germany, but before it had run its course, it had involved much
of what we now call the EU. Dates for the conflict are difficult to pinpoint exactly,
depending often on whether it is being described as a Protestant–Catholic conflict,
or a series of fights for the defining of national boundaries. Of course, disputes over
religion and real estate combined have been a common feature of war and have
had (and continue to have) an immensely negative impact on public health, but
these factors have been especially significant in the history of Europe generally.

The legacy of the Thirty Year War was almost a century of economic disloca-
tion, insecurity and negative impacts on public health. Those negative impacts
reflected themselves in two principal ways. Firstly, there was the direct impact of
the battles themselves on the general population. It is in the Thirty Years War that
we first note the huge shift of this impact from the actual participants in the battles
(the soldiery of both sides) to the civilian populations. This shift has continued
to the present day, as we shall later see when we consider figures from the war
in Iraq. Secondly, it was in the Thirty Years War that the use of mercenaries first
became systematised and this, likewise, is a development which continues today.

Frequent wars, of course, generate easily marshalled mercenary forces, because once one war is over, the released veterans are still young and fit enough – and often less well trained for anything in civilian life – to be hired for some other conflict, if it comes along soon enough! As the Wikipedia account details, traditional armies, along with marauding bands of mercenaries, rampaging over large areas of the countryside create an ideal milieu for the spread of disease. They destroy housing and other civic infrastructure, interfere with the prosecutions of agricultural pursuits and – above all – create levels of anxiety and aggression that noticeably increase the incidence of mental illness.

So the impacts on health of the Thirty Years War have been analysed by a legion of historians in the hope of throwing some light on how such impacts can be lessened. They have not been outstandingly successful! There is general agreement in all of the encyclopaedia accounts consulted by the author, including the Wikipedia, that the most noticeable impact was a disastrous reduction in the civilian population in the areas affected, by figures ranging from a third to a half – even more in some areas. Thousands of entire towns and villages were completely obliterated. Some modern historians now argue that, in the area that is now Germany, the death rate may have been only half that priorly estimated, but it was still hugely significant in its subsequent impact.

Likewise, as with all wars since, both morbidity and mortality due to disease and injury even exceeded parallel figures caused by military activity alone, such as gunshot wounds, bombings, etc. By 1625 these more general impacts on public health were becoming conspicuous in the Thirty Years War, when Denmark became involved. Those soldiers seemed to have carried some contagious disease with them, because, soon after the Danish forces arrived, outbreaks of typhus increased and spread rapidly to surrounding areas. Then, when French forces engaged Hapsburg forces in Italy, bubonic plague broke out. Sieges of cities constituted ideal contexts for the spread of disease and numerous accounts tell of similar events when the Swedish armies attempted to seize Nuremberg in 1632. In that case, both scurvy and typhoid carried away many on both sides.

Bubonic Plague (Black Death) skulked in those corridors of war for some years, infecting the populations of Dresden and Munich starting as early in 1634 and continuing until a year or so after the final shots had been fired.

And this says nothing at all about the medium- and long-term political effects. The aforementioned Treaty (or 'Peace') of the Westphalia, for instance, laid the groundwork for 19th century nationalism – and the origins of both the Second World War and of the recent conflict in former Yugoslavia. As the author has argued in previous books, it not only has proven an obstacle to global mediation of conflict through the UN and its agencies,[7] but also has enabled narrow corporate interests to effectively undermine health equity worldwide.[8]

HEALTH AND FINANCIAL COSTS OF THE FIRST WORLD WAR

Much has already been written about this and details are not needed here. The horrors of trench warfare and its impact on both the physical and mental health of the soldiers involved during the actual war years have made (one hopes) an indelible impact on cultural values worldwide. The impact on civilian health tends to be less understood internationally. The great 'flu pandemic' was doubtless rendered far more lethal (and far more quickly) because of massive troop movements over the earth's surface. In all of the countries involved, mental health institutions are to this day still coping with the direct effects of that war.

The financial costs of the First World War amounted to US$125 690 417 000 for the Allies and US$60 643 160 000 for the opposing forces. These figures can be accessed at Spartacus Schoolnet.[9] Almost any analysis of the war itself shows how easily it could have been averted! A resurgent sense of expansionist desire among the German states proved threatening to the large and powerful French and British Empires and – as we now know – adroit use of existing banking arrangements could have obviated the need for conflict if the more well-established corporate interests had been prepared to suffer a temporary reduction in profits, making room for some of the newer corporate players to increase their share.

The conduct of the First World War was in some ways incipient in the Franco–Prussian War of 1870, in its widespread and almost random destruction of civil society, along with an increasing mechanisation of the conflict between the armies themselves. And, of course, the First World War set the pattern for an exponential development of both in the Second World War – and in numerous wars since.

Among the unforeseen consequences of the First World War, was the erosion of power of various European empires; the collapse of the Romanov administration of Russia (and the establishment and gradual growth of the Soviet Union); the wholesale massacre of the Armenians in Turkey; and the increasing resort to armed uprisings in many colonial areas. Improvement in levels of literacy and the development of increasing numbers and types of media led to a greatly increased appreciation among 'the common people' of the futility of international armed conflict.

At the European national level, this led to popular demands for more participatory forms of government and a number of European thrones tottered and fell. Communism (of a sort) was developing in Russia and also, under various 'social democratic' aegis, socialism was becoming increasingly expressed in political party terms. Some have argued that this general weariness with the politics of war led to the development of the League of Nations – especially under the encouragement of the US President Woodrow Wilson. But back in 1864, the Geneva Convention first put forward what could be seen as an international code of conduct in time of war and in that spirit also the Red Cross – with its particularly robust advocacy of universal health rights and interventions designed to promote them – came onto the scene.

Again one cannot in this book deal with the many twists and turns taken by these encouraging developments, but it is important that readers inform themselves of these issues if they are to understand the arguments that follow and be able to act on them. For instance, the collapse of the League of Nations was instrumental in accelerating the development of Japanese, German, French and British preparations for international war.

THE WARFARE STATE

The Second World War and the corporate/banking advocacies which financed it and – on the whole gained from it – presented us with many of the same problems as the First World War, except that parallel advances in weapons technology has very much increased the rates of injury and death among civilians in all wars since, phrases such as 'surgical strikes' notwithstanding. One has only to think of nuclear arms, bacteriological weapons, nerve gases and the like.

WAR AS FOREIGN POLICY SINCE 1945

Surely only very few thinking people believed that the end of the Second World War, and the 'peace' – largely based on the twin ideas of 'nuclear deterrence' and 'Mutually Assured Destruction' – which followed, actually solved any of the major international problems that were outstanding before 1939 and which have arisen (in their multitudes) since.

In terms of advances in healthcare, war did appear to confer *some* short-term legacy of good – for example, the development on a large scale of antibiotics such as penicillin to fight infection. But attempts – by setting up the UN in 1944 – to actually promote health and other human rights globally has not fulfilled its promises to the degree which it was expected to. We know that unless we take immediate steps to close the yawning chasm of health inequities we will continue to be set back and dehumanised by more wars, the negative impacts of which will be increasingly exacerbated by the environmental crisis.

Therefore, given that continued, and almost reflex, recourse to war represents one more obstacle to equity in global access to healthcare, we need raise at least two questions:

1 War, as state Foreign policy, is widely unpopular. How, then, and why is it increasingly applied?
2 What can 'ordinary people', i.e. the broad electorates in conventional 'democracies', do about it?

There is no shortage of recent or ongoing wars to draw on as source material in attempting to ask these questions. The second one will be accorded analysis in the final chapter, but at present we shall try to answer the first. Basically, war is good business. An encouragement to engage in war is an obvious and profitable result of the manufacture and sale of arms of all types. The UK plays a leading rôle in the international arms trade. Indeed, one of the key arguments raised against pacifism as foreign policy is the negative impact it would have on employment.

The author lived and worked in Nottingham in 1981–82 and was struck by the joy and eagerness among local unemployed people at the outbreak of war in the Falklands. Men, even in their thirties and forties, who had become unemployed, had visions of increased openings in arms manufacture. More surprising was the eagerness of younger males, say 17–25, to actually go and fight! The old catch cries of 'Queen', 'honour', and 'courage' – seemed to work its magic almost as well as it did in the First World War. On asking a group of teenagers outside a recruiting station where the Falkland Islands *were*, only one seemed to know – and he said: 'Just off Scotland, sort of!' This was all rather disheartening for one who had optimistically thought that perhaps we were outgrowing war.

But the class of people who *really* stood to gain had absolutely nothing to lose – and a whole lot to gain. They were largely male, but too old for recruitment, so – unless Argentina invaded the UK – they could not be in danger of enemy fire. Additionally, they either held leading positions in arms manufacture and supply, or were linked to investment in such enterprises.

All of this becomes very clear when we look at the war in Iraq.

WHAT IS THE WAR IN IRAQ COSTING?

Even if we concentrate only on financial costs, the question is difficult to answer. Steve Schifferes, an economics reporter for the British Broadcasting Corporation, has published an analysis of it online which concentrates mainly on the costs from the US point of view.[10] He concludes that the war's cost has already far exceeded the US government's anticipated costs back in 2003.

But controversy still rages over the ultimate size of the bill for the war, with some suggesting the cost could reach $3 trillion ($3000 billion or £1500 billion). According to the non-partisan Congressional Budget Office, the direct costs of the war on terror, which include operations in both Iraq and Afghanistan, have so far have reached $752 billion, if the current year's appropriation of $188 billion is included.

About 80% of that cost has been spent in Iraq. By the end of 2009, the direct cost to US Treasury will be over $1 trillion. The war has been far more costly than planned because it has continued for so long. That has led to growing spending on procurement, to replace ammunition and vehicles, as well as higher costs for the large numbers of troops on the ground. In fact, the yearly cost has doubled since the 2003 appropriation of $74 billion – which the Bush administration expected to be the total cost of the war.

Schifferes' report goes on to try to compartmentalise the costs in terms of health costs and economic costs, but the data does not make this an easy task. Beginning with President George Bush's assertion that whatever the war is costing in terms of lives lost (presumably Iraqi lives don't count because he has no data on them) and of treasure lost (The Iraqi National Museum does not count, nor does its library), *it is worth it*. Why? Because if the Iraqis were allowed to win, the cost (to America!) would be much higher!

Clearly Schifferes is not overwhelmingly impressed by President Bush's analysis and quotes various Democrat Party sources to the effect that it would have been more to the point to have devoted that money to rectifying social problems at home. He quotes presidential-hopeful Hilary Clinton as asserting that the trillion dollar cost would be enough to provide healthcare for all 47 million uninsured US citizens, and still have enough over to provide high quality pre-school childcare for every child of the appropriate age group in the country; to solve the housing crisis once and for all, and as well, to make a college education affordable to every US student.

The higher cost of the war has also contributed to the US budget deficit, which could rise further if the economy slows down, and has reduced the fiscal headroom to put in place a bigger economic stimulus package. The Bush Administration insisted on funding the war as an 'emergency appropriation' each year, which means it has not been included in the official calculation of future budget deficits.

He then addresses the economic impact by pointing out that many economists argue that the indirect costs of the war are even greater. For instance, a study by the Nobel Prize economist Joseph Stiglitz, of Columbia University, and Linda Bilmes, a budget expert from Harvard, concludes that the cost could be at least $3 trillion. The figure is so large because, Professor Stiglitz says, it includes costs that official estimates do not, such as the cost of the lifetime medical care for 65 000 injured American personnel.[11]

Stiglitz also says that 100 000 of the 750 000 combat troops who have been discharged so far have been diagnosed with mental health problems. On the strength of evidence from previous conflicts, he said, still others will have various health and mental problems in the future. There will be disability pay and health-care costs to the US budget that will continue for several decades. Altogether, he estimates these costs could add another $600 billion to the price of the war.

Calculation of the health costs is more problematic. His figures also include the loss to the economy from injured people being unable to contribute as productively as they might otherwise would have done, and the cost of sending hundreds of thousands of National Guard troops who would otherwise have had worked at their civilian jobs – which he says amounts to around $400 billion. More controversial are the attempts to add up other economic costs of the war.

Professor Stiglitz – who served in the Clinton administration and is a former World Bank chief economist – says it is right to add the interest that the government will have to pay on its borrowing to his cost calculation, which will amount to another $600 billion. He also brings in the cost of higher oil prices, which he says are partly due to the conflict.

Schifferes goes on to argue that the US government is paying for the war by deficit financing, and as a result of this the US economy could soon be in trouble because the long-term, macro-economic cost to the economy could be as high as $1.9 trillion. And he says the overall cost of the Iraq War is approaching that of the Second World War, which cost the US $5 trillion in today's money.

His calculations on the broader impact of the war are similar to those in 2002 by Yale economics professor William Nordhaus. And they also echo the concerns expressed by Lawrence Lindsey, President Bush's first economic adviser, who was sacked in December 2002 for warning that the Iraq war could cost $200 billion.

Schifferes' views are by no means unique and, whatever happens in the Presidential elections (I write these words in April 2008), the issue of the costs of the war in Iraq will remain a focus for worry for millions of US citizens for years to come as the country skirts the brink of recession. And sombre as Schifferes' analysis is, the reader must remember that it has centred on the immediate cost to the United States – and costs due to deaths only.

A wider and more comprehensive view, was given in March 2007 in an article in the British weekly, *New Statesman*, by Andrew Stephen.[12] He points out that, even in the US itself, the costs of the war will not only be in terms of dead servicemen. It is the wounded who will drain the Treasury of millions for years to come. The reader, therefore, is asked: 'If that is true for US forces, is it not even *more* true for Iraqis – both armed forces *and* civilians?' When one remembers that in most Iraqi cities, water reticulation systems, for example, have been destroyed, hospitals bombed and ambulance services decimated – and that what hospital staff have survived are fleeing the country in droves – to be injured at all badly is often a slow death sentence. But – according to Stephen – the Pentagon is intent on trying to silence US economists who are critical. They generally predict that the long-term care of wounded US personnel would amount to at least US$2.5 trillion.

Andrew Stephen's analysis is worthy of attention because he nicely contrasts the US government's adulation of military service to encourage youngsters to do the idealistic thing and join up (The old 'Dulce et decorum est' argument that the Romans used!), with the way that they are treated when they return home physically or mentally damaged. It has always been the same dreary tale down through the ages, but there is always a new crop of youngsters to swallow the line and lay down their lives for corporate bank balances.

As press reports point out, the US military's own hospital, Walter Reed Military Hospital, is a medical disgrace – underfunded, unhygienic and generally indifferent to the real welfare of its patients. But on top of this, Stephen's article points out how the machinery of information production, controlled by the government, effectively keeps US citizens from finding out the truth about what is really taking place – what is being done in their name.

Yet the story of the US wounded reveals another deception by the Bush administration, masking monumental miscalculations that will haunt generations to come. Thanks to the work of Linda Bilmes, and some other hard-working academics, we have discovered that the administration has been putting out two entirely separate and conflicting sets of numbers of those wounded in the wars.

This might sound like chicanery by George W Bush and his cronies – or characteristic incompetence – but Bilmes and Stiglitz have established not only that the number wounded in Iraq and Afghanistan is far higher than the Pentagon has been stating, but that looking after them alone could cost present and future US taxpayers a sum they estimate to be $536 billion, but which could get considerably larger still. Just one soldier out of the 1.4 million troops so far deployed who has returned with a debilitating brain injury, for example, may need round-the-clock care for five, six, or even seven decades. In present-day money, according to one study, care for that soldier alone will cost a minimum of $4.3 million.

However, let us first backtrack to 2002–03 to try to establish why the administration's sums were so wildly off-target. Documents just obtained under the Freedom of Information Act show how completely lost in Neverland the Bush administration was when it considered Iraq: Centcom, the main top-secret military planning unit at Donald Rumsfeld's Pentagon, predicted in its war plan that only 5000 US troops would be required in Iraq by the end of 2006!

Rumsfeld's deputy, Paul Wolfowitz, was so astute at the economics of it all that he confidently asserted that Iraq would 'really finance its own reconstruction'. Rumsfeld himself reported that the administration had come up with 'a number that's something under $50 billion' as the cost of the war. Larry Lindsey, then assistant to the president on economic policy at the White House, warned that it might actually soar to as much as $200 billion – with the result that Bush did as he habitually does with those who do not produce convenient facts and figures to back up his fantasies: he sacked him.

From official statistics supplied by the non-partisan Congressional Budget Office, we now know that the Iraq war is costing roughly $200 million a day, or $6 billion every month; the total bill so far is $400 billion. But, in their studies, Bilmes and Stiglitz consider three scenarios that were not even conceivable to

Bush, Rumsfeld, Wolfowitz *et al.* back in 2003. In the first, incurring the lowest future costs, troops will start to be withdrawn this year and be out by 2010. The second assumes that there will be a gradual withdrawal that will be complete by 2015. The third envisages the participation of two million servicemen and women, with the war going on past 2016.

Estimating long-term costs using even the second, moderate scenario, Bilmes tells me: 'I think we are now approaching a figure of $2.5 trillion.' This, she says, 'includes three kinds of costs. It includes the cash costs of running the combat operations, long-term costs of replenishing military equipment and taking care of the veterans, and (increased costs) at the Pentagon. And then it includes the economic cost, which is the differential between reservists' pay in their civilian jobs and what they're paid in the military – and the macroeconomic costs, such as the percentage of the oil-price increase.'

Let me pause to explain those deceptive figures. Look at the latest official toll of US fatalities and wounded in the media, and you will see something like 3160 dead and 23 785 wounded (that 'includes 13 250 personnel who returned to duty within 72 hours', the *Washington Post* told us helpfully on 4 March 2008). From this, you might assume that only 11 000 or so troops, in effect, have been wounded in Iraq. But Bilmes discovered that the Bush administration was keeping two separate sets of statistics of those wounded: one (like the above) issued by the Pentagon and therefore used by the media, and the other by the Department of Veterans' Affairs – a government department autonomous from the Pentagon. At the beginning of this year, the Pentagon was putting out a figure of roughly 23 000 wounded, but the VA was quietly saying that more than 50 000 had, in fact, been wounded.

As though that is not bad enough, Stephen's article cites various media releases to the effect that the US government is complicit in under reporting casualty rates to minimise the adverse effects on voter behaviour in the coming elections.

To draw attention to her academic findings, Bilmes wrote a piece for the *Los Angeles Times* of 5 January 2007 in which she quoted the figure of 'more than 50 000 wounded Iraq war soldiers'. The reaction from the Pentagon was fury. An assistant secretary there named Dr William Winkenwerder personally phoned her to complain. Bilmes recalls: 'He said, 'Where did you get those numbers from?'' She explained to Winkenwerder that the 50 000 figure came from the VA (US Department of Veterans' Affairs) and faxed him copies of official US government documents that proved her point. Winkenwerder backed down.

Matters did not rest there. Despite its independence from the Pentagon, the VA is run by Robert James Nicholson, a former Republican Party chairman and Bush's loyal political appointee. Following Bilmes' exchange with Winkenwerder – on 10 January 2008, to be precise – the number of wounded listed on the VA website dropped from 50 508 to 21 649. The Bush administration had, once again, turned reality on its head to concur with its claims. 'The whole thing is scary,' Bilmes says. 'I have never been conspiracy-minded, but watching them change the numbers on the website – it's extraordinary.'

What Bilmes had discovered was that the tally of US fatalities in Iraq and Afghanistan included the outcome of 'non-hostile actions', most commonly vehicle accidents. But the Pentagon's statistics of the wounded did not. Even troops incapacitated for life in Iraq or Afghanistan – but not in 'hostile situations' – were not being counted, although they will require exactly the same level of medical care back home as soldiers similarly wounded in battle. Bilmes and Stiglitz had set out, meantime, to explore the ratio of wounded to deaths in previous American wars. They found that in the First World War, on average 1.8 were wounded for every fatality; in the Second World War, 1.6; in Korea, 2.8; in Vietnam, 2.6; and, in the first Gulf War in 1991, 1.2. In this war, 21st century medical care and better armour have inflated the numbers of the wounded-but-living, leading Bilmes to an astounding conclusion: for every soldier dying in Iraq or Afghanistan today, 16 are being wounded. The Pentagon insists the figure is nearer nine – but, either way, the economic implications for the future are phenomenal.

So far, more than 200 000 veterans from the current Iraq or Afghanistan wars have been treated at VA centres. Twenty per cent of those brought home are suffering from serious brain or spinal injuries, or the severing of more than one limb, and a further 20% from amputations, blindness or deafness, severe burns, or other dire conditions. 'Every person injured on active duty is going to be a long-term cost of the war,' says Bilmes. If we compare the financial ramifications of the first Gulf War to the present one, the implications become even more stark. Despite its brevity, even the 1991 Gulf War exacted a heavy toll: 48.4% of veterans sought medical care, and 44% filed disability claims. 88% of these claims were granted, meaning that 611 729 veterans from the first Gulf War are now receiving disability benefits, and a large proportion are suffering from psychiatric illnesses, including post-traumatic stress disorder and depression.

More than a third of those returning from the current wars, too, have already been diagnosed as suffering from similar conditions. But although the VA has 207 walk-in 'vet centres' and other clinics and offices throughout the US, it is a bureaucracy under siege. It has a well-deserved reputation for providing excellent healthcare for America's 24 million veterans, but is quite unable to cope with a workload that the Bush administration did not foresee.

As for injured veterans who cannot even access appropriate medical care, there is now a waiting list of in excess of 400 000 cases. Stephen quotes Frances Murphy, the US Veterans Administration health spokesperson, as saying that claims will reach 930 000 by the end of 2008. Casualties sent back from Iraq for admission to Walter Reed Hospital now outnumber those already there from previous recent wars by a ratio of 17 to 1. There are so many, in fact, that many have to be put up in nearby motels! Suicide attempts are increasing, and conditions are so bad that it is routine for the less seriously wounded to have to look after their more seriously injured colleagues.

But there are many other hidden costs – unemployment, depression, desperate recourse to drugs and alcohol, family violence and breakdown, all impose local community costs – to say nothing of the non-financial human costs. Mentioned above was the projected US$ 2.5 million costs and that included non-medical equipment replacement costs. According to media reports cited in Stephen's account, nearly 40% of the US army's equipment is now being used just in Iraq.

Significant quantities of equipment are being destroyed, too. Media reports say that in December 2007 the army alone has lost more than 280 000 major pieces of equipment in the combat zones; the Army Times reported as long ago as February 2007, that 20 M1 Abram tanks, 50 Bradley fighting vehicles, 20 Stryker wheeled combat vehicles, 20 M113 armoured personnel carriers, 250 Humvees, hundreds of mine-clearing vehicles and the like – plus more than a hundred aircraft, most of them helicopters – have been lost. Those figures have increased considerably since then, as fighting has intensified. Add something between $125 billion and $300 billion for these unanticipated long-term costs, say Bilmes and Stiglitz.

Yet another gargantuan White House miscalculation was over the price of oil. Before his departure, Larry Lindsey told the *Wall Street Journal* (*WSJ*) in September 2002 that 'the successful prosecution of the war would be good for the economy'; the *WSJ* echoed his thoughts in an editorial the same day, arguing that 'the best way to keep oil prices in check is a short, successful war on Iraq'. In 2002, the average cost of a barrel of oil was $23.71; today, it is hovering around $100. Dick Cheney's chums in firms such as his own Halliburton – or ExxonMobil, Shell, BP and Chevron – have profited enormously, but Bilmes estimates that even if only $5 of the oil price increase can be attributed to the Iraq war, that alone adds $150 billion to the cost of war.

There are also countless imponderables that add to the bill. The deployment of hundreds of thousands of reservists depletes the economy. At present, 44% of US police forces, for example, have members deployed as reservists in Iraq, and their duties have to be performed by others in America. The same goes for firefighters, medical staff, prison wardens.

Then there are the future illnesses that may well unfold. For instance, nobody knew that the notorious Agent Orange defoliant, used by the US in Vietnam from 1961–71, would turn out to have had carcinogenic and other effects on US troops. Needless to say, its impacts on Vietnamese people is not worthy of consideration! Today, there is mounting evidence that exposure to depleted uranium – used for firing anti-tank rounds from US M1 tanks and A-10 attack aircraft – can cause cancer, diabetes and birth defects. Many veterans are returning to the US with their health apparently in ruins from adverse reactions to anti-anthrax injections and/or consumption of experimental pills to counter chemical warfare agents. The other costs reflect to an even greater degree the level of human degradation and loss of dignity involved. For instance, some of the people being treated at Walter Reed have been asked to take part in the testing of drugs being developed to counter the effects of chemical warfare. This often incurs ancillary costs for psychiatric side effects.

Costs continue to spiral in a sort of ripple effect. For instance, spouses of soldiers killed are supposed to receive US$100 000, so the extra cost to the US economy of its young soldiers being killed is about US$6.5 million.

BRITISH COSTS

Britain, as a close ally of the US in prosecuting the war in Iraq, has also been racking up debts which detract from funding social policies that actually work – such as medical care and education. By 30 April 2008, *direct* expenses – just the cost of actual military activity – are expected to reach £5.6 billion. This does *not* take into account costs involved as a result of soldiers being wounded. So far, 4800 have had to be evacuated due either to physical injury or mental breakdown. But that is only the military estimate. Many more are being treated as ordinary NHS patients and the NHS is unable to provide data on that. The author has tried various sources without success. This is not due to any official 'cover-up' operation, but solely the response of a very much over-used and under-staffed government agency.

It is interesting to note that 2123 serving British troops have so far (March 2008) been diagnosed as having serious mental problems – but this author has also been informed that such cases can take more than a decade to manifest themselves. It would appear, then, that the costs of our involvement in just this one war will continue to accumulate for some time to come.

GLOBAL CULTURAL COSTS

So far we have barely mentioned the cost of the war to Iraqis. Before considering the obscenely high estimates of the number of Iraqi soldiers and civilians actually killed or wounded, what about the destruction of Iraqi civilisation itself – the irreparable damage done to its many cultural sites, its national museum, libraries and schools? In historical terms, the sacking of the library at Alexandria in Egypt nearly 2000 years ago is often held up to us as constituting a serious and lasting assault on our shared heritage as humans, wherever we live.

But what has happened in Iraq is much worse and much more total – and could have been either prevented or at least greatly modified. Louise Witt describes it in the following words:[13]

The sacking of Iraq's museums is nothing less than the lobotomy of an entire culture, according to art experts. And these same experts had repeatedly warned the Pentagon of this possibility months before the war took place.

In so many respects a visit to Iraq, even under the rule of Saddam Hussein, represented the opportunity to experience more fully what it means to be human. Truly, that region of the world is the source of many of our cultural values. Its casual, and even cynical, destruction was an act of the grossest philistinism – a frontal attack on the very roots of our consciousness. The damage done is largely irreparable and there is no question but that today the human race is much poorer than it was before the war. How much information and forewarning did the US actually have prior to the invasion?

Witt's article makes the claim that on 24 January 2003, a corps of leading archaeologists and art curators met with Joseph Collins at the Pentagon. Collins, we are told, reports directly to the Deputy Defence Secretary, Paul Wolfewitz. Included at that meeting were four other Pentagon officials. They discussed the crucial importance of preserving these valuable documents and artefacts and how they could and should be protected once an invasion took place. But what happened?

On 10 April 2003, a day after Saddam Hussein's regime collapsed and Baghdad was in the hands of US military forces, the National Museum of Iraq was ransacked. In a matter of hours, thousands of Iraqis, some thought to be working for art dealers, clambered into the museum that had been closed to the public for years. After two days of looting, almost all of the museum's 170 000 artefacts were either stolen or damaged. Ancient vases were smashed. Statues were beheaded. In the museum's collection were items from Ur and Uruk, the first city-states, settled around 4000 BC, including art, jewellery and clay tablets containing cuneiform; considered to be the first examples of writing. The museum also housed giant alabaster and limestone carvings taken from the palaces of ancient kings.

Records and artefacts going back 5000 years were wantonly pillaged – many randomly destroyed and thrown on the floor with smashed pottery and figurines. US archaeologists and historians called it an incredible crime. But it was a crime that continued without significant official let or hindrance. Witt goes on in her account to describe how, after Baghdad's museums had been so desecrated, the city's libraries were attacked. At the National Library, a treasured repository of the earliest written records of medical, mathematical and other intellectual development – which had provided much of the basis for subsequent human history and development – many of the holdings were actually burned to ashes and not even stolen for profit. Pure vandalism reigned.

What tells us so much more about what the exercise of unregulated brute force does to people's minds was the reaction of some US military officials to the scandal. For instance, US Secretary of Defence Donald Rumsfeld, when told of the outrage, made it clear that he did not regard the protection of our historical and cultural roots as a priority. He even went on to blame the media's reporting of the crime and was quoted (by Witt) as saying:

> The images you are showing on television show pictures of one person after another walking out of some building with a vase. You see it 20 times and think: My goodness. Were there that many vases?

The sheer ignorance and insensitivity of these comments outraged thinking people worldwide, not least in the US itself.

Because hostilities are still underway in Iraq, the full impact of this attack on civilised values has not yet been felt. But close to home has been the profligate sacrifice of the lives and human rights of Iraqi civilians through the conduct of this war. In this book, space permits only a discussion of Iraq, but the implications are far wider. All such wars represent a serious assault on the health and other rights of the civilians caught up in them. For instance, the International Committee of the Red Cross (ICRC) issued a report in March of 2008 in which it commented on the degree to which civilian life in Iraq had become dangerously degraded. The lack of reliable access to good drinking water alone has created enormous health problems.

THE ICRC 2008 REPORT ON IRAQI CIVILIAN LIFE

Various media carried reports on the ICRC's findings. A particularly complete comment on it appeared in the UK's *Morning Star* newspaper.[14] In the report the ICRC pointed out that, whatever one says about 'progress' being made in bringing peace to Iraq by virtue of the so-called surge in US forces, the fact is that life is becoming increasingly difficult for individual citizens and their families. The report, entitled 'Civilians Without Protection', reveals that increasing violence has forced nearly a million people from their homes. The majority of those fleeing the danger are professional people – doctors, teachers, and so on – the very people needed to help make life bearable for the less well trained. This alone has caused the situation to worsen as some of the better educated try to find refuge in Jordan. The water reticulation system was ruined by the Coalition Forces' bombing and the electricity grid is rarely able to operate for more than a few hours – if that – a day.

The result has been a crisis in sanitation and waste disposal, and even hospitals are having to cope with limited access to electricity to operate diagnostic equipment, air conditioning and adequate lighting.

In fact, as the report goes on to say, healthcare facilities are stretched to the limit just at the time that, because of the rapid increase in crime driven by desperation and violence, the food shortage has led to widespread malnutrition. As of the end of 2007, over 30% of the population now live in poverty, with about 5% in extreme poverty. Unemployment and poverty levels are both increasing and daily more and more families are forced to rely on government help simply to meet their basic needs. The ICRC report describes the level of suffering among many citizens as having become unbearable.

Anyone involved in any of the array of national anti-war campaigns in existence today is, of course, aware that the anti-war movement predicted these catastrophes in chilling detail, but it made little discernible difference in the conduct of the war. In every sense, the civilian population of Iraq are paying dearly – and even dying in unbelievable squalor – in order to promote US corporate greed for oil, with the UK serving as a docile ally in the crime.

Estimates of actual Iraqi civilian deaths directly due to the armed intervention of the coalition forces have been extremely difficult to obtain. The US Defence Department stated quite clearly that they do not take any account of Iraqi dead. Therefore, various statistical techniques have been used. These lead to figures varying from 500 000 people to 650 000 people. A well-documented source quoted in the *Washington Post* by one staff writer, David Brown, puts the 'excess deaths' among Iraqi civilians at 655 000 in October 2006.[15] It obviously has exceeded that by now (April 2008), but the author's choice of that estimate is based on its thorough reliance on sound statistical and epidemiological practice. But before dealing with it, the reader needs to be clear about what epidemiologists mean by 'excess deaths' over a particular time interval. It simply means that, based on deaths *before* the time period in question, how many more (or fewer) died during the period examined. In this case, the period was March 2003 – June 2006 (39 months). By counting it this way, the figure includes people actually killed outright by military action *plus* all others who died, say, of illness, injury, lack of access to water, destruction of electricity supplies and who (presumably) would *not* have died had the invasion not happened.

The survey was conducted by a team of Iraqi and US epidemiologists and involved interviewing random examples of residents' of households throughout every region of the country. The results of this scrupulously careful analysis pro-duced a figure more than twenty times the 30 000 civilian deaths favoured by President Bush. It is also more than 10 times a British estimate of 50 000 civilian deaths made by their 'Body Count' research group. But the latter was based on direct body counts after specific military actions.

The surveyors said that they had found a steady increase in mortality since the invasion, with a steeper rise in 2003 and that appeared to reflect a worsening of violence as reported by the US military, the news media and civilian groups. In the year ending in June 2007, the team calculated Iraq's mortality rate to be roughly four times what it was the year before the war.

Of the total 655 000 estimated 'excess deaths', 601 000 resulted from military violence and the rest from disease and other causes, according to the study. This is about 500 unexpected violent deaths per day throughout the country.

The survey was done by Iraqi physicians and overseen by epidemiologists at Johns Hopkins University's Bloomberg School of Public Health. The findings have been published in various reputable journals. The same group, in 2004, estimated that roughly 100 000 civilian deaths accrued in the first 18 months after the invasion in March 2003. This, the study discussed, puts the Iraqi excess civilian deaths since September 2004 and up to 1 October 2006 at 500 000. Both of these studies deserve a far higher level of credibility than many others because they are the only ones (so far) to have used rigorous statistical/epidemiological methods. The technique used is not novel in itself. It has been used widely to estimate mortality in large-scale natural disasters and is technically referred to as 'cluster sampling'.

As well, scientists scrutinising the data were strongly re-assured by the fact that the great majority of the deaths were also substantiated by death certificates.

The reader, appalled by these findings, may derive some comfort by a statement made by Colonel Mark Ballesteros, a Defence Department spokesman to the *Washington Post*:

> The Department of Defence always regrets the loss of any innocent life in Iraq or anywhere else. The Coalition takes enormous precautions to prevent civilian deaths and injuries.

BUT THE WAR OBSTACLE GROWS!

What we have said so far in this chapter might give the impression that, although humankind seems to have lived with military conflict since the beginning, warfare is becoming worse. And that would be right. It is becoming relatively more expensive, more destructive, involves more and more collateral damage – including civilian deaths – and has an exponentially increased capacity to actually destroy the very foundations of civilised values. In a sense, humans can be perceived as having incredibly subtle scientific and artistic insights, to be able to create what are acknowledged as 'great' civilisations and to express what we might call virtues, such as love, to a degree that marks us out as being unique in the animal kingdom. But they also seem to have some kind of wired-in behaviour pattern leading to war. Thus people and entire societies are pulled in opposite directions by these two inbuilt tendencies. The two have been able to coexist for millennia, but only because the military side has been fairly limited in the extent of its power.

As this author has suggested above, we reached a tipping point in the balance, perhaps in the Franco Prussian War or, more likely in the First and Second World Wars. Since then technological developments have greatly increased the power of totalitarian regimes and of military action. Britain itself plays a dominant rôle in using the global arms trade to bolster its economy. So the obstacle of war – probably the most threatening of all – is growing quickly indeed. It, along with climate change, will no doubt prove our undoing if we cannot surmount it and close the global health equity gap – itself a continuing cause of war.

But in closing this chapter, the author would like to address one more issue intimately linked with war: how the strength of the 'war tendency' in our make-up can gradually change our social psychology and weaken our capacity to oppose it. One important example is provided by our attempt to 'tame' war for limited use. Just as we were preoccupied for some centuries with the need to incorporate war in our socio-ethical evolution (for example, elaborating doctrines for 'just wars'), we have tried to prevent some of the excesses caused by use of better war technology by agreeing on 'rules for war', such as the already mentioned Geneva Convention.

By and large that document has been honoured over the last two centuries – with certain glaring exceptions – but the power of war over industry and finance has now reached the point where many of the power brokers are prepared to discard those parts of the Geneva Convention which interfere with corporate interests.

Take Guantanamo Bay as an example. Even as late as the 1960s, enemies of 'the West' had a sort of grudging respect for British and American commitment to 'democracy' and 'rule by law'. The idea of openly funding and operating a prison in which people from all over the world could be placed without some specific charge – and held indefinitely – would have been regarded as probably a totalitarian idea and/or as some kind of perverse science fiction – as recently as, say, 1965.

When and how did large numbers of decent democratic citizens decide that it was OK? A simple answer would be 'after the horrific events of September 11'. But to make such an idea psychologically acceptable, we had to scare people. The 'War on Terror' was a brilliant idea in that context, partly because 'terror' cannot be pointed at in an atlas and it could even be beside you in work or behind you in a bus queue! The idea has frightened people and frightened people rarely make rational decisions.

So, perhaps a bit uneasily, we have come to live without too much protest, with Guantanamo Bay. But then there is that delightful phrase 'extraordinary rendition'. It sounds as though it refers to a spectacularly good performance of a demanding piece of violin music! In use of language, as in love and war, 'All's fair!' We have even learned to live without serious protest with the idea of the US Central Intelligence Agency (CIA) being allowed to pick up anyone anywhere and to fly them to imprisonment in Guantanamo Bay.

And what happens to the people in Guantanamo Bay? Well, among other things, they are interrogated. But what does one do if they won't answer usefully? Our Western liberal-democratic tradition, which in any case says they shouldn't even be there, also responds to another fear. 'What if he/she knows where a huge nuclear or germ-warfare bomb is located; when it is going to go off and who will set it off? We have no proof that the person did anything or knows anything, but that doesn't prove that he or she doesn't! Do you put the entire planet in jeopardy just because your liberal-democratic conscience is too squeamish to use a bit of torture?'

Most of us cannot answer questions like that, so it makes it more logical just to leave it up to our leaders. After all, they know more than we do – how many times has *that* been said in history? But it is the casual acceptance of the idea that war (one of the most irrationally destructive of human activities) is a legitimate extension of diplomacy that has led us to this predicament. It is comparatively easy to identify that small group of people who benefit financially from war and even to realise that most of us lose by it. Hence the issue does require serious and constructive thought and action.

The medium-term danger if we do nothing is that we will all be destroyed. The short-term danger is that, unless we coherently address the task of removing the obstacle of war, we will find ourselves huddled into small protective caves – both physical and metaphorical – weak and sequestered in mutual fear and hatred of all the other groups.

Once we toss out our slowly accumulated mantle of civilisation by equivocating on such things as the Geneva Convention and agreeing to 'a bit' of torture here and there, we have started on that path to what Morris Berman has called a new dark age.[16] The Preface to his book is available online and worth reading.

OTHER ISSUES

One could devote an entire book to war as an obstacle to global health equity. We have had to make do with one chapter. Most of our attention has been focused on the Iraq War, but that is only because data related to it is readily accessible and because it has stimulated a worldwide anti-war movement. So far, there are few books about such current examples, such as Israel's activities in the Occupied Palestinian Territories, the developing situation in the states making up former Yugoslavia, and Chinese emerging power in international trade.

And yet, destructive, violent and irrational as it is, military conflict draws about it a whole psychology, what this author refers to as 'the Warfare State'. The impact of this as a style of diplomatic and economic thinking is becoming increasingly pronounced and pervasive as time passes. It is rather like some sinister Wagnerian 'Gotterdammerung', which constitutes a matrix that now enmeshes us all. The next chapter deals with it.

REFERENCES

1 Johnson J. *Morality of Contemporary Warfare*. New Haven Connecticut: Yale University Press; 1999. p. 45.

2 Aquinas T. *Summa Theologica Vol II – The Just War*. Notre Dame, Indiana: Ave Maria Press; circa 1251.

3 Durant W, Durant A. *The Lessons of History*. London: Simon and Schuster; 1968.

4 Euripides. *Euripides*. (Translated by Kenneth McLeish). New York: Penguin; 1998.

5 Thucydides. *The Peloponnesian War*. (Translated by Rex Warner). New York: Penguin; 1998.

6 Wikipedia. *Thirty Years' War*. http://en.wikipedia.org/wiki/Thirty_years_war (accessed 18 Mar 2008).

7 MacDonald T. *Health, Human Rights and the United Nations*. Oxford & New York: Radcliffe Publishing; 2007.

8 MacDonald T. *Sacrificing the WHO to the Highest Bidder*. Oxford & New York: Radcliffe Publishing; 2008.

9 Spartacus Schoolnet. *Financial Cost of the First World War*. Available at: www.spartacus. schoolnet.co.uk/FWWcosts.htm (accessed 7 May 2008).

10 BBC News. *The Iraq War: counting the cost. An analysis by Stephen Schifferes*. Available at: www.news.bbc.co.uk/2/hi/business/7304300.stm (accessed 7 May 2008).

11 Stiglitz J, Blimes L. *The Three Trillion Dollar War: the true cost of the Iraq conflict*. London: Penguin; 2008.

12 Stephen A. Iraq: hidden costs of the war. *New Statesman*, 12 Mar 2007. Available at: www.newstatesman.com/200703120024 (accessed 9 May 2008).

13 Witt L. *The end of civilisation*. Available at: http://dir.salon.com/story/news/ feature/2003/04/17/antiquities/ (accessed 18 Mar 2008).

14 Roberts A. Red Cross warns on humanitarian crisis. *Morning Star*, 12 Apr 2007. p. 1.

15 Brown D. Study claims Iraq's excess death toll has reached 650 000. *Washington Post*. Available at: www.washingtonpost.com/wp-dyn/content/article/2006/10/10 (accessed 10 May 2008).

16 Berman M. *Dark Ages America – The Final Phase of Empire*. Available at: www. bullnotbull.com/archive/dark-ages-america.htm (accessed 10 May 2008).

Chapter 6

A world mortgaged to war

THE WARFARE STATE – END GAME FOR NEOLIBERALISM

Although the contents of the previous chapter certainly make clear the cardinality of war itself as a barrier to closing the global equity gap in access to healthcare, what the author wishes to argue in this chapter is that hardly any war is a one-off independent barrier to universal health. The fact of the matter is that human psychology not only exhibits a propensity to engage in war, but – as a species – we have evolved an increasingly tight matrix of war, politics and trade so that any one major war is linked through international relations with the others. As time passes, neoliberalism becomes more efficient at using warfare as a mechanism for self-actualisation. In a sense, we can feel so inexorably caught up in it that, like the dinosaurs of old – powerful though they were – we can only wait to be snuffed out by forces we cannot control.

But we are not dinosaurs and it is not beyond human imagination to work out a less disastrous approach to social organisation. The Iraq War represents a good example to illustrate the point. For instance, none other than the widely regarded Joseph Stiglitz (a former President of the World Bank) commented – just after the attack on Iraq began – that the war was not started *only* because Iraq's territory lay on top of a major source of the earth's oil, but that it was daring to trade in Euros rather than US dollars!

A full account of how the global trading mechanism became dominated by the US dollar in the first place can be accessed by consulting the author's *Third World Health: hostage to first world wealth*.[1] Suffice to say here that all World Bank and all IMF loans have to be paid off in US dollars, which immediately puts the poor debtor nations at the economic mercy of First World trading requirements, and as the author shows, requires each debtor nation to pay an enormous price for the transition in terms of the healthcare of its own people. Thus, if Iraq began to drift away to trade in Euros instead of US dollars, it would sabotage the financial hegemony over world trade by US banks. That had to be stopped, at virtually any cost, in order to deter other nominally dependent countries from following suit. But where else does that warfare matrix drive us as we struggle for global dominance?

As a letter by Michel Boncza to the *Morning Star* pointed out, for years before the assault on Iraq, increasing EU confidence in their own Euro was giving them ideas above their station.[2] By 2000 the EU was feeling its strength and its rapid development had a global impact on trade that was undermining the global pre-eminence of the US dollar. The latter was also increasingly seen as too unstable to be an ideal currency for international trade. US actions against Serbia's economic integrity at this time were, the public were asked to believe, entirely coincidental.

COINCIDENCE OR CUNNING?

Indeed, though, the US instigated an attack on Serbia because it would not submit to having its economy controlled by US banks through the IMF and its SAPs. The effect of this (very much welcomed by US banking interests) was that the Euro collapsed in international value.

Let us look even further abroad. The Chinese economy has not been easy for US corporate interests to live with. The US economy has over-invested in war. China's growth exacerbates collapse of the already debilitated US economy, which is rapidly being assaulted by huge and mounting military expenditures. Its recent banking problems have not helped and many doom-mongers even predict a 1929/30 style general depression, possibly foreshadowed by events in the sub-prime lending fiasco in US banks that toppled the Northern Rock Bank in Britain.

But the US propaganda machinery was ready for action to not only put a gloss on it but to try to undercut China. Boncza's letter recognises this as an effectively opportunistic masterstroke of diversionary tactics, as a well-oiled worldwide campaign exploded out of nowhere with unprecedented saturated media coverage of supposed Chinese misdeeds. The corporate-owned media have been able to exploit the Tibetan issue in such a way that it could have become the basis of a boycott of the 2008 Olympics. China holds US$ 1430 billion, a figure that is growing by the day, and its Premier, Wen Jiabao, voiced concerns about the increasing difficulties posed by the steady decline of the US dollar and the managing of these vast reserves.

Moreover, we are not speaking here of a moral matter, or even of 'trading ethics'. To think of China as a society practising 'communism', or anything approaching it, or of Tibet as being 'a gentle innocent victim', are simplifications too far. But what we are witnessing is the determined struggle of two great powers – one to gain trading ascendancy and the other to preserve its own power – by economic means, with a war or two thrown in, if they are perceived as worthwhile. If China could be checked in its ambitious moves toward global financial hegemony by rendering its management of the Olympic Games as an embarrassment it just might give US bankers the temporary strategic advantage they need.

But this represents only a small part of the warfare matrix. China needs Iraq's oil and the US – as the accustomed broker of Middle East Oil (the Israel/Palestine dispute being only another coincidence!) – also wants to control that resource at the global level. The global warming crisis could put a brake on this, but as we shall see, there are ways around that problem! And what may appear as mysteriously different UN moral responses to very similar wholesale breaches of human rights are all easily understood if, instead of considering a response to the human rights abuse (say, rape, murder or torture) itself, we focus instead on what is good for the US dollar.

This epigrammatic statement, in fact, is well summed up by Michel Collon in the following:[3]

> What are the exact rules that govern the right to secession and, more generally, self-determination of peoples?
>
> Some tell us these rules are confusing. And if we believe the corporate media, we might think that:
>
> In Asia, Tibetans have that right, but not Iraqis, nor Afghans.
>
> In the Middle East, Israelis have this right. But neither Palestinians nor Kurds do.
>
> In Africa, the gangster generals of the East Congo have this right, but not Western Sahara.
>
> In Latin America, wealthy and right-wing provinces of Bolivia and Venezuela have this right, but not the indigenous peoples of Chile, or of Mexico, etc. . . .
>
> In Eastern Europe, Albanians of Kosovo have this right. But not the Serbs of Kosovo, nor those of Bosnia and, of course, not the Transnistrians.
>
> In Western Europe, the Flemish might have this right, but not the Northern Irish, nor the Basques.
>
> Complicated, indeed. How can it be simplified? Like this: only those people who are 'with us' are entitled to self-determination, and no-one else.
>
> And as long as we're here, let's replace the word 'democratic' with the words 'with us'. And let us replace the word 'terrorist' with the words 'against us'.
>
> That's politics. Simple when you know how!

DISTORTING THE MANDATE OF THE IAEA

For instance, consider the honourable attempt during the 1980s made to decrease the likelihood of nuclear war in the Nuclear Non-Proliferation Treaty (NPT). Soon after the advent of nuclear war (in other words, the dropping of two A bombs on Japan in 1945) another UN agency was set up. It was the International Atomic Energy Agency (IAEA), and its overall mandate was to monitor all future developments and applications of nuclear energy in order to forestall its application in international war. After Hiroshima and Nagasaki, the need for such an agency was obvious.

Perhaps for that very reason, the IAEA was rather ignored by the media and allowed to quietly address itself to its noble task. Among these tasks was to act as the UN's watchdog should any country embark on a nuclear programme. The general rule was that if a country's only interest was to use nuclear energy for, say, medical applications as in oncology or to generate power for domestic and normal industrial use, there would be no objection. The UN could send in an IAEA team of inspectors to oversee the installation and to report their findings to the UN if they suspected military use for it was being planned.

If the IAEA's report to the UN is such as to raise suspicions that a nation is developing nuclear power for military use – provided it is not one of those nations already equipped for nuclear warfare – then the UN is supposed to step in to protect the world community from such an undertaking.

In 1969 there were only five states armed with a nuclear warfare potential. The IAEA set about the task of developing a UN document, the NPT, designed specifically to prevent the further spread of the capacity for nations to carry out nuclear warfare.[4] Accordingly, the NPT was drafted under the UN Charter, and it obliged the five nuclear-armed states (the United States, Russian Federation, United Kingdom, France, and China) not to transfer nuclear weapons, other nuclear explosive devices, or their technology to any non-nuclear-weapon state.

Non-nuclear-weapon States Parties must undertake not to acquire or to produce nuclear weapons or nuclear explosive devices. They are required also to accept safeguards, allowing the IAEA to detect any diversions of nuclear materials from peaceful activities, such as power generation, to the production of nuclear weapons or other nuclear explosive devices. This must be done in accordance with an individual safeguards agreement, concluded between each Non-nuclear-weapon State Party and the International Atomic Energy Agency (IAEA). Under these agreements, all nuclear materials in peaceful civil facilities under the jurisdiction of the state must be declared to the IAEA, whose inspectors have routine access to the facilities for periodic monitoring and inspections. If information from routine inspections is not sufficient to fulfil its responsibilities, the IAEA may consult with the state regarding special inspections within or outside of the declared facilities.

The Treaty was opened for signature on 1 July 1968, and signed on that date by the United States, the United Kingdom, the Soviet Union, and 59 other countries. The Treaty entered into force with the deposit of US ratification on 5 March 1970. China acceded to the NPT on 9 March 1992, and France did so on 3 August 1992. In 1996, Belarus joined Ukraine and Kazakhstan in removing and transferring to the Russian Federation the last of the remaining former Soviet nuclear weapons located within their territories, and each of these nations has become a State Party to the NPT, as a non-nuclear-weapon state. In June 1997 Brazil became a State Party to the NPT.

The NPT is the most widely accepted of all arms control agreements. As of early 2000, a total of 187 states were Parties to the NPT. Cuba, Israel, India, and Pakistan were the only states that were not members of the NPT. Of these, Cuba is, as of 2008, the only one which has not developed nuclear power for military use.

In accordance with the terms of the NPT, on 11 May 1995, more than 170 countries attended the 1995 NPT Review and Extension Conference (NPTREC) in New York. Three decisions and one resolution emanated from NPTREC. First, the NPT was extended for an indefinite duration and without conditions. Second, Principles and Objectives for Nuclear Non-Proliferation and Disarmament were worked out to guide the parties to the Treaty in the next phase of its implementation. Third, an enhanced review process was established for future review conferences. Finally, a resolution endorsed the establishment of a zone free of weapons of mass destruction in the Middle East.

There is no confirmed instance so far of State Party governmental transfers of nuclear weapon technology or un-safeguarded nuclear materials to any non-nuclear-weapon state. However, some non-nuclear-weapon states, such as Iraq, were able to obtain sensitive technology and/or equipment from private parties in states that are States Parties to the NPT. South Africa conducted an independent nuclear weapons production programme prior to joining the NPT. However, it dismantled all of its nuclear weapons before signing the Treaty. In 1994, the United States and North Korea signed an 'Agreed Framework' bringing North Korea into full compliance with its non-proliferation obligations under the NPT. North Korea affirmed its NPT member status and committed itself to allow implementation of its IAEA safeguards agreement.

NEOLIBERALISM AND NUCLEAR POWER

As we have already seen, neoliberalism accords corporate control of prominent sources of finance a high priority, and the nuclear power industry therefore represents an important arena for neoliberal involvement. Older readers will probably recall that for a short time after the wartime use of nuclear weaponry on Japan there was widespread fear of its dangers and – at least initially – a reluctance to consider domestic applications of it. But this soon passed, especially in developed countries, as the huge potential for peaceful uses of nuclear energy became appreciated.

The events at Hiroshima and Nagasaki gradually became seen as bizarrely inappropriate uses of the technology. The threat, of course, of genetic damage created a rash of fears and wild speculation. All of these factors created further barriers to widespread acceptance of the use of nuclear power for domestic purposes. There was considerable popular debate about the health and safety issues in the media and nuclear power stations were built in various countries. The advantages of nuclear power became widely known – its cleanliness in particular – but also its comparative aesthetic unobtrusiveness and its comparatively low cost to the consumer.

Generally, people were becoming comfortable with the idea, until such nuclear accidents as the Three Mile Island partial meltdown in the US and the Windscale radiation leakage in the UK, re-awoke the old fears. The nuclear industry was very quick in these cases to provide reassurances. For instance, in the case of the Three Mile Island incident, it was pointed out that the fact that the warning instrumentation had alerted staff and thus prevented a real disaster indicated just how safe nuclear energy could be. Additionally, an intensive advertising campaign financed by the nuclear lobby drew people's attention to the fact that conventional coal-fuelled power stations can themselves be extremely hazardous to health and safety.

All in all, many people began once again to feel that, on the whole, nuclear power as a source of electricity was the way forward – and with the distinct advantage that it did not require having to cosy up to unpredictable foreign regimes to source oil or gas supplies. That was probably the biggest attraction of the nuclear option in the popular mind and many people tended to dismiss from their minds concerns about how to safely dispose of spent rods. Of course, this was fine with the large and wealthy corporate enterprises which built, owned and rented out nuclear power stations. The 'nuclearisation of neoliberalism' was rapidly becoming a fait accompli.

But the nuclear accident at Chernobyl in the Ukraine (at that time in the old Soviet Union) was in a different league altogether. The author dealt with this event at length in a previous book but in outline it can be described as follows.[5]

CHERNOBYL, THE IAEA, NEOLIBERALISM AND THE UN

The Soviet authorities had been running a large nuclear power plant in the Ukraine, just outside the town of Chernobyl, for over a decade. It was an immensely valued piece of infrastructure – providing employment to a large corps of scientists, engineers, technicians and thousands of less skilled people. Chernobyl was a peaceful and prosperous community and the reactor complex in no way represented a negative feature in the environment. That could never have been said of a conventional fossil-fuel reactor. But it all changed in the early hours of 26 April 1986, when Reactor Number Four suffered a meltdown.

During the first few days after the event there was a distinct difference between the way the situation was reported in the Soviet Union and in the EU, US, and some other 'free-enterprise' countries. The old USSR tried to play down the seriousness of what had happened and they initially even denied that a meltdown had occurred – despite satellite photographic evidence to the contrary. The news services in the 'West', on the other hand, were only too pleased to show the USSR in a bad light. They broadcast initial reports of hundreds killed, thousands injured and of whole populations having been exposed to levels of radiation that could inflict genetic damage on them for generations to come.

Even areas of the UK reported fallout and a sudden rise in radiation levels. What appeared odd at the time was the reluctance of Soviet authorities to accept offers of medical aid from the 'West'. They accepted equipment, medicines and food – but tended to draw the line at personnel. Then, within a month, the USSR officially announced the death toll. They claimed that only 56 people had died!

This was such a derisory figure, given the physical impact of the blast and the subsequent fires, that few believed it. As the author makes clear below, such scepticism was not confined to the 'West', but also characterised the response of several eminent medical figures in the region. But within the week, US President Reagan announced the same figure! Their findings tallied with those of the USSR in all important respects.

Of course, one rôle of the WHO is to immediately play an active part in responding to such a large-scale health emergency. But, as the author reported in his book cited above some WHO personnel trying to gain accurate health data arising from the event, found themselves blocked. It was even stated that the IAEA itself had pressured WHO to cooperate in not giving too much public prominence to the situation.[6] We are entitled to ask what had really happened.

HAS THE IAEA BEEN SUBORNED?

The Chernobyl accident, along with the lurid way in which much of the media reported it, re-awakened popular concern about the safety of nuclear reactors as a source of power – quite apart from possible military implications. As evidence of an impending environmental disaster led by global warming gradually attracted growing public concern, people began to move away from accepting the nuclear option and to place their hope in exploiting such renewable sources as wind, wave, and geothermal energy.

It is noticeable that no major government threw themselves wholeheartedly into researching this option, though. Our leaders have strongly moved in support of the nuclear option. Indeed, Britain is even being led by its government to re-place much of its nuclear arsenal, especially the Trident missile-firing submarine fleet. If this does not itself constitute a breach of the NPT, it is difficult to see what does.

But it is all perfectly consistent with a government policy that accords business acumen and entrepreneurship such high esteem. The recent actions of the IAEA have also indicated an eagerness to comply with a neoliberal agenda and this is reflected in some respects in Michel Collon's somewhat waggish comment cited above. For instance, an important part of the IAEA's founding mandate was that it would assess the nuclear development of countries newly embarking on such activities. What has it done in this regard, remembering that development of nuclear power for non-military domestic/industrial use is permitted under the NPT?

It has sent observers to assess the nuclear development situation in Iran. Whatever our suspicions might be, the Iranians have always claimed that their nuclear programme is intended for peaceful domestic development only. Corporate interests, in the US in particular, are anxious to control the vast oil resources of both Iraq and Iran – and of the Middle East generally – and it would be in their interest for the UN to undermine Iran by the threat of economic sanctions (if not of military action). The IAEA has accordingly been reporting to the UN that while they have no direct proof, indications are that Iran *could* be also establishing a nuclear arms capacity. That was enough for the US to prompt the UN Security Council to raise sanctions against Iran. But the IAEA has raised no objections through the UN about Pakistan's and India's *actual* (not just *suspected*!) nuclear developments. The US has never called on the UN to impose sanctions on those two countries. Another anomalous example is provided by Israel and its nuclear development.

Part of the answer, of course, is that the NPT is not really the protective apron it was intended to be, simply because not every member state of the UN has signed it. Prominent exceptions, as noted earlier, are: Cuba, India, Israel and Pakistan. In fact, countries which have not signed the NPT are, under UN regulations, not even regarded officially as being nuclear states! The IAEA has no control over them at all. Does not this state of affairs represent a barrier to global equity in access to healthcare? Even if we only consider the original five nuclear powers (USA, Russia, China, France and the UK), they possess sufficient nuclear warheads to wipe out the world several times over![7] In light of the above, then, the IAEA has become less a supporter and promoter of global health than an aide to corporate enterprises, and especially the international nuclear industry, in undermining equity in health in promoting corporate neoliberal interests.

This illustrates how tightly the 'war industry' is tied into the UN itself and exemplifies the issue of how war (as described in Chapter Five) cannot be seen as a separate barrier to be overcome in our quest for global equity in health. Today, war cannot meaningfully be separated from that matrix of neoliberal interests which also controls the effectiveness of our ultimate guardian of global health rights – the WHO. To analyse this complex of issues systematically, we must revisit the Chernobyl accident and consider how the IAEA has interacted with the nuclear industry corporations.

RÔLE OF THE IAEA IN REACTING TO CHERNOBYL

As mentioned above, initial reports after the accident itself painted a much grimmer health-impact picture than did later accounts. The most authoritative reports came from a medical reporter who was only 24 kilometres from Chernobyl when Reactor Number Four erupted. She is Alla Yaroshinskaya and was certainly among the first qualified medical reporters at the site. Initially she wrote only about what she heard and observed, but before long began to report in a more epidemiologically analytical fashion. It was at this point that the Soviet authorities realised that what she was saying seriously conflicted with the official view, and every attempt was made to dismiss her work as 'rubbish!'

Powerful political voices close to the US government chimed in in this attempt to destroy her scientific credibility. This aroused her suspicions and she researched even more intensively. In 1990 she came across significant documentation of a cover-up. As well, there had developed an officially sanctioned policy of calculated misinformation – an elaborate web of official lies.

The state and party leadership had knowingly played down the extent of the contamination and offered a sanitised version to the outside world. In 1991, five years after the accident, a series of laws was adopted to protect the victims of radiation. Scientists have now begun to find serious flaws in these, too. As recent studies show, the human and environmental damage shows no sign of abating.[8]

One of the facts that she uncovered was that despite its rapidly developing nuclear energy programmes, particularly those associated with nuclear weapons, the former Soviet Union was the only nuclear power in the world that lacked any nuclear safety laws! But the USA and the UK had adopted such laws in 1946, and a year earlier France had done so. Only in 1984 did the former Soviet Union get round to it, but it was never implemented due to bureaucratic inertia, even after the Chernobyl accident! Also, under Soviet Law, there was never any legal entitlement to compensation, even if the law had been enforced. Yet in the Soviet Union, dozens of nuclear accidents had occurred annually, at both military and civilian nuclear establishments. None of these were ever reported.

Thus it was quite natural, in the Soviet context, that neither the national government, nor the local authorities, were prepared to take legal responsibility for the ecological, social and other problems caused by the Chernobyl accident

– even though Gorbachev's policies of glasnost and perestroika were already in place. However, the scale of the accident and the changes that had taken place in society by that time made it impossible to conceal the fact of the accident altogether. People in the affected territories repeatedly demanded the introduction of legislation to cover their health problems, as well as to compensate for the ecological damage and for material losses arising from the accident. And yet these were problems the very existence of which both the Soviet Union and the US were vigorously denying! As Yaroshinskaya explains:[9]

> In April 1990, the Supreme Soviet reviewed the situation concerning the consequences of the liquidation of the now unusable Chernobyl nuclear facility, and noted the discrepancies. Yaroshinskaya points out that the accident at the Chernobyl nuclear power plant is, in terms of its consequences, the gravest disaster of modern times, affecting the destinies of millions of people residing in a vast territory. The ecological effect of the Chernobyl accident has made the country face the necessity of solving new, exceptionally complex, large-scale problems that affect virtually all spheres of social life, many aspects of science and manufacturing, culture, ethics and morality.
>
> It appears that the government of the former Soviet Union was more anxious to protect its people from information than from nuclear health risks! Legislation was slow in being enacted, was very limited and that most Soviet citizens were not widely aware of it. In fact, the author was surprised, on a brief visit to Russia in 1991, to find that educated civilians to whom he spoke informally about Chernobyl were not aware of how they stood legally with regard to any possible future nuclear accident.
>
> One law actually authorised a programme in 1991–92 for immediate measures to deal with the Chernobyl aftermath. It assigned the Council of Ministers the duty of drafting a 'Law on the Chernobyl Catastrophe' and submitting it to the Supreme Soviet in the fourth quarter of 1990. This law was intended to define the legal status of the catastrophe victims, the participants in containment and clean-up operations, persons living and working in the affected areas, and those compulsorily resettled. It would also cover the 'legal regime of the disaster area, discipline of population, their housing and activities, military service, formation and functioning of state administrative bodies, and public organizations in the affected area'.
>
> However, as the next relevant decree of the Supreme Soviet on 9 April 1991 noted: 'There has been no possibility at present of adopting the Law on the Chernobyl Catastrophe and the Law on Nuclear Energy Use and Nuclear Safety, due to the delay in submitting the drafts of these laws.' Only in 1991, five years after the accident, were fully adequate legislative acts adopted defining the

responsibility of the government for the damage inflicted on citizens by a nuclear enterprise adopted in the former Soviet Union.

However, these laws applied primarily to the affected population and only dealt indirectly with environmental problems. Compared to the legal vacuum of the previous five years, however, they were a significant step forward. This is all the more important, as no society had ever faced such social and environmental problems before. Nuclear accidents in other countries, such as Three Mile Island in the US and Windscale in the UK, could not be compared to the far-reaching consequences of Chernobyl.

Only almost 20 years after the Chernobyl accident, did scientists, specialists, and ecologists begin to question the 'Chernobyl' laws of Russia, Belarus, and Ukraine. A great many studies have exposed the current system of social-economic and medical measures to harsh criticism, particularly with respect to calculations of the dose of radiation delivered to the population, which still constitute the basis for compensation and assistance.

At this point we need to again bring in the rôle of the IAEA.

THE IAEA AND THE CHERNOBYL FORUM

As the welter of conflicting accounts about the effects of the event continued to mount, and as voices within the WHO raised questions and sought to carry out exhaustive epidemiological research, the IAEA sought to control the situation by establishing a supposedly 'neutral' group, called the 'Chernobyl Forum'. Its rôle was to address the panic and uncertainty existing at the local level and stemming from the fact that, even 18 years after the accident, the affected population had been given little guidance on radiation impacts on health. The Chernobyl Forum, as set up in 2003, was intended – it was claimed – to serve two purposes:

1 To give affected local people balanced and practical information allowing them to cope more effectively with the aftermath of the meltdown of Reactor Number Four and the elevated levels of radiation.
2 To provide both adjacent countries worried about radiation fallout, and even more widespread foreign communities with coherent details of the event.

The Forum – comprising eight United Nations organisations and Belarus, Russia and the Ukraine – met in Vienna on 10–11 March 2004 at IAEA headquarters. IAEA Director of Radiation and Waste Safety, Mr Abel González, said conflicting information had caused tremendous confusion and suffering.[10]

González went on to say that:

People living in the affected villages are very distressed because the information they receive – from one expert after another turning up there – is inconsistent. People living there are afraid for their children. The aim of the Forum is not to repeat the thousands of studies already done, but to give them authoratative, transparent statements that show the factual situation in the aftermath of Chernobyl.

The Forum was set up in 2003 following discussions between IAEA Director General Mohamed El Baradei and the Prime Minister of Belarus. It is part of broader efforts to help implement the UN strategy on the 'Human Consequences of the Chernobyl Nuclear Accident – A Strategy for Recovery'.

At its meeting in Vienna in March 2004, initial reports were presented by the Forum's expert groups for 'health' (led by the World Health Organization) and the 'environment' (led by the IAEA). It was expected that the Forum would issue its findings at an international conference to be held in 2005 or 2006, but that conference has not yet taken place (as of 2008).

Another key aspect of the Forum's work is to advise on, and help to implement, programmes that mitigate the accident's impact. For example, this could include:

- ❐ Remediation of contaminated land
- ❐ Special healthcare of the affected population
- ❐ Monitoring long-term human exposure to radiation
- ❐ Environmental aspects of decommissioning the Chernobyl nuclear reactor and the shelters erected for the clean-up crews
- ❐ Addressing environmental issues related to radioactive waste from the accident.

The UN organisations involved in the Forum include the IAEA, Food and Agriculture Organization, UN Office for the Coordination of Humanitarian Affairs, UN Development Programme, UN Environment Programme, UN Scientific Committee on the Effects of Atomic Radiation, the WHO and the World Bank.

What is important for the reader to appreciate is that the Chernobyl Forum was put forward by the IAEA as the only authoritative voice on the accident and its aftermath, and this was accepted by both Russia and the US. Administratively, research groups operating from within the WHO were compelled to accept this view. This author, in 2006 and 2007, met with several people in WHO who had been affected career-wise by this stifling of contrary views, as described above.[11]

But this left several other loose cannons out in the open, including the aforementioned Alla Yaroshinskaya. She had to be silenced and rendered uninfluential and this was the tactic adopted.

NEUTRALISING IMPACT OF CONTRARY VIEWS

From 1992, when she first wrote a book about the cover-up, Yaroshinskaya found herself not only *persona non grata* in her own country, but also widely and vociferously discredited in the West. To her very great credit, she vigorously rebutted many of these criticisms.

She was prevented from publishing what she found out during the Gorbachev era, despite the so-called Glaznost. When Yeltsin took over, Yaroshinskaya was elected a member of the Russian Parliament, the Duma, and during those years she became the Chairperson of the Chernobyl Investigation Commission, which obtained access to even formerly top secret Politburo reports on what happened in Chernobyl. Those were truly massive and terrible events.

As a 20-year anniversary memorial to Chernobyl's appalling effects, Yaroshinskaya published a follow-up version of her earlier book, called *The Big Lie*, in which she once again documents these 'forbidden truths', largely showing that the vast number of deaths and mobility, which were caused in the former states of the Soviet Union, are far higher and more extensive than the Western press and even the UN reports will admit.

One of dozens of attacks on her credibility follows. It can be found in a Department of Public Information of New York report (a UN report), and is datelined as from Washington and under the authority of the IAEA, the WHO and the UN Development Programme. One could hardly ask for stronger UN support than that for the following resume of the report's 'findings', roundly rebutting Yaroshinskaya's views. The report claims that, after nearly two decades, only 4000 people (at the very most) would eventually die of the effects of the accident, and that this figure was reached by an international team of 100 scientists. Very few non-UN nuclear scientists agree with these findings. After stating that up to 4000 people *could* die, only 50 had done so as of mid-2005! This is so unbelievable that this author wonders why they picked such an unlikely figure, for even with careful monitoring by former Soviet Union security personnel, dozens of foreign reporters had – by interviewing bereaved Ukrainians – determined much higher figures. Moreover, the WHO report goes on to state that of these 50 deaths, almost all of the cases had been highly exposed rescue workers.

The new figures are presented in a landmark digest report, *Chernobyl's Legacy: health, environmental and socio-economic impacts*, just released by the Chernobyl Forum. The digest, based on a three-volume, 600-page report and incorporating the work of hundreds of scientists, economists and health experts, assesses the 20-year impact of the largest nuclear accident in history. The Forum is made up of eight UN specialised agencies, including the IAEA, the WHO, UN Development Programme (UNDP), Food and Agriculture Organization (FAO), UN Environment Programme (UNEP), UN Office for the Coordination of

Humanitarian Affairs (UN-OCHA), UN Scientific Committee on the Effects of Atomic Radiation (UNSCEAR), and the World Bank, as well as the governments of Belarus, the Russian Federation and Ukraine.

'This compilation of the latest research can help to settle the outstanding questions about how much death, disease and economic fallout really resulted from the Chernobyl accident,' explains Dr. Burton Bennett, chairman of the Chernobyl Forum and an authority on radiation effects. 'The governments of the three most-affected countries have realized that they need to find a clear way forward, and that progress must be based on a sound consensus about environmental, health and economic consequences and some good advice and support from the international community.'

'This was a very serious accident with major health consequences, especially for thousands of workers exposed in the early days who received very high radiation doses, and for the thousands more stricken with thyroid cancer. By and large, however, we have not found profound negative health impacts to the rest of the population in surrounding areas, nor have we found widespread contamination that would continue to pose a substantial threat to human health, except within a few exceptional, restricted areas.'

The Forum's report aims to help the affected countries understand the true scale of the accident's consequences and also suggests ways the governments of Belarus, the Russian Federation and Ukraine might address major economic and social problems stemming from the accident. Members of the Forum, including representatives of the three governments, are to meet September 6 and 7 in Vienna at an unprecedented gathering of the world's experts on Chernobyl, radiation effects and protection, to consider these findings and recommendations.

But, says Dr Michael Repacholi, Manager of WHO's Radiation Program, 'the sum total of the Chernobyl Forum is a reassuring message.'

He explains that there have been 4000 cases of thyroid cancer, mainly in children, but that except for nine deaths, all of them have recovered. 'Otherwise, the team of international experts found no evidence for any increases in the incidence of leukaemia and cancer among affected residents.'

The international experts have estimated that radiation could cause up to about 4000 eventual deaths among the higher-exposed Chernobyl populations, i.e., emergency workers from 1986–1987, evacuees and residents of the most contaminated areas. This number contains both the known radiation-induced cancer and leukaemia deaths and a statistical prediction, based on estimates of the radiation doses received by these populations. As about a quarter of people die from spontaneous cancer not caused by Chernobyl radiation, the radiation-induced increase of only about 3% will be difficult to observe. However, in the most exposed cohorts of the emergency and recovery operation workers some increase of particular cancer forms (e.g., leukaemia) in particular time periods has already been observed. The predictions use six decades of scientific experience with the effects of such doses, explained Repacholi.

Repacholi concludes that 'the health effects of the accident were potentially horrific, but when you add them up using validated conclusions from good science, the public health effects were not nearly as substantial as had at first been feared.'

The report's estimate of the eventual number of deaths is far lower than earlier, well-publicised speculations that radiation exposure would claim tens of thousands of lives. But note that the figure of 4000 does not vary all that much from the estimate made back in 1986 by Soviet scientists. And despite the huge amount of contrary material, expensively produced and lavishly distributed by the Chernobyl Forum, it is significant that the majority of scientific assessments support Yaroshinskaya's estimate.

Many people in the Ukraine itself would profoundly condemn the Chernobyl Forum's report as little more than propaganda. Yaroshinskaya unhesitatingly categorised the entire report as 'a lie'.[12] She reports that official Ukrainian government figures show that 142 000 people died within ten years of the Chernobyl meltdown. And this figure did not include deaths in Belarus, Russian and other affected areas. Current estimates for Chernobyl-related deaths in the Ukraine are around 620 000 deaths and millions suffering long-term radiation exposure and acute re-exposure events, also from Chernobyl. The death estimates for Belarus' 1986 population of 10 million will be about 2 million, because at least 25% of the land of Belarus was too contaminated for safe habitation – indeed much of it will remain so for years to come – and represents far worse contamination of Belarus than of any other state. Thus, if the situation is bad in the Ukraine, it is far worse in Belarus, which lies just over the border from Chernobyl – a mere 10 kilometres in fact. The initial radioactive clouds of smoke from the burning reactor blew north for days – carrying the worst radioactivity – directly over Belarus. Kiev is about 70 kilometres south of Chernobyl.

The deaths in Belarus were not even reported by their hard-line, soviet-style officials in Minsk, thus preventing the data from being made public. There the situation is clearly much worse than in the Ukraine. One sees no play given to that fact in the press, either. If the number of deaths caused by the Chernobyl accident were about 620 000 in the Ukraine, then in Belarus the corresponding figure was about 1 million by 2006. This is also consistent with ongoing population declines in the region. Yaroshinskaya also reported the deaths of 100 000 of the 650 000 clean-up workers associated with the building of the 'sarcophagus' and the initial attempts to stop the graphite fires at Chernobyl. She also documents, from official records at the clinics and hospitals, how the number of deaths was 'officially' reduced by not allowing autopsies and by artificially changing the 'radiation-level' exposures. Those people who did not die in hospitals were 'sent home', where they died and thus did not officially meet the criteria for treatment for radiation. Their illnesses were attributed to 'other causes', which also acted to cover up the true mortality and morbidity statistics.

In other words, it is clear to this author that the official Soviet figures are highly suspect, not only because the very low death and morbidity figures belie so much of what we already know about nuclear radiation, but so neatly fit in with the commercial needs of the nuclear power corporations. As Yaroshinskaya states in her own book, *The Big Lie* 'You can believe UN officials, or you can believe the actual, on-ground, onsite events.' The author prefers primary sources, as most thinkers do, for the reason that they are more closely tied to real and direct data than such official 'lies' are.

The UN, the WHO, and Soviet, Russian and US media reports are simply wrong. They even ignored the massive North American radioactive fallout over Idaho and also in New England, which caused a significant rise in thyroid problems in children there just after Chernobyl. Sadly, ignoring the evidence of these Soviet and current denials of events is simply part of the cover-up. Yaroshinskaya's books seek to 'redress this grievance' by showing more of the whole truth, which happened at the time and is still continuing, including such unheralded events as the Sonsnovy Bor reactor accident. This also involved a major nuclear reactor accident, but was not picked up by major global media outlets. One need only read the voluminous relevant documents and citations, a major source of which is cited below, to recognise that such a sea of evidence cannot be ignored by thinking people.

And, of course, those horrendous health implications continue to this very day and will do so for long into the future. Back in 1996, one Walter Huda, published a bibliography of medical and epidemiological commentaries on Chernobyl.[13] Huda himself is a medical physicist, who gained a doctorate in physics from Oxford University and a medical physician doctorate from Hammersmith Hospital in London. He is now Director of Radiological Physics at the Oncology Unit at the Montreal General Hospital in Canada. His native country is the Ukraine and he returns there frequently.

FUTURE IMPLICATIONS OF NUCLEAR ENERGY

It then goes without saying that, as long as conditions persist for such accidents to happen, and for their impact to be covered up for personal and/or corporate gain, we cannot speak meaningfully of closing the global health inequity gap. How we can prevent – or greatly reduce the likelihood of nuclear reactor accidents is an issue that must be addressed transparently and under international supervision.

The time may well come when the scientific community can broadly agree on a safe method decommissioning reactors, in which case we may well be in a position to maintain an environmental sustainability far more easily than we can at the moment. But, as of the first decade of the second millennium, we must break free of the warfare matrix with which both neoliberalism and the nuclear industry are irretrievably enmeshed. These issues will be considered in the final chapter.

THE WARFARE MATRIX EMBRACES ALL CIVIL LIFE

But let us be aware that world health equity is mortgaged by war in many respects other than the nuclear industry. And virtually all of these are caused by the distortions to financial allocation caused by war. It is in many ways a classical manifestation of a biofeedback mechanism. Within that biofeedback cycle one can easily identify various sub-cycles, for example, wars use up oil so wars need oil; but this implies the necessity to control oil supplies leading to wars. And in 2008 we started to become aware that even in the First World we are on the cusp of a serious food crisis.

Space does not permit the author to even begin to address these collateral issues as a whole. Therefore, let us consider the issue of the impact of war on the health of children. There are literally hundreds of relevant studies from which to draw evidence. The horrors of the war in Iraq continues to throw up huge amounts of detail on the issue, but the author will focus only on two areas with which he has had field experience – Palestine and Mauritius.

Let us first consider an analysis by three midwives of the situation in Gaza, in the Palestine Occupied Territories.[14] Their account was published in the *Journal of Clinical Psychology and Psychiatry* in 2005 and was made available online in 2007. Their work centred on interviewing Palestinian children (aged 6–11) of both sexes, and their mothers (aged 21–55 years). A resume of their findings follows:

The aims of this study were first to examine how exposure to war trauma, maternal neuroticism and psychological distress are associated with child psychological distress and second, whether good maternal mental health and low neuroticism can moderate the negative impact of war trauma on child mental health. Third, they investigated as to whether, and to what degree, mother–child dyads' psychological distress was dependent on who was the main war trauma victim in the family: the mother, the child or both. Fourth, they tested whether mother-child dyads express similar or different symptoms. The sample consisted of 121 Palestinian children (aged 6–16 years; 45% girls and 55% boys) and their mothers (aged 21–55 years) living under conditions of military violence and war in Gaza. Child psychological distress was measured using the CPTS–RI (child-reported), the Rutter Parent Questionnaire (mother reported) and mothers' mental health was measured using the SCL-90-R.

The results failed to show any moderating effect of good maternal mental health or low neuroticism in protecting child mental health from negative impact of war trauma. The main effects showed that the child's young age, war trauma and poor maternal mental health were associated with children's internalised symptoms; and that male gender, maternal neuroticism and poor mental health were linked with children's externalising symptoms. There were gender differences in psychological distress depending on whether the mother, the child or both were the main war trauma victim in the family. Girls showed particularly high psychological distress when their mothers were exposed to war trauma (family systems model) whereas boys showed high levels of distress when both they themselves, along with their mothers, were exposed to war trauma (accumulative impact model). Similarities were confirmed in dyadic symptom expression: significant associations were found between mothers' depressive and children's internalising symptoms, and between mothers' hostile and children's externalising symptoms.

In other words, the people of the occupied Palestinian territories would only experience comparatively short-term social tranquillity in trying to re-establish normal civil life should the Israelis unilaterally withdraw tomorrow! The longer Israel continues to use military means to achieve their purposes in the region the greater will be the accumulated heritage of people who are psychologically traumatised as children and less capable of facing normal social challenges in later life.

This must be true, of course, in any warfare situation. For instance, during the Vietnam War, people in the war areas themselves often spoke to the author (he was working in Hanoi) about 'when peace comes, we will all sing and dance'. But more than thirty years since the end of hostilities there is still not much evidence of singing or dancing! Peace may have come militarily, even victory, but it has made little difference and psychological peace is conspicuous by its absence. What continues to amaze this author – who has returned to the region several times since 'peace' was restored, leading groups of teachers, medics and other professionals on four-week tours, is how children, now only 14 or 15 years old are so badly affected. After all, we are speaking here of people who were born at least 15 years after the last shot was fired and who can have no personal memory of bombs going off.

What amazed me most was the degree to which these children had developed a capacity to avoid empathy. Their reactions to having been brought up in a society in which such normal emotions as affection, concern for the less able in society and an easy-going optimism had been placed 'on hold' during actual warfare was to continue blocking off overt expression of those emotions. For instance, in 2006, the author spoke briefly to a class of fifteen 11-year-old Vietnamese children (13 boys, 2 girls) at an English as a Foreign Language School in Sussex. By definition these children were from the more privileged economic backgrounds and were expected to return to Vietnam when the three-month course was completed in order to enhance and expand family businesses; but it soon became clear that in their world there could be little room for sentiment or family values. Among opinions expressed by them were:

1 If children refused to learn in school, they should be either starved until they were willing to study or put to work in unskilled positions where they would die off due to accidents.

2 There should be no pensions. Once a person was too old to work effectively, he/she should be humanely destroyed.

And these were children who only the evening before had been laughing hysterically with me in child-like innocence at the film, *Chitty Chitty Bang Bang*. Only two of them had a pet dog or cat back home.

Never say that we can calculate the cost of war! And let us never say that if we come to our senses and stop it as a matter of international survival logic the problems of the human race will be over!

NEGATIVE IMPACT OF WAR ON CHILDREN'S HEALTH

On 5 September 2002, the UN General Assembly held a special session in which speakers were asked to address the issue of the negative impact of war on children's health.[15] A few of the comments made at that meeting by the leaders of various countries are summarised below.

President Yahya Jammeh of Gambia said that as long as wars and violence sparked by greed and hatred continued, one might think that world leaders were the true enemies of children. Urging the international community to say 'yes' to children and 'no' to violence, he said the problems afflicting the children of Africa, and indeed the world, could not be tackled without confronting poverty, war and terror.

President Alejandro Toledo of Peru, reaffirming his commitment to reprioritise public expenditure on education, health and nutrition, said his government had decided to reduce its military expenditure and redirect those funds towards investment in children. Addressing businessmen, he said, 'Don't give them fish, but teach them how to fish. Don't give them food, but open your markets, because with markets, we can generate employment and income.' He suggested that the technology and knowledge of private enterprise be used to generate more social projects directed towards children.

President Levy Mwanawasa of Zambia said that the ghastly shadows of poverty and protracted conflicts further darkened the future of African children. Zambia was a 'plateau of peace' and had therefore become home to many refugees fleeing war and strife in other countries. He appealed to the United Nations and other humanitarian organisations to help Zambia share that burden.

The President of Bahrain's Supreme Council of Women said that by condemning all offences perpetrated by the Israeli occupying forces the international community would be taking a moral and humanitarian stand that could end Israel's aggression against the Palestinian people. Events in the occupied Palestinian territories not only violated international law and the Fourth Geneva Convention, but also constituted a breach of all civilised human values.

The observer for Palestine said that the lives of Palestinian children were marked by the systematic denial, by Israel, of even their most basic rights. Hundreds of them were illegally detained in Israeli prisons, tens of thousands had had their educations disrupted and thousands had been rendered homeless. However, although Palestinians did not exercise sovereignty over their land, this had not prevented the Palestinian Authority from endorsing and implementing the provisions of the Convention on the Rights of the Child.

Comments were also made by various European political figures as follows:

Georgia's Minister of Foreign Affairs said that conflicts, separatism and ethnic cleansing in Abkhazia, Georgia, and elsewhere in the world had brought tears and hardships to hundreds of thousands of children. 'How could the international community accept the fact that the separatist regime in Abkhazia denied the right of the children there to study in their own tongue and to use books written in Georgian?' he asked. Just as in the 20th century, indifference remained the foremost enemy and sin of mankind.

The Minister of Labour and Social Insurance of Cyprus said the continuing occupation of nearly 37% of the country by a neighbouring state had prevented the implementation of a plan of action that would benefit all Cypriot children. For Cyprus, creating a world fit for children would require a political settlement that would allow all Cypriot children – whether of Greek, Turkish, Armenian, Maronite or Latin origin – to have equal access to services and basic human rights, including the right to associate freely with one another.

The head of Ukraine's State Committee for Family and Youth Affairs, noting that general morbidity among children had increased threefold since the Chernobyl nuclear disaster, said her country had demonstrated resolve to prevent the recurrence of such tragedies in the future by voluntarily renouncing its nuclear military arsenal and by fully decommissioning the Chernobyl plant.

Germany's Federal Minister for Family Affairs, Senior Citizens, Women and Youth said her country could not stand by while 250 million children between the ages of 5 and 14 years were subjected to ruthless exploitation and even enslavement. She added that despite increasing awareness of the commercial sexual exploitation of children, the number of victims, especially those exploited in connection with child trafficking and child prostitution was growing worldwide.

Addressing the session, Willemijn Aerdts, Youth Representative of the Netherlands, said that her intervention meant that youth participation was taken seriously, but the fact that she was only one of the few youth representatives doing so implied that it was not taken seriously enough at the national level.

With such a vast panoply of opinion converging on such a crucial issue one has to wonder how and why it has not yet led to a course of definitive action. That question will be dealt with again in the final chapter, but as this author looks back on decades of experience in poorer countries, he is increasingly conscious of the global significance of that global health equity gap. No country is immune from its malign influences.

THE SITUATION IN MAURITIUS

One of the many smaller countries in which this author was privileged to serve for a short time was Mauritius and it was their Prime Minister Anerood Jugnauth who spoke. Mauritius, he asserted, could easily be an exceedingly peaceful community in the sense that it can – to a high degree – meet all of its sustenance needs locally and it is blessed with an exceptionally congenial climate. It is a republic and includes in its heritage three main experiences of European colonialism – Dutch, French and British.

But the author, while in Mauritius, was never aware of many of the usual resentments against Europeans that such a background often produces. However, plenty of inter-ethnic tension exists between the descendents of large numbers of indentured labourers brought in by the various colonisers to carry out the heavy agricultural labour that the locals could not be induced to do. Thus, the Dutch (1598–1710) brought in boatloads of Javanese, Africans of various types and others to do agricultural work. Then the French were there 1715–1810 (having defeated the Dutch in yet another war) and they imported at least two huge drafts of slaves from West Africa to run the now prosperous sugar cane plantations. About one third of Mauritius' population is now derived from these roots, calling themselves Creole French.

Then the British, as a result of one of its defeats of the Napoleonic forces, took Mauritius in 1810. They abolished slavery, thereby creating another large indigenous sub-population. To replace the slaves, they brought in corps of Indian indentured labourers, whose descendents now account for about 67% of the Mauritius population. Tension between these ethnic groups lead to periodic clashes – but rarely what could be called war.

Therefore, the author was especially interested in what the Prime Minister of Mauritius would say with respect to war and children's health. As things happened he addressed most of his remarks to the situation prevailing in continental Africa. Much of this author's own work has been with respect to HIV/AIDS in sub-Saharan Africa, and Anerood Jugnauth's comments centred on the children thus affected by the various wars in the area. He noted, importantly, that very young children, especially from the Middle East and from Africa, were often victims of unspeakable atrocities. He attributed this to the fact that such children routinely witnessed public displays of brutality and torture and were encouraged to participate, first of all through torturing bound adult prisoners by piercing them using poles with sharpened ends.

As they developed further expertise with such hideous practices as gorging out eyes and amputating tongues, they were armed (often with AK47s almost as tall as they were) to execute designated victims. Obviously, there is no way in which the children's mental health would not have been seriously undermined by such experiences. In both Liberia and Côte d'Ivoire, the author often spoke to both boys and girls who had been trained as soldiers – often from 7 or 8 years of age – and then, in their early teens, expected to re-adapt to a life of peace and rational behaviour. What I noticed, in particular, was how many of them relied heavily on alcohol and tended to be social isolates – not even fraternising with other former child soldiers.

Prime Minister Jugnauth was empathetic in his observations that this was not 'someone else's problem' but had to be addressed by all of us.

It was his view that government institutions, non-governmental organisations (NGOs), community-based organisations and parents had participated in his country's successful launch of the 'Say Yes to Children' campaign. More than 230 000 people, including children and adolescents, or 22% of the population of Mauritius, had participated in the vote to determine the priorities. The vote had identified three top priorities: educate every child; care for every child; and stop harming and exploiting children.

The government had created a special portfolio in the Ministry of Women's Rights and Family Welfare to address child development. Children enjoyed free access to all levels of education. Since 1995, primary education has been compulsory. Public healthcare services were free and easily accessible through an extensive network of hospitals, healthcare centres and community health centres, which provided comprehensive healthcare, including prenatal and early child development.

He said the Government had taken effective steps to contain the negative side-effects of rapid socio-economic development on children without jeopardising its strategy for economic progress. To encourage increased accessibility to information and communication technology, it had launched a major school information technology (IT) project. Conscious of the negative impact of the Internet culture on children and youth, Mauritius was taking bold steps to shield its children from harmful exposure to it.

One could present much more data on this distressing aspect of war, but the good sense of much of what the Mauritius Prime Minister had to say indicates the sort of transnational controls that we must put in place as a preliminary to the reforms he suggests.

In closing this chapter, especially with respect to the impact of war on children, the reader should be reminded of the international trade in child trafficking. This is very much one of the results of military assumption of control over civilian life in large numbers of countries. Myanmar is a prime example, as this author has detailed in a previous book, and as the aftermath of the disastrous cyclone that so grievously battered that country in May 2008 made abundantly clear.[16]

REFERENCES

1 MacDonald T. *Third World Health: hostage to Third World wealth.* Oxford & New York: Radcliffe Publishing; 2005.

2 Boncza M. Stiglitz' Valuable Insight. [Letter] *Morning Star,* 7 Apr 2008, p. 7.

3 Collon, M. *Keep it Simple.* Available at: http://michelcollon.info (accessed 22 Mar 2008).

4 United Nations. *The Nuclear Non-Proliferation Treaty (NPT).* Available at: www.fas.org/nuke/control/npt/ (accessed 12 May 2008).

5 MacDonald T. *Sacrificing the WHO to the Highest Bidder.* Oxford & New York: Radcliffe Publishing; 2008. pp. 172–9.

6 *Sacrificing the WHO to the Highest Bidder,* op. cit. pp. 172–7

7 BBC Radio 4. *The World's Nuclear Arsenal.* Available at: www.news.bbc.co.uk/1/hi/world/733162.stm (accessed 22 Mar 2008)

8 *Sacrificing the WHO to the Highest Bidder,* op. cit. pp. 175–7.

9 Yaroshinskaya A. *The Big Lie: the secret Chernobyl documents.* Available at: www.eurozine.com/articles/2006-04-21-yaroshinskaya-en.html (accessed 14 May 2008).

10 IAEA News Centre. *Chernobyl: clarifying consequences.* Available at: www.iaea.org/NewsCenter/News/2004/consequences.html (accessed 12 May 2008).

11 *Sacrificing the WHO to the Highest Bidder,* op. cit. pp. 177–9.

12 *The Big Lie: the secret Chernobyl documents.* op cit.

13 Huda W. *Annotated Chernobyl Bibliography.* Available at: www.brama.com/Ukraine/chernibib.html (accessed 14 May 2008).

14 El Sarraj E, Punamaki R, Quota S. *Mother-Child Expression of Psychological Distress in War Trauma.* Available at: www.cat.inst.fr/?aModele=afficheNscpsidt=16720207 (accessed 14 May 2008).

15 UN General Assembly. *Negative Impact of Armed Conflict on Children.* Special Press

ת

Releases from the 27th Special Session of the General Assembly 5 Sep 2002. Available at: www.un.org/News/Press/docs/2002/ga10019.doc.htm. (accessed 22 Mar 2008)

16 MacDonald T. *Health, Human Rights and the United Nations: inconsistent aims and inherent contradictions.* Oxford & New York: Radcliffe Publishing; 2007. pp. 51–66.

Chapter 7

Imperialism and global health

THE PSYCHOLOGY OF IMPERIALISM

When this author first came to Britain in 1957, he was struck by the vigour and moral certainty evident in comments about the old British Empire. Very roughly, the views expressed could be broken down into three broad categories:

1 The 'empire' was something about which all decent people should feel ashamed. The British Empire had been built on huge assumptions of racial arrogance (white supremacy, no less), pillaging and looting other less well-armed countries for their possessions and through the development of an enormously profitable international trade out of capturing people for slavery.

2 Throughout history empires have come and empires have gone, but the British Empire was by far the most enlightened and least rapacious. Its subject peoples widely benefited from its internationally acclaimed educational system, the impartiality of its laws and its capacity to organise trade and commerce and such infrastructures as road systems and railways to keep it running efficiently.

3 The British Empire gradually lost power and influence most dramatically in the post-1945 years, when India, Pakistan and several African nations achieved independence. The sun had been able to set on the British Empire by 1950!

What was often missing from these views was much sense of what imperialism was *for*. Its purpose is/was to gain power and advantage by exploiting another country's resources, including its people. No empire ever arose as some kind of social experiment, although that aspect sometimes entered the equation later, but did so in order to increase the relative strength of the imperial nation with respect to others. There has rarely been any question but that imperialism decreased the relative strength of the 'captive' nation or people.

Because we no longer sell boat-loads of West African slaves for profit or send out District Commissioners or other administrators to run various trading arrangements, people tend to think that classical European imperialism is pretty well finished. But that is far from true.

In this chapter, then, we shall be doing two things. First, we shall show how the classical model of imperialism has been used in poaching medical personnel from poor countries to augment the medical facilities of First World countries. Second, we shall consider and evaluate the various mechanisms derived to finance healthcare initiatives globally under neoliberal auspices. It will become evident that the 'poaching medical staff' aspect is but a symptom of the deeper problem of trying to fund healthcare globally – and at a profit – in a neoliberal context.

What we are referring in this first issue, broadly speaking, is the practice of staffing the health provision needs of First World countries by regularly hiring cohorts of doctors, nurses and other ancillary healthcare workers from many of the less developed countries (LDCs). By doing this, First World countries make great savings financially because they have been spared the time and expense of training their own personnel. A number of First World countries have been engaged in this activity for several years and some have developed elaborate methods of varying the intake of such personnel to prevent serious competition with internal markets.

The countries primarily considered in this chapter are: the UK, the US, Canada and Australia. Before considering the individual impacts of these countries' recruitment activities we need to consider some of the general effects of this 'brain drain' on the countries that are being deprived.

NEGATIVE IMPACTS OF THE BRAIN DRAIN ON THIRD WORLD COUNTRIES

If we go back as far as 2000, according to material analysed by this author in 2006 and again in 2007 one can immediately see the direct effect of the advantages gained by the NHS (and private hospitals) in the UK through the huge proportion of medical personnel from places like the Philippines, Sri Lanka, India and various African countries.[1,2] What is the impact of the loss of these valuable people from their own countries? In terms of personnel losses we know that between 1988 and 1995 a full 60% of Ghana's medical graduates left. Most came to the UK and have stayed; others went to Australia and the US. In Zimbabwe, though, the situation was far worse. For instance, just in the decade from 1990–2000 their medical school produced 1200 graduates and 840 of them left.

Of course, in Zimbabwe the 'push' factors, encouraging doctors to leave, probably exceeded the 'pull' factors of better working conditions elsewhere. Many of them migrated across the border to South Africa where, in 1999, nearly 80% of doctors in the rural areas had been trained outside of South Africa. In the year 2001 alone, 2114 South African trained nurses migrated to the UK. And it was the UK, with its ever staff-hungry NHS, that soon became the largest exploiter of health professionals trained abroad.

The *British Medical Journal* (*BMJ*), in one of its editorials in 2002 drew attention in detail to the analysis mentioned above. As that editorial pointed out, not all of the loss was due to foreign recruitment.[3] Trained medical staff tended to shift from one country to another within Africa, sometimes to avoid legal or emotional entanglements in their own. But in 2000, data from South African medical schools indicated that about 43–46% of their graduates went further abroad, usually to English-speaking countries. And even back then the steady and growing loss of fully trained nurses was much greater. The editorial recalls that in 2002 150 000 Filipino and 18 000 Zimbabwean nurses were working overseas.

In England, London was for a long time the favoured target for foreign medics and nurses coming to the UK. But in the UK as a whole, 31% of its doctors and 13% of its nurses were from overseas. In London those figures (in 2000) were 23% and 47%. As the *BMJ* editorial (cited above) points out, it is not only medically trained people who are being lured away from their countries, but in this chapter we shall concentrate only on health imperialism.

It is not only 'pull' factors (such as better pay and working conditions in the country chosen) that operate, but such obvious 'push' factors as lack of social status, unavailability of reasonable equipment and political violence. This latter varies in intensity from one county to another and from one unsolved political crisis to another. As indicated in the previous chapter, military activity tends to drive doctors and nurses away in large numbers.

And these factors operate whatever the actual local health needs are. The disease burden of HIV/AIDS, for instance, in sub-Saharan African countries – as of 2007 – involves one in eight citizens, with young women being the hardest hit.[4] In fact, the same data showed that one in five South African nurses were HIV positive! Even if generic copies of the appropriate antiretrovirals could be provided, their correct administration would require a much greater increase in the number of available nurses. As a matter of priority, one step in trying to solve this problem is to establish effective transnational barriers to health imperialism.

As things stand now in Africa, we can say with confidence that health access in that continent is declining and the health inequity gap widening. There are a host of proximal reasons, such as failure at the local level to address non-clinical health determinants – secure and comfortable housing, work satisfaction and access to education – and this impacts negatively on health status. There is a declining per capita spending on healthcare leading to lack of availability of medically trained personnel, lack of drugs needed for specific conditions and insufficiency of petrol to move people to hospitals and/or clinics. On top of all of that, further pressure is brought to bear on slender resources by the energetic promotion (through the IMF and the WTO) of such health sector 'reforms' as health insurance and SAPs impacting on local communities, because of various trade agreements in which the country as a whole may have become involved.

The above-cited *BMJ* editorial tends to see some cause for optimism in the fact that some LDCs have had the foresight to improve domestic conditions and have thereby started to draw their migratory medical personnel back home. For instance, Thailand and Ireland have set up 'reverse brain drain' strategies, offering more research funding and more opulent working conditions. But this author has rarely seen this happen as a result of individual LDCs reassessing their values. It only occurs if huge donations from outside – either from individuals or governments – can provide the cash required.

And this exemplifies the point, which the author will make in greater detail below, that imperialism can never regard the state to which it is applied as an 'equal partner' in the enterprise. The 'colony' is there to be exploited. When its resources (for example, medically trained people) are required, they will be taken. But as economic changes take place in the imperial country, it may have to stop recruiting from abroad and even divest itself of many of the foreign graduate doctors being given training (at the host country's expense) to prepare them for an incorrectly anticipated need for consultancy posts. Various ways are routinely found of terminating previous agreements and sending the people back home under the strict immigration rules increasingly applied by First World countries.

In the UK, this started to happen with a vengeance in 2007; before that, however, another important change took place. In 1998/99 various conferences were held at which complaints against the UK's NHS were made. The NHS stood accused of solving its own staff shortages by actively recruiting nurses and doctors who had recently qualified in certain Third World training institutions. As can be imagined, the quality of nursing and medical training can vary immensely from one teaching facility or hospital to another. In some, one can virtually buy a degree. But some training facilities have their standards regularly vetted by such agencies as the British Medical Association and the American Medical Association, and their students sit essentially the same examinations to qualify as do their British or American counterparts. Of course, to become employable in Britain a foreign-trained graduate may require a short term of instruction including language training, and this is followed by various broad examinations, both written and practical.

But the NHS prior to 1998 had been finding it worthwhile to sign on foreign medical staff as soon after graduation as they could, and then providing them with the appropriate top-up training in a British hospital. They were also paid to work on the wards under close supervision, and were thus regarded as staff members. Their pay was somewhat lower than that of people whose entire training had been in the UK, but that usually meant a considerable economic gain on what they would have earned if they had not been recruited.

If one were a patient at a British hospital, especially in London, one became quickly aware of the large proportion of medical staff who had grown up abroad and with some of whom the language barriers meant that ordinary discourse – say, filling in the form of a patient's personal details – could sometimes be amusingly difficult.

But the NHS stopped such direct recruiting in 1999. That being the case, why does one (especially in London) still encounter that earnest and friendly phalanx of Tagalog (and various other language) speakers when one is admitted as a patient? The answer is that, although the NHS no longer actively recruits abroad for staff, privately run hospitals and clinics still do. And their staff then often register with nursing agencies in the UK for temporary placements on weekends and on their regular days off.

These 'agency nurses', as they are called, are in constant demand in the NHS especially in the busy London hospitals, and since the NHS did not itself recruit foreign nurses for their own use there is no barrier to them using them on an 'agency nurse' basis. It turns out to be an exceedingly costly way for the NHS to meet its staffing needs, even though they (the NHS) did not have to train them. In February 2008 the most radical shake-up in NHS pay structures since the NHS itself was established in 1948 was ushered in by what became known as the 'Agenda for Change'. Under this mandate, a hospital had to pay the agency about £36 an hour for an agency nurse, of which the nurse got about half.

All of this suggests a growing realisation that the problem of meeting First World health staffing needs by relying on foreign recruits is not that simple and cannot be sustained long term. This will become clearer as we consider the experience of other First World countries with the same issue.

US FORAYS INTO GLOBAL HEALTH IMPERIALISM

The whole issue of whether or not it is defensible for First World nations to recruit medical staff, whose training they have not paid for, from poorer countries is discussed at length in an excellent editorial by Amy Hagopian.[5] She considered the issue primarily with respect to medical doctors only, and from the US perspective. It confronts many of the same moral ambiguities already encountered in our consideration of the British experience, but – unlike the case in Britain – the real healthcare staff gap in the US is in the ranks of GP's and family doctors.

For, in the United States, there is *great* reluctance on the part of medical graduates to go into general practice. This is not entirely unnatural, because during the last two years of the medical course the students are acquainted with various choices of specialisation such as obstetrics, gynaecology, paediatrics, surgery and general practice is in there too. Each student does a rota of about three months in the various areas and, during each, is addressed by specialists in the area, telling them the career advantages of their specific specialisation.

This author, while assistant dean at a medical school, listened to a number of these 'pitches' for recruits and many of them were highly amusing, as well as informative. For example, obstetrics and gynaecology is very good. Only rarely does anything go wrong, the mother does all the work and then gives the obstetrician all the credit and thanks. One enthused: 'They think you're Jesus Christ or something, and for some reason they often bake you a cake on the baby's first birthday, so you get plenty of cakes!' Commented another: 'Cosmetic surgery is the ticket. It is generally safe, you can charge like a bull and you are hardly ever going to get called out at nights or on the weekends,' and so on.

The UK reader must bear in mind that medicine is a private business in the US and medical graduates charge individual patients for their services. At annual reunions at medical schools, there is considerable competition between graduates with respect to how much they are earning. One's worth as a medical graduate is often judged by one's bank balance and it is in this regard that general practice (family medicine) fails in the popularity stakes. It is not respected as highly by 'customers' and the wealthier people prefer to pick a specialist. A general practitioner's request is *not* a requirement for a visit to a consultant (specialist) in the US, so for a patient to go to a general practitioner is regarded as a sign that he/she is not as well off as his/hers neighbours. A general practitioner earns a lot – even by US standards – but not as much as medical graduates who have gone into a more high profile speciality. A lot of status considerations come into the equation.

Meeting that perpetual demand for a sufficient number of general practitioners is the main reason for the recruitment of foreign-trained doctors. Hagopian's editorial, cited above, discusses this topic in depth, pointing out that as of 2007 US medical graduates displayed their continuing disdain for family medicine, as shown by the results of the 2007 National Resident Match Program. US graduates filled only 42% of the family medicine residency slots available (2621 total slots), with the rest coming from other countries (1206) or going unfilled (308).[6]

Studies of the origins of medical personnel bear this out with respect to foreign-trained physicians landing on American shores to provide primary care. Indeed, more than 28% of US primary care doctors have been trained abroad, typically in countries with poor health indicators and shortages of physicians (although in previous generations medical immigrants tended to be from Europe).[7]

Physician migration patterns reflect thousands of individual and family-level choices, based on judgements of economic, social, professional, and other interests. Article 13 of the 1948 Universal Declaration of Human Rights asserts that 'everyone has the right to leave any country'. Social justice and immigration rights advocates endorse that well-established human right. But what if the person leaving his country wants to take with him the assets of others he leaves behind? What if those remaining in the home country experience, as a result of that person's right to emigrate, an appreciable decline in their own circumstances? Dr Hagopian explains the moral dilemma clearly.

In the case of persons with a tertiary education – say, those who have been prepared for professional service by 15 to 20 years of education and training – their emigration takes with them the expensive training afforded by the institutions and governments of their home countries. Those investments are made, in part, to improve the living conditions of the collective citizenry of the country. Educational investments are afforded by a collective contribution of taxes and donations, both from the country's citizens and from individuals and granting agencies abroad. In almost no university or medical school anywhere, do the fees paid by students meet the total costs involved. We are therefore faced with trying to balance the right (under the UDHR) of an individual citizen with the rights of his/her community as a whole (also guaranteed under the UDHR)!

As well, the recruit is themselves not morally uninvolved. They are not mindless commodities but are capable of autonomous action. Dr Hagopian argues that US citizens must understand that physicians trained in low-income countries are as rational as anyone else when it comes to deciding their futures. In the summer of 2006, she conducted a study of health worker motivation, satisfaction and intent to stay for the Ministry of Health in one of the East African countries most commonly used as a source of recruits. She surveyed conditions of practice in the home country and then held focus groups with hospital-based physicians working there. She heard repeatedly that working conditions were so dismal, compensation was so low, and opportunities for advanced training so stunted, that physicians cannot help but be lured by the greener pastures, as they call them, in wealthier countries. These physicians described domestic circumstances in which the hospital had no electricity (and, for example, no operating room lights) for long periods. One large regional public hospital had not had a working x-ray machine or ambulance for more than a year. Running water was not even available in a number of hospitals. Fewer than one-half said access to drugs, equipment, and supplies was adequate. One physician said her hospital had a single oxygen tank, requiring daily decisions about which patients would be selected to live and which to die.

When foreign-trained physicians come to the United States, they almost always are required to complete a US residency training programme as a condition of state licensure. Many have already completed residencies in their home countries, but even a residency position in the US earns more money than a medical faculty position at home, so graduates have little reluctance to repeat the training. Many participate in the post-match scramble, relegating them to the specialty choices that remain after US graduates have had their pick. Now that primary care residencies are so unpopular, they are more available to international medical graduates (IMGs).

The above account of the United States' involvement in the 'poaching game' reflects some differences in detail and orientation from what we have seen of the British experience, but still rests on traditional imperialist assumptions – mainly that the strong have a natural right to exploit the weak for their own convenience. That is perfectly consistent with neoliberalism and is all too often supported by 'moral' justifications that have their philosophical parallels in disquisitions about the 'white man's burden' and even religious arguments in favour of the slave trade!

MODERN APOLOGISTS FOR IMPERIALISM

A particularly fine example of such an up-to-date rationalisation of what amounts to nothing more than robbery of other countries' resources, was reflected in a recent article by Kerry Howley in the *Los Angeles Times*.[8] He argues that medical journal editorial boards, various think tanks and moral issue groups have been deceiving us into feeling guilty about a trading relationship that is perfectly legal. To him it is all part of an upsurge of 'human rights twaddle' and other left-wing sophistry and that we should be strong enough to withstand it and stand by the dictum that what is good for America is ultimately good for everyone else. The author recalls the general media approval in 1943 when the then President of General Motors (US) made the confident statement: 'What is good for General Motors is good for America!'

How right it seemed to people at the time and yet how bitterly the comment must ring today as Detroit's unemployed try to survive day by day on short-term jobs (if they can get one at all), low pay and union rights abrogated under NAFTA (North American Free Trade Agreement) and other blossomings of neoliberalism. But Kerry Howley is worth quoting:

> Is Ephraim Dagadu stolen goods? The Ghana-born and trained physician, who runs a successful family practice in Maryland, does not speak like a man who has been ripped from his rightful home and forced to toil in the Baltimore suburbs. His visage appears on no milk cartons; no cross-continental Amber Alert calls for his return. But according to a recent piece in a prominent British medical journal, a caring U.S. would have done more to keep Dagadu from encountering opportunity abroad. He, goes the argument, belongs to Ghana.

'Active recruitment of health workers from African countries is a systematic
and widespread problem throughout Africa and a cause of social alarm: The
practice should, therefore, be viewed as an international crime,' Edward J.
Mills of the British Columbia Centre for Excellence in HIV/AIDS and nine co-
authors write in the Lancet. They go on to suggest a place to nail those who
tell Ghanaians, Kenyans and Malawians about jobs available elsewhere: The
International Criminal Court.

While Mills' 'off with their heads!' approach is uniquely spirited, he is giving
voice to a conviction broadly held in the development community. In Kenya,
there are 14 physicians for every 100 000 people. In the United States, there are
256 serving the same number. How cruel, then, when a fresh-faced American
recruiter alights in Nairobi, luring away precious human resources with juicy
promises of good pay and better hours. (This is sometimes called 'poaching,'
which suggests educated African men and women are some kind of exotic prey;
tellingly, MSNBC and American Renaissance News are equally fond of this
phrasing.) Shouldn't we round up these deadly sirens and ship them to The
Hague?

He then goes on to claim that we have been bamboozled into believing that such
a drain of medically trained people from a country adversely affects that country
from sustaining its own healthcare needs. His evidence is that the medical schools
in those countries produce so many medical graduates that the more of them who
leave, the more that are produced to replace them. But he ignores the issue of who
pays to train the replacements!

Even more outrageously, he argues, First World recruitment strategies involve
advertising in the country's newspapers, sending emails and text messages to
medical graduates – and that such strategies can easily be countered. He uses
Malawi as an example. As the reader is aware, Malawi is one of the most sorely
disadvantaged countries in sub-Saharan Africa; it is rife with both HIV/AIDS
and TB, and administered by one of the poorest economies in the world. What is
Howley's considered advice to this community? Simply ignore the inconvenient
fact that Malawi has a per capita GDP of US$596 (approx. £298), its HIV/AIDS
crisis and endemic corruption at every level of government – ignore all that – and
ban those pesky recruitment emails and newspaper advertisements!

The reality is that countries like Malawi, Kenya and even countries as large
and well equipped as South Africa, and those as small and poorly equipped as
Mauritius, train huge corps of doctors and other medical workers. The aim of
most such students is not to work locally because facilities are scarce, research
opportunities few and far between, equipment shoddy and professional life
harassed by corruption and low pay. On graduating from medical school – or

often one year before – they sit exams to qualify for entry to medical schools and hospitals in the First World. Those who pass leave while the others stay behind. It is left to the reader's imagination as to what the impact of this is on the health needs of the home country.

THE WHO'S RESPONSE

In complete contradiction to Howley's rationalisations, the World Health Organization has spoken decisively on the matter. This was discussed in 2006 by Olivia Ward,who reports the WHO as declaring the practice 'deadly'.[9] She wrote her article to mark World Health Day 2006, and points out that while Canadians may complain about a doctor shortage in their own country, people in Third World countries suffer really life-threatening gaps in their medical services and that this is caused almost entirely by the 'brain drain' of their trained personnel to Canada.

Canada's rôle in global health imperialism is partly engendered by the fact that the largely urban-educated, middle-class students at Canadian medical schools are reluctant – and often poorly prepared – to serve in remote areas of the country where there is a chronic need for medically trained people. Overseas medical graduates are often only too glad to fill this need, so it is not at all uncommon – even when visiting arctic areas of Canada – to run across doctors from Sri Lanka, India, Pakistan and various African countries. Some of them find the climate so trying they pack up and go home, but many stay, to the immense gratitude of the communities concerned. The author met one such doctor in the bleak grey surroundings of Resolute Bay, where the Ghanaian doctor cut an exotic figure among crowds of barking husky dogs and awe-struck Inuit children. In his flat, he showed me about a dozen highly colourful flower-patterned short-sleeved party shirts. His sorrowful comment was that most of the year it was too cold to sport such gear, and when it was warm enough the mosquitoes 'ate you alive', unless you wore white long sleeved shirts!

The WHO's 2006 report, *Working Together for Health*, cites a crisis in 57 of the least-developed countries which, using 2006 figures, identified a need for 24 million health workers of all types – doctors, nurses and midwives.[10] The WHO Report goes on to state that globally at least 4.3 million health workers are needed to meet the needs of more than 1.3 *billion* people lacking any kind of access at all to the most rudimentary healthcare. For these people even a minor illness is often the prelude to death. But Canada's rôle as a medical imperialist is compounded by the fact that the country also serves as a conduit for American recruits south of the border.

Meanwhile, WHO reported Canada, Britain, the United States and New Zealand import a quarter or more of their physicians from other countries, including Africa, which faces serious medical challenges. On average, a quarter of all African-trained doctors have migrated to the world's wealthiest nations.

The organisation has called on rich countries to stop 'poaching' medical personnel, and urged both poor and wealthy states to work on ways of solving the problem. It called for immediate investment in recruiting and training new workers in needy countries, as well as making it worthwhile for graduates to remain at home.

In an article for the online newspaper of the Canadian Medical Association, its president Ruth Collins-Nakai said the report had an 'important message' for Canada because it showed that global competition will only intensify for qualified personnel in the future. But, she said at the University of Toronto's Joseph L Rotman School of Management, Canada itself is the target of a medical recruitment drive.

The US needs large numbers of foreign doctors to fill its workforce gaps, and Canada is a net exporter of healthcare professionals, with the 'cumulative new loss of MDs to the US more than 4000 from 1991 to 2004.' Only last year was there a 'meagre gain' of 55 physicians.

Training doctors is expensive, and importing them saves millions of dollars a year, WHO points out. But freeloading at the expense of developing countries has deadly consequences when needy countries are left with no doctors and nurses to carry out vital immunisation services, community healthcare and basic medical services for women and children. However, points out the Canadian Medical Association's senior communications editor Steve Wharry, the medical personnel who migrate here may not even work as doctors, and often end up doing other jobs: 'The issue in Canada is less about poaching and more about getting graduates (from foreign countries) credentialed to work in the Canadian system.'

RÔLE OF PUSH AND PULL FACTORS

As pointed out earlier, though, recruitment of people trained as medical personnel in the Third World to fill posts in the First World does *not* depend only – or perhaps even primarily – on the blandishments by eager recruiters of the 'good life' abroad. The issue is complex and involves an interplay of push and pull factors. In the report, the WHO acknowledged that doctors in the poorest countries have strong incentives to leave, including the lure of better pay and a higher standard of living. In their homelands, doctors face 'unsafe conditions in the workplace, poor pay and working conditions, low morale and motivation, lack of supportive supervision,' and too frequently, 'death from the very diseases they work to cure.'[11]

The World Medical Association drew up 'ethical guidelines' for international recruitment of physicians three years ago and the Canadian Medical Association has worked with them to endorse principles of social justice and international cooperation while recognising the right of medical workers to choose their own destinies.

The WHO said it was important to remember that poor countries suffer disproportionately from a lack of qualified personnel, and in countries where the medical systems have collapsed there are global implications, such as the spread of SARS (severe acute respiratory syndrome) and avian flu. Dangerous psychological conditions that can lead to violence also tend to go untreated. Africa, which has 11% of the world's population, has 25% of its disease burden and only 3% of its health workers.

US citizens control more than 50% of the world's financial resources, while Africa has less than 1%, the report adds. 'The global population is growing,' said WHO Director-General Lee Jong-wook, 'but the number of health workers is stagnating or even falling in many of the places where they are needed most.'[12]

Despite frequent vigorous campaigns on the part of countries like Australia and New Zealand to attract doctors and nurses from poorer countries, the US remains by far the main recipient, with Canada as a convenient accessory. There are various reasons for this that can be considered internal to the workings of the US economy. As the author has already explained, it is the more economically deprived patients who general practitioners/family doctors usually see. Financially speaking, US citizens have to have access to considerable wealth to consult any level of the medical system, but the general practitioners represent the cheaper end of the cost spectrum.

According to a paper by Robert Ferrer, the evidence shows that family physicians were consulted by nearly 50% of those US citizens who attended any kind of medical care in 2004.[13] They are the only medical speciality that regularly works with large numbers of the less affluent. It follows that as a declining proportion of those general physicians are domestically trained, and as crowds of exotically foreign physicians fill those rôles, the US will continue to widen the global health equity gaps.

In fact, the US Council on Graduate Medical Education predicted (in 2006) that the USA will be in need of about 85 000 more physicians than its colleges can produce by the year 2020.[14] The Association of American Medical College responded to these findings by recommending that medical school intakes be increased in size. However, this costs money and – as of 2008 – not one state legislature has agreed to meet that need. As has always been the case, imperialism has a distinct appeal to bursars and bookkeepers!

IS IT INEFFICIENCY OR CRIME?

In drawing this discussion of healthcare imperialism to a close, let us briefly consider the question of the fundamental ethics involved. The reader will recall

Kerry Howley's view that the so-called 'poaching' of medically qualified people from the Third World is 'morally neutral', a sort of natural working of market forces with which we should not interfere. This, of course, is quintessentially the correct neoliberal view. But we should be reminded of just how antagonistic it is to the general evolution over the centuries and millennia of human society and morality.

For instance, the book of Psalms in the Old Testament – itself a rather recent corpus of writings in terms of the entire gambit of human history – avers that, 'The Earth is the Lord's and the Fullness thereof' (Psalm 24: verse 1). Even more recently (but before neoliberalism's step was heard on the staircase of history!), the philosopher Immanuel Kant in 1784 made the following groundbreaking ethical assertion, 'common ownership of the Earth entitles all of the world's citizens to the right to free movement'.[15] It would, of course, be convenient if they were quite content to stay where they were born, but geography does not provide for equity in access to food, so mobility becomes a necessity, as well as a human right.

As we shall see, then, when in the final chapter we address ways of overcoming the various barriers to global health equity, we must – as a matter of urgency – address our attention to allocating the basic causes of global poverty and resolve them as a global community. Our global village has become so small, and our extinction, if we fail to confront these issues, so certain, that we have no choice. If we address poverty, then we address health, unemployment, natural disasters, war and all the rest. In the long run – or maybe not all that long – the only realistic option (or the first of a series of them) is to aim for global equity in access to healthcare – and this will involve us in the issue of how to fund it.

So we come back to the issue: do our present health imperialistic approaches (such as recruiting health workers from poor countries for the good of rich countries) constitute a crime? A group of public health researchers, from Canada and other countries, strongly argued in 2008 that the practice should be classified as an international crime.[16] That, technically, is a rather tricky proposition to uphold, but the group, led by an epidemiologist, Edward Mills, argues that the practice violates Article 13 of the UN's Universal Declaration of Human Rights. Whatever the legal issue, the figures they cite are certainly arresting. For example, there are more Malawian physicians in the city of Manchester in England than there are in all of Malawi itself. Yet Malawi faces more critical health problems right now, especially with HIV/AIDS levels among the highest in the world, and associated with AIDS, higher levels of tuberculosis. Malaria also stalks the country, robbing many a cradle – although it can affect people of any age.

The view that the practice of this sort of 'poaching' constitutes an international crime can be argued as follows. Countries such as Canada, the United States, Britain and Australia are home to thousands of doctors, nurses and pharmacists from Africa. Some decided to immigrate independently, but many have been lured to their new homes with offers of an enormous increase in pay, moving expenses and help to navigate the visa and citizenship processes.

The number of doctors from sub-Saharan countries alone who are working in the four countries is staggering – an estimated 13 272. Mills himself was on an operating table in South Africa last year after suffering an accident. He said the physician's cell phone buzzed several times throughout the procedure. The doctor told him later that the calls were from recruiters!

When Canada, or any other another wealthy country, recruits in South Africa – as the Shoppers Drug Mart chain was attempting to do in search of pharmacists in 2007 – the effect is like tumbling dominos. South Africa, in turn, fills its vacancies by recruiting from other, less-affluent African countries. The problem in many countries is dire, with completely untenable doctor to patient ratios. In Malawi, there is one doctor for every 50 000 people, while in Canada there is one for every 500.

While the battle to get affordable antiretroviral drugs to Africans with HIV/AIDS is paying off, the healthcare workers needed to deliver the drugs don't exist. For example, he noted that in Northern Uganda, nurses, aides – people with a year or two of training – are now being trained to undertake the delicate task of starting HIV-positive infants on antiretroviral therapy. It's a job best performed by paediatricians, but there are none to do it.

Many of the plundered countries have taken to training healthcare staff to sub-optimal levels – medical officers instead of doctors – so they are less desirable to foreign recruiters, Mills said, noting it is the only way they can hang onto personnel. He and his colleagues argue that the impact of this poaching of Africa's healthcare professionals constitutes an international crime that is contributing to the deterioration of essential healthcare services on the continent.

However, Professor Amir Attaran, who teaches in the University of Ottawa's Institute of Population Health and the Faculty of Law, sympathises with the general thrust of the argument. But he said he does not agree with the position that poaching health professionals is a crime under international law.

'I don't have any difficulty saying that it would be lovely and I would prefer to live in a world where it were criminal,' said Attaran. 'But their argument is that already customary international law tells us that this recruitment should stop. That is an incorrect understanding of what customary international law is.'

Professor Attaran co-authored an article published in January by the *Canadian Medical Association Journal* which denounced Shoppers Drug Mart for recruiting in South Africa. He said Canada's policy in the early 1990s to cut back enrolment numbers in its own medical schools created a situation where this country can't now – and won't be able in the foreseeable future –meet its own need for doctors.

'If you want to look at it over a course of two decades, our management of health systems in this country has gone from nearly negligent to morally reprehensible,' he wrote. 'The negligent decision was we wouldn't train, and it would save us a few dollars here and there. The reprehensible one is we go: "Oh, we should have trained. We didn't. Gosh. Well, let's just poach."'

Experts in international law disagree as to whether or not this outrageously imperialistic approach to the problem of securing medical staff for First World hospitals and other medical facilities actually constitutes a 'crime' – prosecutable, say, at the International Court of Justice. This author has discussed the matter with over a dozen professionals in the field. But that is not really the issue. This issue is that the systems we now use are not uniform, are under no international media- tion, and above all, greatly widen the global health inequity gap. Since that latter is the basic problem we have set out to solve, it must be addressed.

It is not as though the problem has not been a focus of international concern for over three decades. Indeed, this author has, in a previous book, considered some of the approaches put into place in an attempt to address it.[17]

But all of the systems attempted so far have been strictly within the limits set by neoliberalism – with various countrywide health insurance schemes favoured. As might have been expected, such systems tend to be hugely divisive – requiring some contributions even from poverty-stricken individuals. But there are various models of them. This chapter will end with an analysis of some of these.

HOW CAN HEALTHCARE BE FUNDED?

The issue of how to actually fund healthcare in various countries has become increasingly acute since 1988, as the WHO itself became increasingly entangled in the neoliberal web of finance initiatives imposed through IMF and World Bank Structural Adjustment Policies and, later, by the impact of WTO regulations, TRIPS, and others. Out of all this arose a number of local attempts to rationalise the necessary funding under this growing web of constraints. The World Bank has been assiduous in promoting various private health insurance schemes – some obligatory – under which minimum levels of protection can be made available to the poorest citizens. But, whenever this has been tried, there have always been people who are so poor that even the most modest premiums are beyond their resources, and so they effectively are not protected by the system.

Another approach that has attracted a lot of debate in government circles is simply for the very wealthy to fund the very poor. There are various ways in which this might be mediated. The G8 Summit of 2005, spurred on by such initiatives as the Bob Geldof Live 8 programme and the Make Poverty History Campaign, brought pressure to bear on the governments of some of the world's most powerful nations to commit themselves in two ways: by modifying the severity of their loan demands – even writing off some loans altogether for the very poorest nations; and also by contributing 0.7% of their respective GDPs to a fund for healthcare supplements to many of the Third World countries. Neither of these has worked particularly well so far. The idea of the wealthy helping the poor directly (such as Bob Geldof's Live 8 initiative) created considerable enthusiasm for a short time, but could not be relied upon as a systematic or long-term solution. As for each of the G8 nations dedicating a very small proportion of their national budgets, this generated a plethora of promises from grand-standing world leaders, but none of the countries concerned reached even that modest target. Indeed, as this author has shown, some other countries – such as Norway – which were not even in the G8, did achieve the stated targets![18]

FUNDING HEALTHCARE LOCALLY UNDER NEOLIBERALISM

As stated above, there has arisen a host of local attempts at funding healthcare, none of them without serious internal flaws and none of them completely inclusive. The basic reason that none of these adequately come to grips with the real problems of global inequity is not simply that they vary locally, but also because of the requirement to meet neoliberal financing criteria as promoted both by Structural Adjustment Policies and the WTO policies which impact so adversely on local health. These attempts can be briefly summarised as follows.

It is important for the reader to realise that these methods are still in use and continue to contribute to the widening global health equity gap. The WTO, under its present neoliberal dominance, has endorsed such strategies to be applied locally, at least in part to obviate the need for a gross worldwide redistribution of wealth.

A number of commentators have attempted to systematically list these strategies and among them, one of the most comprehensive of such attempts has been that by Sara Bennett and Lucy Gilson, in a publication by the Department for International Development (DFID).[19]

Clearly, reforms in health financing can be the only basis for even beginning to act on the question of health equity globally. Eventually, this author argues, these must involve global redistribution of funds. But in this chapter let us concentrate on the DFID analysis. They argue that the current international concern must move away from massive movements of money from the first to the Third World in direct aid. They even state that 'equity is largely a secondary issue'.

The various strategies adopted for local funding will diverge widely over different Third World nations. See Table 7.1, from Bennett and Gilson (2001).

MAKING LOCALLY FINANCED POLICIES 'PRO-POOR'

What does it mean for a health financing system to be pro-poor? The most important dimensions are that the system should:

❐ Ensure that contributions to the costs of healthcare are in proportion to different households *ability to pay.*

❐ Protect the poor (and the nearly poor) from the *financial shocks* associated with severe illness.

❐ Enhance the *accessibility* of services to the poor (particularly with respect to perceived quality and geographic access).

For that reason, of course, how the funds for healthcare are raised is a pivotal issue. It also has to be done in a way that adequate pro-poor funding can be delivered. This raises problems, if it is to address global inequities, of international policing of these local initiatives and so far this has not been provided.

Consider the data in Table 7.1, which itself comes from the DFID report cited above.

TABLE 7.1 Major trends in healthcare financing

Trend	Objectives	Countries reforming in this way
Introduce or increase use fees to tax-based systems	Raise more revenues Encourage more efficient use of resources Create greater accountability to the consumer	Many countries in sub-Saharan Africa
Introduce community-based health insurance in systems currently based on user fees and tax revenues	Reduce financial barriers created by use fees Encourage more efficient use of resources Raise more revenues	Large-scale activities in Thailand and Indonesia; numerous small-scale efforts in many other countries, e.g. Zambia, Tanzania, Uganda, India
Shift from tax-based to social health insurance type systems	Create independent, sustainable source of health finance Raise more revenues	Thailand, many countries in the former Soviet Union and Eastern Europe; proposed but not implemented elsewhere, e.g. Nigeria, Zimbabwe, Ghana
Consolidate multiple state insurance funds	Increase equity and prevent tiering and fragmentation Increase administrative efficiency	Mexico, Columbia and other countries in Latin America

Financing and provision of healthcare are most effective if they are closely linked. Although there are no user fees in a wholly tax-funded system, there are frequently other barriers to accessibility, for example:

❐ If the perceived quality of care is very low, even the poor may prefer to pay more to use higher-quality private sector services.

❐ There may be significant time and transport costs associated with accessing care, particularly for the poor.

❒ Even in a system where there are no formal charges, informal charges for care may be widely prevalent.

Tackling these problems is important to ensure that the mix of financing mechanisms in any country promotes redistribution between the rich and the poor, a central element of pro-poor financing policies. As the reader will appreciate, this moves us into the realm of taking from the poor to help the very poor.

But who are the poor? In many low-income countries, the majority of the population is formally classified as poor. It is important to distinguish between the majority poor and the minority very poor in developing pro-poor policies in countries where this is the case. For example, a user-fee system which succeeds in improving quality of care may benefit the majority poor who can afford to pay the newly introduced fees. But for the minority very poor, fees will create yet another barrier to access to healthcare.

For both the 'poor' and the 'very poor', the most important cost that results from illness derives from the loss of labour associated with illness and/or injuries.

Although some financing mechanisms may mitigate the costs of care associated with such health problems, they do not address the consequences of ill health, whether through loss of income or loss of services provided by unpaid family members. Pro-poor healthcare financing mechanisms can only play a limited rôle in tackling the resource constraints that fundamentally shape the health-seeking behaviour of poorer households and thus their ability to capture the benefits of healthcare. This is a very prominent feature with respect to the growing impact of HIV/AIDS in the Third World.

Box 7.1, overleaf, lists the principal financing mechanisms for healthcare services.

TAX-BASED FINANCING

This is the most widely used form of healthcare financing in most of sub-Saharan Africa and in South Asia. It also used to be employed in the USSR and its European satellites. It is argued that this mechanism is pro-poor because:

❒ Well-run, tax-based health funding is generally 'progressive' – the more you earn, the more you pay.
❒ The poor are most easily ruined by unexpected large healthcare costs.
❒ There need be no user charge at the point of user need.

But counter-arguments are not hard to find. For example:

❒ There is an automatic bias against the rural poor as opposed to the urban poor. The latter are likely to have easier access to a wider range of healthcare facilities.

Box 7.1 Principal financing mechanisms

Tax-based financing: health services are paid for out of general government revenue such as income tax, corporate tax, value added tax, import duties etc. There may be special earmarked taxes (e.g. cigarette taxes) for healthcare.

Social insurance financing: health services are paid for through contributions to a health fund. The most common basis for contributions is the payroll, with both employer and employee commonly paying a percentage of salary. The health fund is usually independent of government but works within a tight framework of regulations. Premiums are linked to the average cost of treatment for the group as a whole, not to the expected cost of care for the individual. Hence, there are explicit cross-subsidies from the healthy to the less healthy. In general, membership of social health insurance schemes is mandatory, although for certain groups (such as the self-employed) it might be voluntary.

Private insurance: people pay premiums related to the expected cost of providing services to them. Thus, people who are in high health risk groups pay more, and those at low risk pay less. Cross-subsidy between people with different risks of ill health is limited. Membership of a private insurance scheme is usually voluntary. The insurance fund is held by a private (frequently for profit) company.

User fees: patients pay directly, according to a set tariff, for the healthcare services they use. There is no insurance element or mutual support. This is the most common way of paying for privately provided services in developing countries, and is also used as a component of financing for public sector services.

Community-based health insurance: as for social health insurance, premiums are commonly set according to the risk faced by the average member of the community, i.e. there is no distinction in premiums between high and low risk groups. However, unlike social health insurance schemes, enrolment is generally voluntary and not linked to employment status. Funds are held by a private non-profit entity.

❐ Although the general income tax might be progressive, much of the funding tends to come from 'indirect' taxation. These taxes are usually raised in the purchase of goods most used by the less poor – petrol, luxury items, and so on. This renders horizontal (countrywide) healthcare provision a less likely option than the vertical planning favoured by many IMF Structural Adjustment Policies.

❐   Since we are discussing this in the context of Third World societies, a tax raised on personal income is not likely to be enough to fund adequate healthcare.

Studies based upon household data suggest that inequitable access to publicly financed healthcare is indeed a substantial problem. Because public primary care services are generally perceived to be of poor quality and the private costs (transport and time costs) of accessing public hospitals are high for the poor (*see* Box 7.2), the poor often prefer to use the services of private doctors. Yet the rich continue to use public hospital care, especially where there are few alternatives. The result is that the poor may use publicly funded services (particularly hospital services) less than do the rich.

Box 7.2 Barriers to accessing publicly financed healthcare services in Sri Lanka

'If we go to the general hospital we would go in the morning and expect to come back in the afternoon. I would not be able to work and get my Rs 200. So after work I go to the private doctor or only the pharmacy – this is easy and costs about Rs 100.'

'It is often easier to go to a private place close by than to the Kalubovila (government) hospital . . . when you consider the time, and what you have to spend for the bus. If we feel thirsty, we need to drink something. And if someone is going to Kalubovila two people have to go – while the patient goes to see the doctor another person has to get a place in the medicine queue, so you have to spend for two people.'

Quite recent work by Wagstaff suggests that, in general, tax revenue financing of healthcare in Third World countries is at least mildly progressive, while funding from direct tax, such as income tax, is even more so.[20] But it is not adequate and, for that reason, not really equitable.

Another variation on the theme is Social Insurance Funding.

SOCIAL INSURANCE FUNDING

This concept is predicated on the principle that if a desperately poor person is suddenly faced with a need for medical care, this can be paid for out of a medical insurance contributed to by the relatively rich in the community. This takes the element of risk out of the issue, so that the poor are not at a psychological disadvantage in that respect compared with the rich.

As the reader is doubtless aware, many of the First World nations – such as the Netherlands, France and Spain – provide health cover through a combination of social insurance funding and income tax. But when it comes to Third World nations, the amount that the relatively rich can pay for social insurance can only finance a meagre healthcare package for each citizen. In many Third World countries, for example, only those in regular employment can draw on the fund. That is, the relatively rich are actually further enriched by the poor in the following ways:

❑ The government may subsidise the social health insurance fund in order to make the new system more palatable to employers and employees. This can be done directly through government contributions or indirectly through the subsidised treatment of members in public facilities. If government resources are limited this may involve withdrawal of some financial support for the basic services provided to the poor.

❑ The development of a social health insurance fund establishes a significant new purchasing power. If the inputs necessary to provide healthcare (such as doctors and nurses) are limited, this may attract inputs away from providing services to the poor.

Ideally, this system should go far to eradicate within-country inequities with respect to healthcare access. However, this presupposes that coverage is universal and in many Third World nations (and even in the US!) this simply is not so. Consider the case of South Korea. The government there successfully expanded its system of social health insurance to the entire population and there was a concurrent expansion in healthcare facilities and health staff to meet the increased demand. Nonetheless, the poor, the elderly and those who live in rural areas still have lower access to healthcare, due to the misdistribution of both health staff and facilities, which tend to be located in urban centres where there is greater demand and more ability to pay.

When only part of the population has coverage, social health insurance is likely to increase the disparities in access between the poor and the rich. The nature of the benefit package to be paid for through the insurance mechanism may introduce differentials in the range of services and quality of care offered to the insured and the uninsured. Most schemes (or proposed schemes) in low and lower middle income countries depend significantly upon government contributions, and government staff represent a large proportion of beneficiaries. In times of economic expansion (as in Thailand during the early 1990s), it may be possible to launch a social health insurance scheme with government financial support, without adversely affecting services for the poor, but when the economy is stagnant, this is unlikely to be feasible. Government resources may be redirected away from the healthcare provided to the poor, and health professionals are likely to be attracted towards the better-funded service.

PRIVATE HEALTH INSURANCE COVER

There is no need to explain in detail how this works. Individuals can take out private cover – of various levels of completeness – but in doing so they have to pay regular premiums. It is routinely used by many people in the First World countries, even if a national health service already exists. In the UK, where the NHS is available to all, private health insurance can provide quicker access to hospital care.

However, only the relatively well off can afford it. In the US, it is estimated that some 30% of the population finds itself entirely unprotected.[21] They cannot afford private insurance premiums and do not qualify for Medicaid or Medicare. It is therefore not difficult to appreciate how inadequate such a scheme would be in a Third World country. Such insurance would only be available to the economically – and probably educationally – well endowed. However, there are some important and noteworthy exceptions to this. Both South Africa and Zimbabwe have routinely run private health insurance for many years and the well off of both countries depend on it.

While well-run systems of private insurance in the First World usually limit claims made for basic services, this is not at all common in many Third World countries. There, private health insurance is often a mechanism by which demands made by privately insured people impact adversely on the health needs of the very poor. In countries with low GNP, it is impossible to raise more than 10% to 20% of delivery cost through mechanisms such as private insurance.

It can be argued, as pointed out in the DFID publication cited above, that private health cover represents a means by which the wealthier will make less use of state provision, thus freeing more government resources for the poor. However, the strength of this argument depends critically on whether any 'freed' resources are actually used to support healthcare for the poor, as well as upon the regulations governing private health insurance and how they interact with the rest of the healthcare system.

❐ It is important to consider whether or not those purchasing private health insurance are allowed to 'opt out' of the primary financing mechanism or whether they must continue to contribute to the solidarity fund. Allowing the middle class to opt out of the primary financing mechanism may not only damage the potential of this mechanism to subsidise healthcare for the poor, but may also reduce political pressure to maintain high standards of care under this scheme if they seek their care outside the public sector.

❐ The tax treatment of private insurance premiums (in other words, whether private insurance premiums are taxable or not) is an important factor. Advocates of private insurance try to argue that making private insurance premiums tax exempt will serve to encourage more people to purchase private insurance thus freeing up more government resources for the poor. However, exempting premiums from taxes will also direct significant subsidies to those already purchasing insurance.

However, private health insurance actually uses significant government subsidies, even if the government does not explicitly subsidise private health insurance. For example, in South Africa not only has the government given tax breaks on private health insurance contributions, but the following additional means of capturing government subsidies have been identified:

❒ Expensive cases are 'dumped' on the public system by insurers once their insurance benefits have been exhausted in private hospitals.
❒ Insured patients frequently claim to be uninsured and thus escape paying for care in public hospitals.
❒ Fees charged by public hospitals to private insurers do not recover the full costs of care.
❒ Poor billing systems often fail to charge and recover fees from insured patients.

In Chile it was also found that higher income persons covered by the private insurance entities (ISAPREs – The Spanish acronym for the Chilean Government's own Health Insurance system, under to which about 25% of the population pay premiums), captured a larger-than-average subsidy from government.

In practice, issues of political economy mean that the regulations governing private insurance cannot ensure that this will be a 'pro-poor' financing mechanism.

USER FEES

It is probably obvious to the reader that in the Third World context such a system would automatically exclude the majority of people seeking healthcare. But the DFID does propose that introducing such a system might well be pro-poor, because:

❒ Tax-financed systems are skewed towards subsidising urban hospital services, at the expense of rural and primary care services. Introducing user fees for select (urban and hospital) services could redirect subsidies to the rural poor.
❒ Increasing resources available for healthcare would allow governments to expand or upgrade their network of rural, primary care services, hence improving accessibility of such services for the poor.

Among the many counter arguments which have emerged are the following:

- Low household income levels mean that the revenue-generating potential of user fees in low-income countries is low, limiting the scope to improve the quality and accessibility of rural primary care services.
- It is often not politically feasible to reallocate government subsidies as desired.
- It is difficult, in practice, to design price discrimination schemes that protect the poor while charging the more affluent.

It is unquestionable, as Jamaica discovered in 1974, that user fees undermine political support for the goal of universal coverage of basic healthcare services.

Wherever user fees have been introduced, there has been an associated decrease in people making use of the service. In other words, the desperately poor do without it! The magnitude of this drop in utilisation was not unnaturally frequently large, and of longer duration, among the poor. Although there is little evidence that the additional burden that fees may place on household resource levels, at a minimum they are likely to act as an additional deterrent to accessing care (especially for the very poor); while catastrophic costs would have much greater impact.

While the effects to date of user fees on the poor appear almost universally negative, in virtually all cases this has been a result of poor design, planning and implementation. Increases in user fees have rarely been accompanied by improvements in quality, and very little attention has been paid to the design and implementation of effective exemption mechanisms. Neither those responsible for implementation nor the wider community have had much involvement in the design of the systems that most immediately affect them.

The DFID maintains that if properly implemented and appropriately designed initially, user fees can deliver benefits to the poor. They look to some very large schemes indeed, such as that in Kenya, to support their view that user fees should not be regarded as automatically suspect by those whose concerns are social justice and equity.

This author's own experience in a wide range of Third World communities has made it quite clear that people on low incomes could not raise much of the necessary healthcare costs. Either the number of services would have to be drastically reduced, and/or this alternative would either reduce the number of user-fee customers, or raise each user-fee cost. The DFID document estimates that it is probably impossible to raise more than 10% to 20% of delivery costs by that means. The issue becomes further distorted by the wealthier areas generating more user fees than the poorer by introducing differentials between localities within the country. This, in turn, might well lead to uneven health provision – clinics, even hospitals – between areas. If health spending is to be efficient there must be an active policy by which the government actually moves money from the wealthier to the poorer areas.

COMMUNITY-BASED HEALTH INSURANCE

In situations in which there is high-user finance of healthcare, community-based health insurance can work well. There are many examples of this to back up the argument, but not many in the Third World's poorest nations. Where such schemes operate, they effectively meet the needs of that particular community's relatively poor.

But, as the DFID report makes clear, the very poor need an infrastructure (transport and communications) to allow them to access benefits. Not many Third World governments are able to bear such a burden, especially if their debt repayments actually supersede the amounts that they can devote to health. Likewise, such systems would – even in the fairly short term – create geographical inequities in the same ways that user fees do.

In China, between 1985 and 1999, community-based health insurance represented the principal source of healthcare financing. The Chinese government quickly found out that this involved them in a quagmire of redistribution programmes. The administration of these was recognised as an unsuitable drain on tight health resources.

None of these schemes address the really crucial issue of how to *guarantee* that access to healthcare for all – including especially the most desperately in need – is achieved. And, indeed, this should not surprise us because the primary purpose of neoliberalism is *not* social justice, but good profit margins for the stockholders.

Of all the Third World countries, Thailand seems to run a much more successful community-based health insurance scheme than most, and this is largely because it is under strong centralised control – an absolute anathema generally to neoliberalism. But even in Thailand the scheme is often spectacularly unsuccessful in meeting its putative objectives, to which this author can bear witness.

IT DOESN'T WORK IN RICH COUNTRIES, EITHER!

In the UK and in various other EU countries there has recently been a strong drive to 'take government out of healthcare'. The argument is invariably based on the idea that a public service is inferior to a private one because the 'customer' (patient) has only a restricted right of choice and because market forces cannot be involved to weed out the inefficient in a publicly run service. This author is amazed at the seeming power of such specious arguments, especially when the 'inefficiency' of the NHS is contrasted with the supposed 'patient-responsive efficiency' of privatised healthcare as practised in the US.

Such views do not prevail among serious public health professionals in the US, though. Steffie Woolhandler and David Himmelstein, both Associate Professors of Medicine at Harvard University, recently had a paper published in the *British Medical Journal*, which – in the context of privatised medical care in the world's most wealthy country – raised many of the issues with which we have been dealing above in Third World contexts.[22]

They raise the rhetorical question: 'Why would anyone choose to emulate the US healthcare system?' After eight pages of careful analysis, they came to some most instructive conclusions. First, they raise the issue of the value of privatisation in providing public health. As they point out:

> Evidence from the US is remarkably consistent; public funding of private care yields poor results. In practice, public-private competition means that private firms carve out the profitable niches, leaving a financially depleted public sector responsible for the unprofitable patients and services. Based on this experience, only a dunce could believe that market based reform will improve efficiency or effectiveness. Why do politicians – who are anything but stupid – persist on this track?
>
> Such reforms offer a covert means to redistribute wealth and income in favour of the affluent and powerful. Privatisation trades the relatively flat pay scales in government for the much steeper ones in private industry; the 15-fold pay gradient between the highest and lowest paid workers in the US government gives way to the 2000:1 gradient at Aetna.
>
> But even more important, privatisation of publicly funded health systems uses the public treasury to create profit opportunities for firms needing new markets. US private insurers used to focus on selling coverage to employer sponsored groups and shunned elderly people as uninsurable. Now, with employers cutting health benefits, insurers have turned to public treasuries for new revenues. And why stop at selling insurance? Why not tap into the trillions spent annually on care in hospitals and doctors' offices?

So, what lessons can other countries learn from the US experience? Their response is absolutely categorical, namely that we let neoliberal double-talk guide us at our peril.

> Market fundamentalists conjure visions of efficient medical markets partnered with government oversight and funding to assure fairness and universality. But regulation is overmatched. Incentives for optimal performance align imperfectly, at best, with the real goals of care. Matrices intended to link payment to results instead reward entrepreneurs skilled in clever circumvention. Their financial and

political clout grows; those who guilelessly pursue the arduous work of good patient care lose in the medical marketplace.

Health systems in every nation need innovation and improvement. But remedies imported from commerce consistently yield inferior care at inflated prices. Instead we prescribe adequate dosing of public funds; budgeting on a community-wide scale to align investment with health priorities and stimulate cooperation among public health, primary, and hospital care; encouragement of local innovation; explicit empowerment of patients and their families; intensive audit for improvement, not reward or blame; a system based on trust and common purpose; and leadership not by corporations but by 'imaginative, inspired, capable and ... joyous people, invited to use their minds and their wills to cooperate in reinventing the system, itself ... because of the meaning it adds to the lives and the peace it offers in their souls.

They end the argument by pointing out that, given the USA's long experience with the privatisation of medicine, and its extensive experience in researching its effects, they can conclude that such research shows that market forces are inimical to the provision of good healthcare. In other words:

The US has long combined public funding with private healthcare management and delivery. Extensive research shows that its for-profit health institutions provide inferior care at inflated prices. US experience shows that market mechanisms undermine medical institutions unable or unwilling to tailor care to profitability. Commercialisation drives up costs by diverting money to profits and fuelling growth in management and financial bureaucracy. The poor performance of US health care is directly attributable to reliance on market mechanisms and for-profit firms and should warn other nations from this path.

The reader, at this point, is surely left with the rhetorical question: What else is there to say?

ARE DONATIONS FROM THE SUPER RICH A SOLUTION?

A recent surge of interest has been generated by the idea of very wealthy private people agreeing to significantly fund such crucial Third World progress as research on the development of vaccines for such scourges as malaria and especially since the industrial revolution, has been ennobled by the generosity of such famous benefactors as Andrew Carnegie, the Rockefeller family and many others.

In fact, long before the industrial revolution, there were frequent incidents of prodigiously wealthy individuals realising, as they approached death, that they couldn't take their wealth with them and so gave it away. In days gone by, the super-rich would try to secure a place in heaven by funding the building of great cathedrals, whereas in recent times (having presumably written heaven off as a lost cause!) they fund the establishment of medical research centres to at least secure the approval of other people.

Dwarfing most of these by a long piece of chalk, though, has been the recent contribution to the fight for global health equity by Bill and Melinda Gates. They have already contributed a higher sum than that allocated by the World Health Organization itself.

THE BILL AND MELINDA GATES INPUT

According to their own account, the Bill & Melinda Gates Foundation (B&MGF) is 'the largest transparently operated charitable foundation in the world. It was founded by Bill Gates and his wife Melinda in 2000 and then doubled in size by a major financial input on behalf of Warren Buffet in 2006.'[23] According to their fact sheet, 'the aims of the foundation are entirely charitable, and are globally to enhance healthcare and reduce extreme poverty, and in the United States, to expand educational opportunities and access to information technology. The foundation, based in Seattle, Washington, is controlled by its three trustees: Bill Gates, Melinda Gates, and Warren Buffet. Other principal officers include Co-chair William H Gates Sr, and Chief Executive Officer Patty Stonesifer. It has an endowment of US$38.7 billion as of 31 December 2007.'

Bill and Melinda Gates, along with the musician Bono, were named by *TIME* as 'Persons of the Year 2005' for their charitable work. In the case of Bill and Melinda Gates, the work referenced was that of this foundation. On 4 May 2006, the foundation received the Prince of Austria's award for International Cooperation according to their own announcements on their website.[24]

THE WARREN BUFFETT DONATION

On 25 June 2006, Warren Buffett (then the world's richest person, now estimated worth of US$62 billion as of 16 April 2008) pledged to give the Foundation approximately 10 million Berkshire Hathaway Class B shares spread over multiple years through annual contributions. Buffett set conditions so that these contributions do not simply increase the Foundation's endowment, but effectively work as a matching contribution, doubling the Foundation's annual giving: 'Buffett's gift came with three conditions for the Gates Foundation: Bill or Melinda Gates must be alive and active in its administration; it must continue to qualify as a charity; and each year it must give away an amount equal to the previous year's Berkshire gift, plus another 5% of net assets. Buffett gave the Foundation two years to abide by the third requirement.'[25] The Gates Foundation received 5% (500 000) of the shares in July 2006 and will receive 5% of the remaining earmarked shares in the July of each following year (475 000 in 2007, 451 250 in 2008, and so on).

As of 2006, the Foundation has an endowment of approximately US$34.6 billion. To maintain its status as a charitable foundation, it must donate at least 5% of its assets each year. Thus the donations from the Foundation each year would amount to over US$1.5 billion at a minimum.

The Foundation has been organised, as of April 2006, into four divisions, including core operations (public relations, finance and administration and human resources), under Chief Operating Officer Cheryl Scott, and three grant-making programmes:

❒ Global Health Program
❒ Global Development Program
❒ United States Program

The President of the Global Health Program is Tachi Yamada. The Gates Foundation has quickly become a major influence upon global health. Indeed, the approximately US$800 million that the Foundation gives every year for global health approaches the annual budget of the United Nations' World Health Organization (192 nations), and is comparable to the funds given to fight infectious disease by the United States Agency for International Development. The Foundation currently provides 17% (US$86 million in 2006) of the world budget for the attempted eradication of poliomyelitis (polio).[26] The Global Health Program also included the selection of a veritable army of trainees for other critical health programmes.

IS THIS SORT OF THING A SOLUTION?

In the face of so much money suddenly thrown at our problems of global inequity, it would seem churlish to look such a gift horse in the mouth. But some experts have done so, and the result is not reassuring. Even if it were, of course, we cannot guarantee that an array of Gates think-alikes will continue to spring up! But, in this case at least, things are not as straight forward as the tooth fairy might have us believe.

One observation, for instance, is that – in exchange for the lavish research funding – recipients of it must agree to share their findings, through the B&MGF, with whatever commercial enterprises (including the pharmaceutical giants) used by the B&MGF. Probably one of the best-qualified health economists to have systematically analysed the B&MGF is Professor Howard Berliner, Professor of Health Service Management and Policy at the New School in New York City.[27] His comments are available online, and are quoted below:

The recent announcement that Bill Gates is stepping down from his Microsoft position to play a greater rôle in his foundation and the subsequent announcement that Warren Buffet is giving $31 billion to the foundation (of which he is a board member) has certainly set the philanthropic world aflutter. It is the largest foundation ever, with more money to distribute than the United Nations and largely focused on areas of public health (both topical and geographic) that get little other support.

In the early 1900s, the gifts of John D Rockefeller to international public health not only created the initial schools of public health (e.g., Johns Hopkins), but also brought new medical discoveries to large segments of the world that had no other way of obtaining them. The initial analysis of the Rockefeller gifts was explained in terms of his religious beliefs and his view that it was the obligation of the wealthy to help the poor, if only to enhance the prospect of their entry to Heaven when they died! Later analyses, by E Richard Brown and this author, among others, looked to the way that the philanthropy eased the inroads of Western business into potentially fertile areas, and how such 'gifts' ultimately led to the expansion of markets.

At the time of the Rockefeller philanthropies, much of the criticism was based on the notion of 'blood money' – the Rockefeller money had been expropriated from workers, many of whom died in the struggle to achieve better and safer working conditions and a living wage. Anyone who used the money had the blood of those workers on them. While this argument never really went away, it never stopped anyone from accepting the money either.

The best arguments against the Gates Foundation money have been laid out by Anne-Emanuelle Birn in her piece in the *Lancet*. But critiques from the left seldom have much weight when contrasted with the clear and vast needs of the populations that will receive the largesse.

One could argue that the Gates money is going to areas that Western philanthropy has long ignored, that the United Nations, IMF and World Bank have little interest in, and for which the governments of the countries affected have few resources to spend. Therefore, the Gates money should be welcomed. But the existence of the Gates money has the paradoxical effect of keeping other potential funding away from the problem. Why should a government waste scarce resources on malaria if the Gates Foundation is willing to step in?

It is hard to ignore the rôle of such funds in a neoliberal universe where NGOs are the rule, yet the consequences of the Gates Foundations could be quite dramatic. As Birn notes in her piece, the Gates approach is to use high technology – find cures for diseases, vaccines, pharmaceutical solutions, as well as less high tech approaches – mosquito netting, for example. Yet, the focus on healthcare issues belies the needs for essential infrastructural development in Third World countries. Without a better base in agriculture, the impact of success by the Gates Foundation (and others working in the same fields) will be to increase the numbers of people subject to starvation. Without better primary healthcare systems, success in any one disease will be mitigated or negated by the inability to deal with more common health problems. In his recent book *Planet of Slums* (Verso, 2006) Mike Davis presents a horrendous picture of the growth of cities without access to basic services and the absence of any systems to provide either jobs or nutrition for residents. The growth of automobile traffic, high levels of air and water pollution from manufacturing industries, substandard housing and inadequate nutrition will all create public health problems that will take greater resources than the Gates Foundation to solve. But who will take on that rôle?

BACK TO PATENTING THE RIGHT TO LIFE

Professor Berliner's analysis is useful indeed, but the basic argument – in this author's mind – goes right back to the whole issue of the morality of TRIPS (Trade Related Intellectual Property Rights) in relation to WHO's mandate. As the author has emphasised in previous writings – patent laws, and the right of individuals to make a financial profit from patents, is unquestionable when it comes to commodities.[28] If I exercise my intelligence to invent a better mouse trap, I am perfectly entitled to make myself rich by it and am under no obligation to share my wealth with the mice that keep me wealthy by mindlessly walking into my super-duper trap.

But basic human rights, such as access to healthcare, are not commodities. Under neoliberalism they have been made so, but that contradicts their classification as 'rights'. So the whole idea of TRIPS, when it is applied to generating protected patents 'owned' by individuals or (more likely) by multinational pharmaceutical corporations, flies right in the face of WHO's mandates, one of which is to promote, defend and protect human rights – especially health.

How does the B&MGF largesse in funding research on some of the major health scourges today assailing humanity fit in with the TRIPS issue or with the idea of 'Intellectual Property' (IP)? The Gates Foundation requires that researchers receiving its grants share their findings with other recipients and the B&MGF works to develop their output through and with 'Big Pharma'. In other words, these grant recipients cannot be certain about the implications of the data-sharing requirement. To what extent, for example, could it create patent conflicts with Bill Gates with respect to IP? This seems to call into question the consistency of Bill Gates' personal views on IP generally.

It would seem that this appearance of an inherent conflict between defence of a strong support of TRIPS and a parallel support for transparently open access is an illusion. This is because the decision to be selective in exercising one's own intellectual property rights is made without regard to how far these rights can extend. Is it not more realistic to suppose that Bill Gates can afford to demand that results be shared for two obvious reasons? These are:

1 The IP that generates the profits (largely for the Big Pharma corporations involved) is totally unrelated to whether or not the long-term goal (for example, creating an effective AIDS vaccine) is ever achieved.

2 The B&MGF controls the cash. Researchers involved must accept the granting terms, or they will lose the grants. But those grants are rarely – if ever – the property of the researcher directly but go to university research centres, and the latter are always desperate for funding!

So, on the whole, the corporate shareholders of Big Pharma make increased profits on the grants, generic copying is prevented and the people who are lowest on the income scale can still end up unable to afford access to treatment.

Leaving moral considerations aside, the whole show is hideously inefficient and it is up to all citizens of the world to work to more effectively marry up great wealth with great need.

The literature is replete with informed criticism of the B&MGF initiative and its real implications and much of that is available online. The important fact to draw to the reader's attention as this chapter closes, is that any methods used to narrow and finally close the global health equity gap must be entirely free of any possibility of regular imperialistic private finance gain and control. It has to be thoroughly grounded in communities at the local level and mediated transnationally, with full access to and by the international community and its elected bodies. These are some of the issues which will be dealt with in the final chapter.

REFERENCES

1 MacDonald T. *Health, Trade and Human Rights.* Oxford & New York: Radcliffe Publishing; 2006. pp. 6–7.

2 MacDonald T. *The Global Human Right to Health: dream or possibility?* Oxford & New York: Radcliffe Publishing; 2007. pp. 66–9.

3 Brain Drain and Health Professionals [editorial] *BMJ.* 2002; **324**: 449–500.

4 MacDonald T. *Health, Human Rights and the United Nations: inconsistent aims and inherent contradictions.* Oxford & New York: Radcliffe Publishing; 2007. pp. 57–63, 120–8.

5 Hagopian A. Recruiting primary care physicians from abroad: is poaching from low-income countries morally defensible? [editorial] *Ann Fam Med.* 2007; **5**: 483–5.

6 Ibid.

7 Ibid.

8 Howley K. The great healthcare robbery. *Los Angeles Times.* 6 Mar 2008, p. 1.

9 Ward O. Stop poaching doctors, WHO tells rich nations. *The Toronto Star*, 8 Apr 2006, p. 11.

10 WHO. *The World Health Report 2006 – Working Together for Health*. Available at: www. who.int/whr/2006/en/ (accessed 10 May 2008).

11 Ibid.

12 Ibid.

13 Ferrer P. Pursuing equity: contact with US primary care and specialist clinics by demographics, insurance, and Health Status. *Ann Fam Med*. 5(6): 492–582.

14 Council on Graduate Medical Education. *Physician Workforce Policy Guidelines for the United States 2000–2020*. Available at: www.cogme.gov/16.pdf (accessed 13 May 2008).

15 Kant I. *Practical Philosopy*. Translated by Mary J Gregor. Cambridge: Cambridge University Press; 1996. p. 720.

16 Canadian Press. *Health workers poaching from sub-Saharan Africa should be deemed a crime: experts*. 22 Feb 2008. Available at: www.amren.com/mtnews/archives/2008/02/ health_workers.php (accessed 13 May 2008).

17 MacDonald T. *Third World Health: hostage to First World wealth*. Oxford & New York: Radcliffe Publishing; 2005. pp. 95–104.

18 MacDonald T. *The Global Human Right to Health: dream or possibility?* Oxford & New York: Radcliffe Publishing; 2007. pp. 70–4.

19 *The Global Human Right to Health: dream or possibility?*, op. cit.

20 Wagstaff A. Poverty and health sector inequalities. *Bulletin of the World Health Organization*. 2000 **80**(2): 40–5.

21 Macdonald T. *Sacrificing the WHO to the Highest Bidder*. Oxford & New York: Radcliffe Publishing; 2008.

22 Himmelskin D, Woolhandler S. Competition in a publicly funded healthcare system. *BMJ*. 2007; **335**: 1126–9.

23 Bill & Melinda Gates Foundation. *Fact Sheet. 2006*. Available at: www.gatesfoundation. org/AboutUs/Announcements/Announc–060504.htm (accessed 15 May 2008).

24 Bill & Melinda Gates Foundation, op. cit.

25 Bill & Melinda Gates Foundation, op. cit.

26 Bill & Melinda Gates Foundation, op. cit.

27 Berliner H. *The Buffet Donation and the Gates Foundation*. Available at: http://leveller. org/index.php?/technoscience/more/6467/ (accessed 15 May 2008).

28 *Sacrificing the WHO to the Highest Bidder*, op. cit., pp. 6–29, 273.

Chapter 8

Global mismanagement of food resources

THE WORLD FACES A FOOD CRISIS

For the first time in several decades, people and governments in the First World are worrying about the availability of food. For people in most of the Third World, though, this has been a problem throughout the last century – and even for considerably longer. A number of causes for this state of affairs have been put forward. The principal ones are:

1 The rapid rise in the cost of oil. This has suddenly caused an immense increase in the prices of various food processing technologies that are fuelled by oil. It has also greatly increased the price of transporting food.

2 The dramatic increase in the use of biofuels. Some of these are directly dependent on crops, such as corn, which would otherwise be used as food.

3 The exponential growth of middle class sub-populations in countries such as India and China has created an increase in the purchasing of meat, with some decline in vegetable consumption. Why should this make a difference? Simply because raising beef cattle, and other meat sources, requires vast acreages of pasture land. But, in energy terms, meat is a prodigiously inefficient source of food energy. For approximately every 9 calories available as food energy from vegetable sources, only 5 calories (roughly) are available to the consumer if they recycle the vegetable product through some animal (like a bull or a sheep) first and then eat it as meat. Another measure to bear in mind is the fact that a steer has to consume about 8 kg of high quality cereal crops for each kilogram of meat it produces! Vegetarianism is definitely more environmentally friendly than a carnivorous, or even an omnivorous, lifestyle!

203

4 The world's population (now just over 6 billion) is expected, if present trends continue, to top 9 billion by 2050. If we have trouble feeding everybody now, how will we cope then?

5 Since 1994, a large number of food growing areas of the world have been adversely affected by drought due to unseasonably long periods of hot weather, and other factors that have caused a marked decline in yields, especially of such grains as wheat and rice.

6 As will be explained in the last chapter, there is a lot of money to be made out of an international food crisis, with the result that such a shortage is welcome to some corporate interests.

These six factors will be dealt with below. However, let us now consider what we know (and what we can control) of the global inequities which exacerbate these six factors.

OUR UNEQUAL WORLD

It is one thing for a working class family in the UK to have to cut down on relatively expensive cuts of meat and to complain about the fact that even bread and common breakfast cereals are rising in cost faster than the wage packet can cope with, and quite another for families in Haiti, to give but one example, to have no food at all and to try to live on dandelion greens. That is, gross inequity stalks the world and thousands of children and elderly people – both groups being the most vulnerable – die horribly and unnecessarily, simply because they live in the wrong country.

And living in a world of such obscene inequities warps the world view of those lucky enough to live within the right borders. Consider the US, for instance. As well as being (at present) the richest nation on earth, some of its own citizens live almost as precariously as do some of the poorest in sub-Saharan Africa. To be able to live and function in such a society requires a certain degree of psychological conditioning. For instance, the consciences of the more fortunate can be put at ease by blaming the poor for their fecklessness, lack of diligence and foresight and for being work-shy. This, in turn, affects how the people's politicians will appeal to them. And this, of course, determines to a large extent how US representatives at various international fora will explain their country to the world at large. Consider the following: on 27 April 2008, the *Washington Post* ran a story based on figures quoted from the *Wall Street Journal* about a large US grain-processing plant known as Archer-Daniels-Midland Company to the effect that its quarterly profits had suddenly shot up.[1] In fact, those profits jumped 42% and the company gloried in a sevenfold increase in a branch devoted to storing, transporting and trading in such grains as corn, wheat and soya beans. This seems somewhat anomalous in a world experiencing critical shortages of food. Some observers argue that financial speculation has helped to increase the prices due to the fact that during the year 2007 wealthy investors flooded the agricultural commodity markets in search of better returns.

The food shortage (only a relative term so far for most First World people) places increased demands on haulage firms to distribute the grains; which fit in nicely with the needs of those corporations currently active in driving up the cost of diesel and of petrol. On the face of it, this seems a highly inefficient way of running an economy, and in some cases, the government has stepped in to demand a more rational use of resources. Of course, such government interventions as directly solving the problem by nationalising the relevant enterprises would be anathema to neoliberal rules. As we know, national leaders such as Evo Morales and Hugo Chávez have carried out such policies and it is significant that some First World leaders have been favourably impressed by that.

For instance, in 2008, even the French agriculture minister warned European Union officials not to place too much trust in the 'free market' on the grounds that, 'We must not leave the vital issue of feeding people to the mercy of market laws and boardroom speculation.'

As implied above, we may not be able to control – nor even predict – national disasters, but not to control markets where and when we can do so surely suggests a level of naiveté and even blind trust that reflects badly on the proposition that people are rational animals!

Corporate interests mediating the sale of oil globally focus their efforts on meeting the expectations of shareholders. But should we let them hoard oil and artificially inflate its price when the effect of doing so condemns people to die of diseases caused by malnutrition? The kindest thing a government can do to them is to insist that the relevant industries be nationalised and their CEOs become civil servants with a considerably reduced salary, but with the morally salutary knowledge that they are performing a valuable community service with global implications, rather than simply making money for themselves.

One can, in the same rational vein, say the same thing for most large corporations and the politicians in their sphere of influence. The foregoing comments are intended to set the stage for a more detailed analysis of those six big problems, with which we began this chapter, and for a discussion of how they are interconnected. Let us begin with the biofuel issue.

BIOFUELS AS A CRIME AGAINST HUMANITY

On 3 May 2008, Jean Ziegler, the UN's special reporter on the right to food, stated that the trade in biofuels – if unregulated – could be classed as a 'crime against humanity'. He called for the suspension of biofuel production altogether until an international agreement could be reached as to how much, what with and where, it should be produced. In making these comments, he argued that at present biofuel production and trade is a major cause for the food crisis we now face, and has already thrown millions of people into poverty.

Speaking at an emergency meeting of the General Assembly in Geneva as he gave his final report as Special Reporter on the Right to Food, he said: 'Biofuels, with today's current production methods, are a crime against a great part of humanity. They're an intolerable crime, and I requested the United Nations General Assembly in New York in my last report to the Human Rights Council that a moratorium be imposed as a five-year ban against this transformation.'[2]

According to Jean Ziegler, the United States burned 138 million tons of corn last year and transformed it into bioethanol and biodiesel. In an interview with Al Jazeera, Ziegler said: 'Burning food today so as to serve the mobility of the rich countries is a crime against humanity.'[3] Ziegler's comments came while the UN held an emergency summit in Switzerland to tackle the global food crisis.

A BIOFUEL DISASTER LOOMS

Only a few years ago, the idea of using biofuels as a significant counter to excessive reliance on such non-renewables as coal, oil and gas was only a topic of academic speculation. But that is no longer so. John James summed the matter up well in a recent Countercurrents online article:[4]

> Biofuel production is pushing huge amounts of land out of food production. One sixth of the grain grown in the US this year will be 'industrial corn' for ethanol. One third of US maize is now used for biofuel and there was last year a 48% increase in the amount of farmland devoted to biofuels. During that time hardly any new land was brought under the plough to replace that lost capacity for food production.
>
> There is only a difference in scale in China, Indonesia and Brazil where primary forests are being cleared to plant energy crops. Yet, after fossil fuel use, deforestation is the largest single source of CO_2.
>
> The competition for water is likely to favour the biofuel producers, as their crop, being subsidised, commands higher prices than corn or soya. Ethanol has roughly 70% the energy content of gasoline while costing 40% more to produce. In Australia, if all our wheat and sugar output was diverted to ethanol it would supply less than 30% of our fuel needs. As these crops now feed 80 million people, what will they eat instead?
>
> It is argued that Australia could increase its biofuel capacity by using marginal land, but Mick Keogh, executive director of the Australian Farm Institute, said: 'A close examination of global biofuel experiences shows they are only viable

with high levels of government support, and have at best a limited capacity to meet future energy needs.'

The attraction of biofuels for politicians is obvious: they can claim they are doing something useful to combat global warming without demanding any sacrifices from business or from voters. For voters the attraction is that they can continue to drive their cars without a thought for the consequences. The attraction for business is that they can make lots of money out of biofuels, and be subsidised to do so.

A straight switch is happening from food to fuel. As oil prices rise – and Peak Oil guarantees they will – it pulls up the price of biofuels as well, so it becomes more attractive for farmers to switch from food to fuel.

On 13 March 2008, the UK Government's Chief Scientific Adviser, Professor John Beddington, strongly endorsed the above comments as reported by Lewis Smith and Francis Elliott, when he stated, 'The rush towards biofuels is threatening world food production and, with it, the lives of billions of people.'[5]

In making these comments, Professor Beddington put himself even more at odds with the UK Government's rather relaxed view towards the issue. After all, the Government has committed Britain to large increases in the use of biofuels for some time to come. But in his first public speech since being appointed as the UK's Chief Scientific Officer, he described the potential impacts of food shortages as being 'the elephant in the room' and a problem that was every bit as crucial as that of climate change.

Beddington went on to say that the world simply cannot sustain the twin tasks of growing enough crops to feed its people adequately while also producing enough of the right kind of crops to produce significant levels of renewable energy. The supply of food is, at the moment, losing out. His comments did not make for agreeable listening for government ministers as he pointed out that by 2030, we would need at least 50% more food just to keep up with anticipated population growth.

Projecting from 2008 figures, though, this author estimates that the amount of land devoted to food production is decreasing so much, because of the land demands for biofuel production, that we would need to double food production on the land actually devoted to it by 2030 just to keep up with population growth. The rush to biofuels, allegedly environmentally friendly, means that an increasing proportion of available arable land is being given over to fuel, rather than food. Already, biofuels have contributed to the rapid rise in international wheat prices and Professor Beddington cautioned that it was likely to be only a matter of time before shoppers in the United Kingdom faced big price rises because of the soaring cost of feeding livestock.

BURNING FOOD WHILE PEOPLE STARVE

When the author was a child in Canada in the 1930s he was twice taken to witness the burning of 'food mountains'. These consisted largely of cereal crops and butter, so they burned easily and quickly. In those days it was done to keep the prices up and great care was taken to keep people – many unemployed and in need of food – from getting close enough to the pyre to actually help themselves to the material before it was set ablaze. It all seemed insane to me then. If people have to starve to maintain a particular political system, why not change to a better one?

Now, about seven decades later, the system is almost equally irrational. As Ben Wikler, of the People's Health Alliance points out, every day 820 million people in the Third World are deprived of enough food to eat.[6] Food prices are rising steeply, and this has caused serious riots – even deaths – in Mexico, Morocco, Haiti and elsewhere, while wealthy countries use up food to produce biofuels as 'environmentally friendly' ways of running vehicles and other machinery.

Specifically, they're using more and more biofuels, such as alcohol made from plant products, in place of petrol to fuel cars. Biofuels are billed as a way to slow down climate change. But, in reality, because so much land has to be cleared to grow them, most biofuels today are causing more global warming emissions than they prevent, even as they push the price of corn, wheat, and other foods out of reach for millions of people.[7]

Of course, some biofuel production is 'good', in that its impact on food use is minimal, while some is grossly bad. Some biofuel use is rational. But sometimes the trade-off is stark: filling the tank of an SUV (sports utility vehicle) with ethanol requires enough corn to feed a person for a year.[8] But not all biofuels are bad; making ethanol from Brazilian sugar cane is vastly more efficient than US-grown corn, for example, and green technology for making fuel from waste is improving rapidly.

The problem is that the EU and the US have set targets for increasing the use of biofuels without sorting the good from the bad. As a result, rainforests are being cleared in Indonesia to grow palm oil for European biodiesel refineries, and global grain reserves are running dangerously low. Meanwhile, rich-country politicians can look 'green' without asking their citizens to conserve energy, and agribusiness giants are cashing in. And if nothing changes, the situation will only get worse.

What is needed are strong global standards that encourage better biofuels and shut down the trade in bad ones. Such standards are under development by a number of coalitions, but they will only become mandatory if there is a big enough public outcry. It's time to move: in December 2007, the 20 countries with the largest economies, responsible for more than 75% of the world's carbon emissions met in Chiba, Japan, to begin the G8's climate change discussions.

What is at issue here, of course, is the conflict in government priorities worldwide between the urgent need to find renewable substitutes for oil-based/

carbon-releasing fuels and to accelerate the rate of food production for a rapidly increasing population. It is important to realise that feeding people itself requires increasing levels of fuel because of transport requirements, but that we have also to find ways of producing fuel that do not exacerbate global warming.

However, even the above summary over-simplifies the problem, for we are beginning to appreciate that even if biofuels could be produced renewably, their production and use itself creates a greenhouse effect. This is bad news indeed, but the careful research of Elizabeth Rosenthal, as reported on the *New York Times* website, leaves no doubt about the matter.[9]

BIOFUELS AS A GREENHOUSE GAS THREAT

Almost all biofuels used today cause more greenhouse gas emissions than conventional fuels if the full emissions costs of producing these 'green' fuels are taken into account, as two recent studies have concluded. The benefits of biofuels have come under increasing attack in recent months as scientists have taken a closer look at the global environmental cost of their production. These latest studies, published in the prestigious journal *Science* and referred to in Rosenthal's article, are likely to add to the controversy. These studies for the first time take a detailed, comprehensive look at the emissions effects of the huge amount of natural land that is being converted to cropland globally to support biofuels development.

The destruction of natural ecosystems – whether rainforests in the tropics or grasslands in South America – not only releases greenhouse gases into the atmosphere when they are burned and ploughed, but also deprives the planet of natural sponges to absorb carbon emissions. Cropland also absorbs far less carbon than any rain forests, or even scrubland, that it replaces.

Together these two studies offer sweeping conclusions: it does not matter if it is rainforest or scrubland that is cleared, the greenhouse gas contribution is significant. More importantly, they report that taken globally, the production of almost all biofuels resulted directly or indirectly, intentionally or not, in new land being cleared either for food or fuel.

'When you take this into account, most of the biofuel that people are using or planning to use would probably increase greenhouse gasses substantially,' said Timothy Searchinger, lead author of one of the studies and a researcher at Princeton University in environment and economics. 'Previously there's been an accounting error: land use change has been left out of prior analysis.'[10]

These plant-based fuels were originally billed as better than fossil fuels because the carbon released when they were burned was balanced by the carbon absorbed when the plants grew. But even that equation proved overly simplistic, because the process of turning plants into fuels causes its own emissions for refining and transport, for example.

The clearance of grassland releases 93 times the amount of greenhouse gas that would be saved by the fuel made annually on that land, said Joseph Fargione, an eniment agricultural land-use authority and now a scientist at the Nature Conservancy. 'So for the next 93 years you're making climate change worse, just at the time when we need to be bringing down carbon emissions'.[11]

The Intergovernmental Panel on Climate Change has said that the world has to reverse the increase of greenhouse gas emissions by 2020 to avert disastrous environmental consequences. In the wake of the new studies, a group of 10 of the United States' most eminent ecologists and environmental biologists sent a letter to President Bush early in February 2008, and the speaker of the House, Nancy Pelosi, urging a reform of biofuels policies. 'We write to call your attention to recent research indicating that many anticipated biofuels will actually exacerbate global warming,' the letter said.[12]

The European Union and a number of European countries have recently tried to address the land use issue with proposals stipulating that imported biofuels cannot come from land that was previously rain forest. But even with such restrictions in place, Dr Searchinger's study shows the purchase of biofuels in Europe and the United States leads indirectly to the destruction of natural habitats far afield.

For instance, if vegetable oil prices go up globally, as they have because of increased demand for biofuel crops, more new land is inevitably cleared as farmers in developing countries try to get in on the profits. So crops from old plantations go to Europe for biofuels, while new fields are cleared to feed people at home.

Likewise, Dr Fargione said that the dedication of so much cropland in the United States to growing corn for bioethanol had caused indirect land use changes far away. Previously, Midwestern farmers had alternated corn with soy in their fields, one year to the next. Now many grow only corn, meaning that soy has to be grown elsewhere.

And the above alarming insights were highlighted a month later by Josette Sheeran, Executive Director of the World Food Programme, when she spoke to the European Parliament and stated that the shift to biofuels has already removed far too much land from food production and caused a serious weakening of the food chain. She asserted, for instance, that prices for palm oil (once a cheap food source) are – as of 2008 – set at fuel prices.[13]

Sheeran warned that booming food prices were hurting the WFP's 'capacity to respond to hunger' by increasing its operating costs, which have risen by 40% since June 2007 alone. The price of many food commodities has soared world-wide to record levels over the last year, due to booming demand in fast-growing Asian countries as well as the increased use of biofuels. Although Sheeran attributed some of the price increase to market speculation, she also said that 'structural factors are part of today's high prices.' 'It may be a bonanza for farmers

– I hope it is true – but in the short-term, the world's poorest are hit hard,' she said.

The 27-nation EU aims to ramp up its use of biofuels in coming years after the bloc's leaders set tough renewable energy targets last year. They committed to increase the EU's renewable energy use by 20% by 2020, compared to 1990 levels, with biofuels to make up 10% of all transport fuels used by then. However, since EU leaders fixed those targets in March last year, concerns have risen about possible negative effects from biofuels, including their impact on food prices and the environment.

Before moving on to a consideration of the rapidly increasing shortage of such food as rice, let us firstly consider climate change as a factor. In fact, as far back as 1996, experts were identifying changes in global weather patterns as constituting a threat to food production.

FOOD CROP REDUCTIONS AND GLOBAL WARMING

In 1995, the message was mixed. Over much of Africa, optimism prevailed. For instance, the UN's Food and Agriculture Organization (FAO) gave a global report that could be summarised as follows:[14]

Throughout Africa, crop production was generally adequate, with only a few countries causing concern. In areas where active military conflict was prevailing, production of food crops was, of course, adversely affected (for example, Liberia and Sierra Leone), but this was to be expected. However, in Madagascar, Malawi and Namibia, cyclones and unseasonably long droughts had also caused a worrying drop in food crop output. Things were not made easier by a succession of very heavy rains in 2005 and 2006. But the rest of the world has not been doing as well.

In Asia, crop prospects remain uncertain in some parts, due to low rainfall. In China, the overall outlook for the dormant winter wheat crop remained uncertain, with the prospect of spring drought in some areas. In Sri Lanka substantially below-normal rainfall since October 2007 was expected to reduce significantly the output of the main Maha rice crop due for harvest in March/April. In the worst affected parts in the north, the rice crop was wilting and production could fall to 50% of the 2006 output. The harvest of the second Yala crop may also be affected by reduced irrigation supplies. More rainfall was also needed in Vietnam, Laos and Cambodia for the developing second season rice crop.

In India, above normal monsoon rains last year increased irrigation supplies and soil moisture levels, favouring the rabi crops, mainly wheat. In Pakistan, scattered light showers in March 2007 over major agricultural areas increased soil moisture levels and favoured the developing wheat crop, for which the target was set at 17.4 million tons. In Indonesia, floods in Sumatra and west Java affected the rice crop, while recent rainfall in October–December 2007 in the Philippines slowed harvesting of the second rice crop. Cereal production in Afghanistan is again likely to be constrained by short supplies of agricultural inputs. In Iraq, area planted is expected to increase, reflecting Government efforts to encourage farmers to produce more grains.

However, yield potential is likely to remain constrained by serious shortages of fertilizers, spare parts for agricultural machinery and other inputs. In Syria and Turkey, the overall prospect for cereal crops remains favourable reflecting generally normal weather conditions since the beginning of the 2007 season. In Saudi Arabia, production of wheat is expected to be less than it was in 2006, as a result of Government measures to limit the use of ground water and cut subsidized production.

In Central America and the Caribbean, harvesting in the 2006 first season crop was completed in most countries. Aggregate cereal production for the sub-region was provisionally estimated at 28.4 million tons, the lowest since 1989, compared to 31.6 million tons in 2007. The decline principally reflected poor production in Mexico, which more than offset a recovery in production in El Salvador, Guatemala, Honduras and Nicaragua, over the drought-affected crops in 2006. In the Caribbean, production has been normal, though significantly below-average output was achieved in Cuba.

In South America, harvesting of the 1995 wheat crop has recently been completed and production is projected to decrease from 15.6 million tons to a below-average 13 million tons. The decline is largely attributable to reduced output in Argentina, the main producer, as a result of dry weather at planting time. Lower production is also expected in Brazil and Chile, while in Uruguay production should be normal. In the Andean countries, output has been above average in Bolivia and Peru and average in Ecuador and Colombia. Planting of the 2008 coarse grain crop has been completed in southern areas where an increase in planting is projected, particularly in Argentina, Chile and Uruguay.

In Europe, early prospects for crops in 2008 are generally favourable. Winter grain plantings have increased (in particular, wheat) in the EC following a reduction in area restrictions and generally favourable weather in the autumn of 2007. Plantings are also reported to have expanded in some eastern countries. However, financial constraints are likely to keep production below potential. In the Baltic States the early outlook for the 2008 grain harvest is satisfactory. Indications are that higher prices and reduced grain availability for export in the CIS (Commonwealth of Independent States) have resulted in a larger area sown to winter grains.

In the CIS, larger plantings and the satisfactory condition of winter grains (mainly wheat and rye) in the major producing states point to a recovery in the

2008 cereal harvest from the poor level of 123 million tons in 2007. However, growing conditions until the harvest and the availability of working capital on farms to obtain essential inputs on time will determine the final outcome. In the European parts of the CIS, market proximity and generally higher cereal prices point to a turn-around in production notably in the Ukraine and the Russian Federation. The outlook is also favourable in Georgia, where state wheat lands have been leased to private farmers. However, efforts to expand grain production in the CIS are being undermined by progressively declining yields due to shortages of credit and essential inputs.

In North America, final United States official estimates for 2007 production put the wheat crop at 59.5 million tons, 3.7 million tons below the previous year and the coarse grains crop at 209.6 million tons, 75.5 million tons down from 2005's record level. The early outlook for the 2007 winter wheat is mixed. Plantings have expanded but crops have come under stress from harsh conditions in January 2008. In Canada, the latest estimate for 2008 wheat output is 25.4 million tons, 2.3 million tons above the previous year and coarse grain production also increased by about 0.5 million tons to 24.3 million tons. For 2008, early indications point to an increase in wheat area; the bulk of coarse grains will not be planted until May to June.

In Oceania, the latest estimate of the 2008 wheat crop is 17.1 million tons, almost double the previous year's drought-reduced crop. The winter coarse grain crop also recovered sharply in 2007. The 2008 summer sorghum crop has, so far, continued to develop well following good rainfall in the major eastern growing areas of Australia in late December and January.

Even if we consider yields from as far back as 1996 we can see that the red flags have been going up for more than a decade; but the matter had to get much worse before most people (even in the First World) were aware of the extent of the crisis. Only as late as 2007/2008 did the mass media become heavily preoccupied with the issue. It did evoke, fortunately, exceptionally high standards of journalism, of which an account given as a feature article by Kate Smith and Rob Edwards in Glasgow's *Sunday Herald* was especially informative and thought-provoking.[15]

The authors link up global warming, rising oil prices and population growth, commenting that together these factors are pushing food prices up beyond levels that many can afford so that humanity faces destruction unless we act. As they see it, the seriousness of the situation is rendered stark, because for once the whole world and not just the Third World faces the same problem. More than 73 million people in 78 countries that depend on food handouts from the United Nations World Food Programme (WFP) are facing reduced rations this year. 'The increasing scarcity of food is the biggest crisis looming for the world,' according to WFP officials.

At the same time, the UN Food and Agriculture Organisation has warned that rising prices have triggered a food crisis in 36 countries, all of which will need extra help. The World Bank points out that global food prices have risen by 75% since 2000, while wheat prices have increased by 200%. Costs of other staples, such as rice and soya bean, have also hit record highs, while corn is at its most expensive in 12 years.

The increasing cost of grains is also pushing up the price of meat, poultry, eggs and dairy products. And there is every likelihood that prices will continue their relentless rise, according to expert predictions by the UN and developed countries. High prices have already prompted a string of food protests around the world, with tortilla riots in Mexico, disputes over food rationing in West Bengal and protests over grain prices in Senegal, Mauritania and other parts of Africa. In Yemen, children have marched to highlight their hunger, while in London, in May 2007, hundreds of pig farmers protested outside Downing Street.

If prices keep rising, more and more people around the globe will be unable to afford the food they need to stay alive, and without help they will become desperate. More food riots will flare up, governments will totter and millions could die.

'Food scarcity means a big increase in the number of people going hungry', says the WFP's Greg Barrow. 'Without doubt, we are passing through a difficult period for the world's hungry poor.' The WFP estimates it needs an additional $500 million to keep feeding the 73 million people in Africa, Asia and Central America who require its help. 'We need extra money by the middle of 2008 so we don't have to reduce rations,' says Barrow.[16] He also points out that age-old patterns of famine are changing. 'We are feeding communities of people we didn't expect to feed,' he explains.

HUNGER IS SPREADING

Barrow asserts that: 'As well as being rural, the profile of the new hungry poor is also urban, which is new. There is food available in the markets and shops – it's just that these people can't afford to buy it. This is the new face of hunger.' Food shortages will also affect Western industrialised nations such as Scotland, Barrow says. 'Scarcity means that some foods will get very expensive, or disappear from supermarkets altogether, meaning a move to seasonal, indigenous vegetables.' Of the 36 countries named in the spring of 2008 as currently facing a food crisis, 21 are in Africa. Lesotho and Swaziland have been afflicted by droughts; Sierra Leone lacks widespread access to food markets because of low incomes and high prices, and Ghana, Kenya and Chad, among others, are enduring 'severe localised food insecurity'. In India last year, more than 25 000 farmers took their own lives, driven to despair by grain shortages and farming debts. 'The spectre of food grain imports stares India in the face as agricultural growth plunges to an all-time low,' warns *India Today* magazine.[17]

The World Bank predicts global demand for food will double by 2030. This is partly because the world's population is expected to grow by three billion by 2050, but that is only one of many interlocking causes. The rise in global temperatures caused by pollution is also beginning to disrupt food production in many countries. According to the UN, an area of fertile soil the size of Ukraine is lost every year because of drought, deforestation and climate instability. In 2007 Australia experienced its worst drought for over a century, and saw its wheat crop shrink by 60%. China's grain harvest has also fallen by 10% over the past seven years. The UN Intergovernmental Panel on Climate Change has predicted that over the next 100 years a one-metre rise in sea levels would flood almost a third of the world's crop-growing land. A recent analysis by the Conservative Party leader, David Cameron, also pinned blame for the 'global food crunch' on the accelerating demand for allegedly green biofuels and the world's growing appetite for meat.

THE FOOD SHORTAGE IS NOT TEMPORARY

As pointed out above, meat is a very inefficient way of utilising land to produce food, delivering far fewer calories acre for acre than grain. But the amount of meat eaten by the average Chinese consumer has increased from 20 kilograms a year in 1985 to over 50 kilograms today. The demand for meat from across all developing countries has doubled since 1980. The world's grain stocks, however, are at their lowest for 30 years. Cameron warns. 'Some analysts are beginning to make some very worrying, very stark predictions. And these analysts say politicians should start to rank the issue of food security alongside energy security and even national security.'[18] Another key driver is the soaring cost of oil. As well as increasing transport costs, oil makes crop fertilisers more expensive.

According to the World Bank, fertiliser prices have risen 150% in the past five years. This has had a major impact on food prices, as the cost of fertiliser contributes over a quarter of the overall cost of grain production in the US, which is responsible for 40% of world grain exports. Tackling hunger has become a 'forgotten' UN millennium development goal, says the bank's president, Robert Zoellick.[19] But increased food prices and their threat – not only to people but also to political stability – have made it a matter of urgency,' he says. Scottish farmers warn that food security is becoming an issue for the first time since the Second World War. 'This is a perfect storm and the effects are being felt right now,' says James Withers, Acting Chief Executive of the National Farmers' Union in Scotland.[20]

'At the same time as demand for food increases, the amount of land we have available to grow food on is reducing,' he adds. 'An area twice the size of Scotland's entire agricultural area has been swallowed up by Chinese towns and cities in the last 10 years.' John Scott, a Scottish Conservative MSP who farms in Ayrshire, goes further. 'It's almost biblical,' he says. 'With all the wine lakes and butter mountains, we've had our 20 years of plenty since 1986.'[21] The prospect of global food shortages is now Malthusian, he suggests. One response from the UK and Scotland should be to grow more of our own food, and to try to reverse the decline in self-sufficiency from 75% in 1986 to 60% now.

It is possible for the UK, and the world, to feed itself, argues Robin Maynard from the Soil Association, but it will require big changes. He invokes the wartime spirit that saw gardens turned into allotments, and 50 mixed farms feeding Britain. 'This is a wake-up call,' he says. 'The choices we make now will determine whether we can feed ourselves in the future. If we get it right we can have a thriving food economy.'[22] Richard Lochhead, the Scottish Government's Environment Secretary, has launched a public discussion to develop Scotland's first food policy. 'I am conscious our generation has not experienced food shortages, but we should never take food for granted,' he says. 'That is why the Scottish government will never allow food security to fall off the national agenda. We recognise the vital rôle of our primary producers in ensuring the long-term capacity and capability of our food supply.'[23]

All of the above comments confront us once again with the trade-offs between the use of agricultural resources to produce biofuels on the one hand, while on the other, the world needs those resources for food. The *Sunday Herald* article (cited above) reminds us that we need to consider far more carefully how biofuel production can be carried out without compromising food supplies. This will require that we research more thoroughly than we have done how to make effective and sustained use of such energy sources as geothermal, wind, wave, and solar. Until now, the US and the EU have strongly advocated the use of biofuels to run vehicles and other machinery, but the evidence is very much that this strategy is contraindicated.

For instance, in 2007, fully 25% of the total US maize crop was converted into ethanol to fuel vehicles and yet the US supplies nearly two-thirds of maize exports. The effect of this, as pointed out by the World Bank, is to put unsustainable pressure on food sources for much of the Third World's people.

'The biofuels surge makes things worse by adding high demand on top of already high prices and low stocks,' said one of the Bank's leading economists, Don Mitchell. 'Ethanol and biodiesel produced in the US and European Union don't appear to be delivering on green promises either, making them very controversial.'[24]

Yet, there are plans by more than 20 countries to boost production of biofuels over the next decade. The US is talking about trebling maize production for ethanol, while the European Union is aiming to make biofuels 10% of all transport fuels by 2020. The dash for biofuels came under fire early in 2008 from the UK

Government's newly appointed Chief Scientific Adviser, Professor John Beddington. In a speech in London, he said that world food prices had already suffered a 'major shock' as a result. Biofuels were often unsustainable, he argued. 'It's very hard to imagine how we can see the world growing enough crops to generate renewable energy and at the same time to meet such an immense demand for food.'

When he was still Professor of Applied Population Biology at Imperial College, London, Beddington argued that large-scale unfettered use of biofuels would quickly lead the world into a 'hopeless situation', and that the idea of cutting down rainforest to clear the land and grow biofuels 'seems profoundly stupid'.

MONETISING FOOD AID

If we could be convinced, though, that all of the food access problems besetting the world were entirely due to 'mistakes' in management (such as relying too heavily on biofuels), the solutions – although difficult – could be considered rationally and implemented. But once again we run up against the inexorable influence of neoliberalism and its impact on politics.

Consider a report which was carried out by IRIN (Integrated Regional Information Network) in 2007 and which dealt with what is termed 'monetised food aid'. This term needs some explanation. The US is one of the few First World countries that routinely tie in 'food aid' with regular marketing procedures. That is, they 'sell' food and – at reduced prices, to be sure – to poorer countries. Most donors give such food directly, or supply cash to UN agencies and NGOs, so that food can then be purchased and distributed. This is in keeping with WTO regulations and is designed to protect free trade, but it has many unintended adverse consequences.

For instance, a well-respected US NGO, CARE, (Cooperation for Assistance and Relief Everywhere), with headquarters in Atlanta, Georgia, but with a remit to provide aid anywhere in the world. made headlines in August 2007 when it turned down 'monetised' food aid from the US government. The issue came out at a meeting of CARE in South Africa on 12 September 2007.[25]

CARE's position was that monetisation risked distorting markets in developing countries and was having an overall negative effect. Monetisation, or monetised food aid, involves food being bought at subsidised prices in the donor country and then sold in the recipient country to generate funds for development projects.

In a two-part analysis, IRIN examines the debate over monetisation and the linked issue of rising demand for food for manufacturing of biofuels – what has become called 'The Iron Triangle'. 'The CARE move is critically important because it marks the end of the so called Coalition for Food Aid of NGOs, which combined with [farm] industry and shipping interests (as the so-called iron triangle) to support US food aid,' said Edward Clay, Senior Research Associate at the Overseas Development Institute, a UK-based think tank.[26] The 'iron triangle' here refers to the coalition of agribusinesses, shipping companies and NGOs that lobby for food aid.

Clay went on to say: 'The US is under considerable pressure in the WTO negotiations to end monetisation and notably, has found little support amongst African governments. Monetisation is not usually used as famine relief, but is an inefficient and trade-distorting form of development aid.'

However, the 15-member Alliance for Food Aid, a group that favours monetisation, including US-based NGOs Africare and World Vision, refuted the claim that monetisation destroyed local agriculture and said the sale of food commodities was conducted in a transparent manner. The food is sold in countries that are poor and depend on imports for a substantial part of their food supplies.

In May 2007, however, the US Government Accountability Office (GAO), an independent investigative arm of Congress and congressional watchdog charged with auditing and evaluating government programmes, reported that the monetisation rate of non-emergency food aid had far exceeded the minimum requirement of 15%, reaching close to 70% in 2001 before declining to about 50% in 2005. CARE's decision came as the GAO report criticised monetisation as ineffective and called for an overhaul of the way food aid is distributed. 'Monetisation entails not only the costs of procuring, shipping and handling food, but also the costs of marketing and selling it in recipient countries,' said the GAO.[27]

'Furthermore, the time and expertise needed to market and sell food abroad requires NGOs to divert resources away from their core missions. In addition, US agencies do not collect or maintain an electronic database on monetisation revenues, and the lack of such data impedes the agencies' ability to fully monitor the degree to which revenues can cover the costs related to monetisation.'

George Odo, a CARE official in Kenya, said that a proposal that 25% of the food aid dispensed by the US Government be in cash to buy food for recipient countries locally or regionally, which the George Bush administration had been promoting for the last three years, also strengthened CARE's position.[28]

'We were also encouraged by the Bush administration's move to push the proposal as part of the 2007 Farm Bill, which is up for review this year ... and even the administration recognises that reforms have to be made to make food aid more effective,' said Odo. The Farm Bill, which determines US agricultural policy and also structures the country's food aid programmes, comes up for review every five years.

FOOD AID DECREASING

CARE's move comes at a time when rising oil prices are driving a growing demand for biofuel, making 'free' food aid increasingly scarce. 'Food aid is getting scarce and expensive; we need to use it strategically . . . where it is needed the most, which is in emergency situations,' said CARE's Odo. 'We have to rethink and reinvent food aid.'[29]

'CARE is absolutely right,' said Christopher Barrett, who teaches development economics at Cornell University in New York and is the co-author of the book, *Food Aid After Fifty Years: recasting its rôle.* He added, 'Increased demand for maize and sugar for biofuel is driving up food prices and making food aid commodities more expensive.'[30]

In their book, Barrett and co-author Daniel Maxwell, a former CARE official, estimate that it costs more than two dollars of US taxpayers' money to deliver one dollar's worth of food procured as in-kind food aid. Barrett told IRIN that since the food aid budget in the US, and globally, 'will not grow by anything approaching the price increases for commodities and the rate increases for freight – if the food aid budget grows at all – the tonnage available for shipment will surely fall. It becomes ever more important to target an increasingly scarce resource to use where it has the greatest impact: in this case, that's emergency food aid.'[31]

What all of this means is that monetised food has given the entire neoliberal agenda a bad name and even the US government is distancing itself from it. These events will almost certainly serve to bring US aid policies more closely into line with those of other countries and perhaps this is to be welcomed.

CARE's decision to say 'no' to monetised aid provided 'additional ammunition' to those attempting to reform US food aid, because 'they are turning down an important source of revenue that funds many of their projects in developing countries,' noted Nicholas Minot, a senior research fellow at the International Food Policy Research Institute (IFPRI), a US-based think tank.[32]

But, in the short term, the strength of agricultural interests in the US Congress, 'in which sparsely populated agricultural states are over-represented, would override any attempts for change. In addition, a basic principle of political economy is that a small group whose members have a large stake in a policy decision (for example, farmers) will have a louder voice than a large group whose members have a small stake in the decision (for example, non-farming taxpayers),' Minot said. And, in the same article, Elspeth Barrett of Cornell University is quoted as saying: 'too early to tell what will emerge, as the Farm Bill has not yet been passed by Congress. It is unlikely, unfortunately, that the Bush proposal for 25% [of cash]. . . for local and regional purchases will go through; there will likely be a smaller pilot programme authorised.'

Clay pointed out that USAID had tried to bring about change five years ago during the last Farm Bill review. Andrew Natsios, the agency's administrator at the time, had proposed that USAID use 25% of food aid funds to buy and ship food procured either locally in the recipient country, or in the region, for famine relief or in an emergency. 'This seemingly reasonable proposal was poorly supported by US NGOs, and was rejected by the US Congress.'[33]

The WTO is another pressure point that could force change. 'WTO members, particularly the EU, consider food aid that is tied to home-country production to be a form of agricultural export subsidy,' Minot commented. According to the WFP, some donors have stopped donating food aid in the form of commodities, providing cash instead, and up to 15 to 25% of all food aid is now purchased in the country or region where it is needed.

John Hoddinott, a senior research fellow at IFPRI and quoted by Odo, cited above, said it would be a matter of the US catching up with global trends. 'The discussions (in the US) have started at a technical level, but have to get to the policy level.'[34] Odo observed that CARE was trying to lobby private donors to make up for the revenue lost for its development projects and hoped that 'we can show a way to other NGOs'. But even if monetised food is no longer used as a device to expedite free trade, the world is still faced with problems of acute shortage of a wide range of foods.

THE RÔLE OF EMERGING MIDDLE CLASSES

Speaking of grain foods generally, a major reason for the recently emerging world shortage of cereal crops is not because our growing population is eating them, but because they are not! This takes some explanation. In both India and China, a middle class is emerging. Their wealth has largely come about through the establishment of business firms with a global outreach, and more specifically, through the sale of finished articles, especially clothing, to the First World. Labour costs are so low throughout most of Asia, that consumer goods can be produced for First World markets at a fraction of the cost that would be possible in highly unionised First World outlets.

This sudden creation of a moderately wealthy middle class in large markets, such as India and China, means that those people can now afford to reflect their new wealth in obvious lifestyle changes. One such lifestyle change has been in eating habits. When this author was working in South India in 1954, almost all of the local people were largely vegetarian. I took this to be mainly an expression of Hinduism. I did wonder, though, why the few very wealthy Hindus I encountered did not seem moved by their religion to shun meat! But, as subsequent development has shown to be so, money available for buying meat was the real cause.

Meats are far more costly to purchase than are vegetables, and one obvious way of demonstrating one's comparative wealth in such a social context is to become a conspicuous meat eater. This has created a vastly increased demand for meat – and hence, of access to land being used for pasturage that used to be used for growing grain. As well, pastured livestock does not subsist by grazing alone, but requires fodder rich in various grains. The more grain in the animal's diet, the better the meat it produces. Thus grain available for food suffers two blows – a considerable portion of whatever grain is produced is now fed to animals destined for the dinner table and, as well, livestock require vast tracts of land for pasturage.

Also, as already pointed out, meat is a far less energy efficient source of food than are cereal grains. For every five calories of energy we get from meat, the animal concerned has had to eat about nine calories of vegetable food.

GROWING DESPERATION

But as the middle classes with their links to business have moved to meat the impact of the sudden scarcity of cereal crops is hitting the lower classes – especially in China and Africa – with a severity about which we in the First World hear little. Robert McKie and Heather Steward wrote a well-documented article in London's *Observer* newspaper, which sums up the issue.[35] They point out, for instance, that as First World people are finding themselves priced out of as much petrol as they would like, millions of Third World people are finding themselves unable to afford sufficient food – moreover, the two phenomena are related. And the disaster is truly global. As McKie and Stewart say:

> Across the world a crisis is unfolding at alarming speed. Climate change, China's increasing consumption and the dash for biofuels are causing food shortages and rocketing prices – sparking riots in cities from the Caribbean to the Far East.

Kamla Devi was one woman they interviewed in a Delhi market. Devi was, above all, angry – a condition which she attributed to her constant pangs of hunger. According to her, she now argues violently with shopkeepers over the ever-rising prices and also quarrels with her husband. Although employed as a labourer, her wages (equivalent to about US$1.00 a day) are no longer adequate to maintain them.

'When I go to the market and see how little I can get for my money, it makes me want to hit the shopkeepers and thrash the government,' she says. A few months ago, Kamla – who is 42 – decided that she and her husband could no longer afford to eat twice a day. The couple, who have already sent their two teenage sons to live with more prosperous relatives, now exist on only one daily meal. At midday Kamla cooks a dozen roti (a round, flat Indian bread) with some vegetables fried with onions and spices. If there are some left, they will eat them at night. The only other sustenance that the couple have are occasional cups of sugared tea.

'My husband and I would argue every night. In the end he told me it wouldn't make his wages grow larger. Instead we went down to one meal a day to cut costs.'

It is a grim, unsettling story. Yet it is certainly not an exceptional one. Across the world, a food crisis is now unfolding with frightening speed. Hundreds of millions of men and women who, only a few months ago, were able to provide food for their families, have found that rocketing prices of wheat, rice and cooking oil have left them facing the imminent prospect of starvation. The spectre of catastrophe now looms over much of the planet.

In less than a year, the price of wheat has risen 130%, soya by 87% and rice by 74%. According to the UN's Food and Agriculture Organisation, there are only eight to 12 weeks of cereal stocks in the world, while grain supplies are at their lowest since the 1980s.[36]

For the Devi family, and hundreds of millions of others like them, the impact has been calamitous, as Robert Zoellick, the World Bank President warned at the latest G7 meeting in Washington.[37] Brandishing a bag of rice, he told startled delegates from the world's richest nations that the world was now perched at the edge of catastrophe.

'This is not just about meals forgone today, or about increasing social unrest, it is about lost learning potential for children and adults in the future, stunted intellectual and physical growth,' he said. Without urgent action to resolve the crisis, he added, the fight against poverty could be set back by seven years.

Not surprisingly, these swiftly rising prices have unleashed serious political unrest in many places. In Dhaka, 10 000 Bangladeshi textile workers clashed with police. Dozens were injured, including 20 policemen, in a protest triggered by food costs that was eventually quelled by baton charges and teargas. In Haiti, demonstrators recently tried to storm the presidential palace after prices of staple foods leaped 50%.

In Egypt, Indonesia, Ivory Coast, Mauritania, Mozambique, Senegal and Cameroon there have been demonstrations, sometimes involving fatalities, as starving, desperate people have taken to the streets. And in Vietnam the new crime of rice rustling – in which crops are stripped at night from fields by raiders – has led to the banning of all harvesting machines from roads after sunset and to farmers, armed with shotguns, camping around their fields 24 hours a day.

But what are the factors that led to this global unrest? What has triggered the price rises that have put the world's basic foodstuffs out of reach for a rising fraction of its population? And what measures must be taken by politicians, world leaders and monetary chiefs to rectify the crisis? Not surprisingly, the first two of these questions tend to be the easier ones to answer. Economists and financiers point to a number of factors that have combined to create the current crisis, a perfect storm in which several apparently unconnected events came together with disastrous effects.

One key issue was the decision by the US government, made several years ago, to give domestic subsidies to its farmers so that they could grow corn that can then be fermented and distilled into ethanol, a biofuel which can be mixed with petrol. This policy helps limit US dependence on oil imports and also gives support to the nation's farmers. However, by taking over land – about 20 million acres so far in the United States – that would otherwise have been used to grow wheat and other food crops US food production has dropped dramatically. Prices of wheat, soya and other crops have been pushed up significantly as a result.

Other nations, including Argentina, Canada and some European countries, have adopted similar, but more restrained, biofuel policies. But without mentioning any countries by name, Zoellick clearly pointed the finger of blame at the US. Everyone should 'look closely at the effects of the dash for biofuels', he said. 'I would hope that countries that, for whatever reason, energy, security, and others, have emphasised biofuel development will be particularly sensitive to the call to meet the emergency needs for people who may not have enough food to eat.'

This point has also been stressed recently by the UK government's chief scientific adviser, Professor John Beddington, already cited. 'It is very hard to imagine how we can see the world growing enough crops to produce renewable energy and at the same time meet the enormous demand for food,' he said. 'The supply of food really isn't keeping up.'

For his part, Hank Paulson, the US Treasury Secretary – recently asked about the impact of US energy policies on food prices – replied dismissively: 'This is a complex area, with a number of causes. The first priority, he added, was to get food supplies to people who need them, before considering the longer term reasons for the rising prices.'[38]

It was not a point shared by the chief of staff in the United Nations trade and development division, Taffere Tesfachew, who flew to London ahead of a vital meeting of the leaders of the world's poorest nations in Accra, the capital of Ghana. Instead of an agenda designed to achieve economic progress in the developing world, the meeting instead focused on the pressing issue of food. Tesfachew said that decades of aid has been skewed to ambitious industrialisation programmes and that the World Bank and others have failed to invest in the agricultural sector. 'We believe these high food prices won't disappear in the next two years, so now is the time to redress imbalances in terms of ethanol subsidies,' he said.

Zoellick was also clear that action was now urgently needed. 'In the US and Europe over the last year we have been focusing on the prices of gasoline at the pumps. While many worry about filling their tanks, many others around the world are struggling to fill their stomachs. And it's getting more and more difficult every day,' added Zoellick, who made an impassioned plea to the world's rich nations to provide emergency help, including $500 million in extra funding to the UN World Food Programme.

This call was backed by finance ministers from the G24, who represent the leading developing countries, who also demanded extra cash to help cushion the poor against the shock of rising food prices. As well as causing hunger and malnutrition, the rising cost of basic foodstuffs risks blowing a hole in the budgets of food-importing countries, many of them in Africa, they argued.

WHEN ADVERSE FACTORS COMBINE

As to the other factors that have combined to trigger the current food crisis, experts also point to the connected issue of climate change. As the levels of carbon dioxide rise in the atmosphere, meteorologists have warned that weather patterns are becoming increasingly disturbed, causing devastation in many areas. For several consecutive years, Australia – once a prime grower of wheat – has found its production ruined by drought, for example. Scarcity, particularly on Asia's grain markets, has then driven up prices even further.

Some campaigners see climate change as the most pressing challenge facing the world while others now say that biofuels – grown to offset fossil fuel use – is taking food out of the mouths of some of the world's poorest people. The net result will be eco-warriors battling with poverty campaigners for the moral high ground.

On top of these issues, there is the growing wealth of China and its 1 billion inhabitants. Once the possessor of a relatively poor and overwhelmingly rural economy, China has becoming increasingly industrialised and its middle classes have swelled in numbers. One impact has been to trigger a doubling in meat consumption, particularly pork. As the country's farmers have sought to feed more and more pigs, more and more grain has been bought by them. However, China has only 7% of the world's arable land, and that figure is shrinking as farmland has been ravaged by pollution and water shortages. The net result has been to decrease domestic supplies of grain just as demand for it has started to boom. Again, the impact has struck worst in the Third World, with wheat and other grain prices soaring.

And finally there is the issue of vegetable oils. Soya and palm oils are a major source of calories in Asia. But flooding in Malaysia and a drought in Indonesia has limited supplies. In addition, these oils are now being sought as biodiesel, which is used as a direct substitute for diesel in many countries, including Australia. The impact has been all too familiar: an alarming drop in supplies for the people of the Third World as prices of this basic commodity have soared.

One such victim is Kamla Devi. For several months she has had to abandon dhal, a central, protein-rich dish of lentils that was a key part of her family's diet. Now even the cooking of fried food – in particular, 'pooris', made of hot, puffed, oil-soaked bread – has had to follow suit, for the simple reason that cooking oil has become unaffordable.

'It has affected my health', she says. 'The rich are becoming richer. They go to shopping malls and they don't need to worry. The problem with prices only matters for the poor people like me.'

HAITI AND THE RICE CRISIS

The most important cereal item for the vast majority of the world's people, though, is rice – especially in Asia. While there have been shortages of rice in various localities in wartime, for instance, or in the case of localised droughts, a worldwide shortage of rice is really not something that we have been familiar with in the last century. But now we are facing just that. One can exemplify the disaster by reference to the situation in a number of countries, but one of the most tragic is Haiti. This author knows Haiti well and has served there a number of times.

Its geographical location has done it no favours and it has experienced French, Spanish and American imperialism in the past couple of centuries. They suffered two particularly prolonged periods of brutal dictatorship in the 20th century, first under Dr Francis Duvalier (1967–71), and then under his son Jean-Claude Duvalier (1971–86). Haiti had always been a poor and badly managed country, but in 1991 – in the country's first reasonably free election – a Haitian priest, Jean Bertrand Aristide was elected as President.

He set up a reform government and was determined not only to bring 'justice to the poor' (i.e. most Haitians!) but to break the severe hold the United States had over its finances, resources, and infrastructure. Very much under pressure from US influences, he was ousted in September of 1991 – less than a year after being elected. From 1991 until 1994, various governments ruled the country, but they were very much under US control. Then, in 1994, the Haitian people again elected Aristide. This time he lasted until 1996, when US banking and corporate interests again organised an internal coup against him. He took up residence elsewhere in Central America, but promised to return and that he did, whereupon he was elected for a third time in 2001. This time he served for three years under almost constant disruption and riots financed largely from the US. In 2003 he was physically removed by US forces, and since then the country has lost many of the social gains ushered in under his administration.

Rioting in Haiti became almost routine between 2003 (when Aristide was removed) and now, but these riots have suddenly been becoming more common since mid-2007, when the global food shortages began to become so acute that even in Port-au-Prince (the capital) cases of children of three and four actually starving to death were noted in the media. As stated above, life has almost always been precarious in Haiti. In 1987, this author was actually handed a tiny baby in a country area by a ragged woman who asked, (in Creole French) 'Are you American?' 'No, Canadian.' I replied. 'Please give me one Canadian dollar and you can keep my son.' Obviously, I was in no position to enter into such a transaction and she quickly vanished. I ran after her to try to organise help with the Canadian Embassy, but was quickly surrounded by a hostile jostling crowd. I have often wondered what happened to her and that baby boy.

Al Jazeera in April 2005, reported a similar series of accounts, one of which concerned a young malnourished woman named Hermite Joseph.[39] She scratched out a precarious living selling out-of-date frozen chicken parts from shack to shack in the Port-au-Prince slums. The three dollars or so she made each day used to be enough to take care of her unemployed husband and three children. Now, she is struggling to stave off starvation.

'Everything has changed,' says Joseph, stabbing at a half-frozen chunk of poul-try with a screwdriver. 'My kids are like toothpicks. Before, if you had $1.25, you could buy vegetables, some rice, 10 cents of charcoal and a little cooking oil. Right now, a little can of rice alone costs 65 cents, and it's not good rice at all. Oil is 25 cents. Charcoal is 25 cents. With $1.25, you can't even make a plate of rice for one child.'

Food prices are rising around the world, sparking protests and riots, but perhaps nowhere have they had such a devastating impact than in Haiti, where around 80% of the population lives on less than two dollars a day.

The price of rice has nearly doubled since December 2007. In March, people began complaining of a hunger so torturous that it felt like their stomachs were being eaten away by bleach or battery acid. In a matter of days, 'Clorox hunger', named after a brand of bleach, was being talked about in slums and villages across the country.

Growing tensions finally exploded on 2 April in the south-western city of Okay, the third largest in Haiti, where demonstrators clashed with United Nations peacekeepers and tore down the walls of a UN military base. Thousands of people from the slums took to the streets, while local leaders demanded that the government end its free market policies and create community shops with subsidised prices.

ANGER WITH THE UN

They also called on the government to fix a date for the removal of the UN peacekeeping mission. Since arriving in June 2004, UN troops have been credited with rooting out armed groups from the slums of Port-au-Prince and help-ing impose a degree of political stability. But the peacekeepers have provoked deep resentment among Haitians, who say they prefer development to security and complain that the mission's $500 million budget is wasted on troops and tanks.

In Port-au-Prince, thousands of protesters set up flaming barricades and threw rocks at the National Palace, burned gas stations and looted businesses. And across the countryside, farmers erected road blockades – one community dragged a vehicle chassis across the road – while residents from a fishing village flipped over a boat.

DEMAND FOR CHANGE

President Rene Preval finally responded. He promised to reduce the price of rice by nearly 16%, while the Haitian senate voted to remove Prime Minister Jacques Edouard Alexis, from office. The moves seem to have pacified the Haitian people, but only for now. Many of those who participated in the protests are vowing to take to the streets again if food prices do not go down rapidly.

'The president needs to hurry,' said Jean Francois Bernard, a student who participated in the protests. 'The mobilisations will continue until we see results. Until now, we haven't seen anything.'[40]

Preval said the price at which importers sell a 110-pound sack of rice would drop from $51 to $43. He also persuaded three major importers to take a three-dollar cut in their profits, and secured three million dollars in international aid to cover the remaining five dollars per sack. But the agreement with the importers is valid for only one month, and it is still not clear how much the price of rice will go down in the marketplaces, if at all. The intermediaries who distribute rice have not yet agreed to also reduce their prices; on the street a sack currently sells for more than $70.

'Reducing the price per sack by eight dollars won't change anything,' said Gerald Baptiste, who sells rice by the can in the poor district of La Saline. 'A little can is still going to sell for three dollars. It's not enough. The price needs to go down to two dollars at the most.' The foregoing was reported to the author by one of his former colleagues in the Canadian International Development Agency (CIDA).[41]

Imported rice has become the most important food staple in Haiti. Decades ago, rice was a luxury in Haiti, grown in the lush Artibonite valley and eaten on special occasions and Sundays. After the removal from power of dictator Jean Claude-Duvalier in 1986, a US-backed military government slashed import taxes, allowing rice and other cheap imports from the US and the Dominican Republic to flood Haitian marketplaces. This, of course, was highly profitable for exporters of US rice, as its production is government-subsidised, but it even further undermined the precarious livelihoods of Haitian rice growers. As well, plans pushed by Washington to transform Haiti's rural economy into an industrial force, capitalising on the country's cheap labour to turn the country into the 'Taiwan of the Caribbean' never bore fruit.

Instead, 20 years later, Haiti has little industry besides a handful of assembly plants where the minimum wage is less than two dollars a day, and the country's agricultural production is mainly subsistence.

'In 1987, when rice began being imported at a low price, many people applauded,' said Preval in a televised speech on 2 May 2008 aimed at stopping the protests. 'But cheap imported rice destroyed (locally grown) rice. Today, imported rice has become expensive and our national production is in ruins. That's why subsidising imported food is not the answer.'

But Preval did just that when faced with the threat of renewed protests if he did not take immediate action to reduce prices. At the same time, Preval promised to relaunch agricultural production by supporting local farmers. He said he hoped to cut the price of fertiliser in half, with the help of the Venezuelan Government, and announced plans to send an official from the Agricultural Ministry to Caracas. Preval's call for boosting national production may have struck right at the root of the problem of high food prices, but it may not be enough to calm tensions in the streets of Haiti.

THE GLOBAL SITUATION

Haiti is but one example considered in some detail, but the problem is truly as international as the UN itself is. For instance, in Pakistan and Thailand, army troops have been deployed to stop food from being seized from fields and warehouses. Prices in these countries for foodstuffs such as rice, wheat, sorghum and maize (corn) have all doubled.

The same source states that the causes range from financial speculation on food, desertification and unregulated population increases. As well, and as we have already noted, both India and China use grains to produce biofuels. The UN's Food and Agriculture Organisation (FAO) is optimistic, though, in that it predicts that world cereal production will increase by 2.6% by the end of 2008. We can only hope that they are right.

As this chapter draws to a close, however, whatever the FAO estimates are, let us briefly look again – but in greater depth – at the main problems with which this chapter opened.

GROWING CONSUMPTION

In January, 2007, Zhou Jian closed down his car spare parts business and launched himself as a pork butcher. Since then the 26-year-old businessman's Shanghai shop has been crowded out – despite a 58% rise in the price of pork in the past year – and his income has trebled.

As China's emerging middle classes become richer, their consumption of meat has increased by more than 150% per head since 1980. In those days, meat was scarce, rationed at around 1 kilogram per person per month and used sparingly in rice and noodle dishes, stir fried to preserve cooking oil.

Today, the average Chinese consumer eats more than 50 kilograms of meat a year. To feed the millions of pigs on its farms, China is now importing grain on a huge scale, pushing up its prices worldwide.

PALM OIL CRISIS

The oil palm tree is the most highly efficient producer of vegetable oil, with one acre yielding as much oil as eight acres of soybeans. Unfortunately, it takes eight years to grow to maturity and demand has far outstripped supply. Vegetable oils provide an important source of calories in the developing world, and their shortage has contributed to the food crisis.

A drought in Indonesia and flooding in Malaysia has also hit the crop. While farmers and plantation companies hurriedly clear land to replant, it will take time before their efforts bear fruit. Palm oil prices jumped nearly 70% in 2007, hitting the poorest families. When a store in Chongqing in China announced a cooking-oil promotion in November, a stampede left three dead and 31 injured.

BIOFUEL DEMAND

The rising demand for ethanol, a biofuel that is mixed with petrol to bring down prices at the pump, has transformed the landscape of Iowa. Today this heartland of the Midwest is America's cornbelt, with the corn crop stretching as far as the eye can see.

Iowa produces almost half of the entire output of ethanol in the US, with 21 ethanol-producing plants. Farmers tear down fences, dig out old soya bean crops, buy up land and plant yet more corn. It has been likened to a new gold rush. But none of it is for food. And as the demand for ethanol increases, yet more farmers will pile in for the great scramble to plant corn instead of grain. The effect will be to further worsen world grain shortages.

GLOBAL WARMING

The massive grain storage complex outside Tottenham, New South Wales, today lies virtually empty. Normally, it would be half full. As the second largest exporter of grain after the US, Australia usually expects to harvest around 25 million tonnes a year. But, because of a five-year drought, thought to have been caused by climate change, it managed just 9.8 million tonnes in 2006.

Farmers such as George Grieg, who has farmed here for 50 years, have rarely known it to be so bad. Many have not even recovered the cost of planting and caring for their crops, and are being forced into debt. With global wheat prices at an all-time high, all they can do is cling on in the hope of a bumper crop next time – if they are lucky.[42] Despite the optimism of the FAO with regard to cereal grain production for 2008, its fact sheet for the global situation does not reflect much cause for such optimism.[43]

FAO'S FACTS ON GLOBAL FOOD SHORTAGES

The following information makes for grim reading, if nothing else illustrating how great a barrier our present procedures for food distribution indeed are to the achievement of global equity to health access. The author makes no apology for including it.

1   GLOBAL HUNGER

☐ Hunger and poverty claim 25 000 lives every day.
    Source: FAO & The State of Food Insecurity in the World, 2006

☐ 854 million people do not have enough to eat. This is more than the populations of USA, Canada and the European Union.
    Source: FAO & The State of Food Insecurity in the World, 2006

☐ 820 million people in developing countries alone are hungry – one in four lives in sub-Saharan Africa.
    Source: FAO & The State of Food Insecurity in the World, 2006

☐ In the 1990s, global poverty dropped by 20%. The number of hungry people increased by 18 million.
    Source: Food as Aid: Trends, Needs and Challenges in the 21st Century

☐ 524 million of the world's hungry live in South Asia. This is more than the populations of Australia and USA.
    Source: FAO & The State of Food Insecurity in the World, 2006

☐ More than 60% of chronically hungry people are women.
    Source: FAO & The State of Food Insecurity in the World, 2006

☐ The number of chronically hungry people worldwide is growing by an average of four million per year at current trends.
    Source: FAO & The State of Food Insecurity in the World, 2006

2   CHILD HUNGER

☐ Every five seconds a child dies because she or he is hungry.
    Source: FAO State of Food Insecurity in the World 2006

☐ Under-nutrition in children under the age 18 affects an estimated 350 to 400 million children.
    Source: Global Framework for Action, 2006

☐ More than 70% of the world's 146 million underweight children under age five years live in just 10 countries, with more than 50% located in South Asia alone.
    Source: Progress for Children: A Report Card on Nutrition (No.4), UNICEF, May 2006

❐ 10.9 million children under five die in developing countries each year.
Malnutrition and hunger-related diseases cause 60% of the deaths.
Source: UNICEF

❐ The cost of under-nutrition to national economic development is estimated
at US$20–30 billion per annum.
Source: Progress for Children, A report card on Nutrition, 2006

❐ One out of four children – roughly 146 million – in developing countries
are underweight.
Source: The State of the World's Children 2007, UNICEF

❐ WFP provided school meals and/or take home rations to 20.2 million
children in 71 countries in 2006.
Source: WFP School Feeding Unit

3   MALNUTRITION

❐ It is estimated that 684 000 child deaths worldwide could be prevented by
increasing access to vitamin A and zinc.
Source: WFP Annual Report 2007

❐ Almost five million children die each year from preventable diseases such as
diarrhoea and measles.
Source: WFP Hunger Facts 2006

❐ Lack of vitamin A kills a million infants a year.
Source: Vitamin and Mineral Deficiency, A Global Progress Report,
UNICEF

❐ Iron deficiency is the most common form of malnutrition, affecting 180
million children aged under four.
Source: WFP Facts and Figures on Child Hunger

❐ Iron deficiency is impairing the mental development of 40–60% of the
children in developing countries.
Source: Vitamin and Mineral Deficiency, A Global Progress Report, p. 2,
UNICEF

❐ Lack of vitamin A weakens the immune system of 40% of under-fives in
poor countries, and can cause blindness.
Source: Vitamin and Mineral Deficiency, A Global Progress Report, p. 2,
UNICEF – WFP Facts and Figures on Child Hunger, p. 2

❐ Iodine deficiency is the main cause of brain damage in the early years of a
child's life.
Source: WFP Facts and Figures on Child Hunger, p. 2

❐ WFP-supported deworming reached 11 million children in 2006
Source: WFP Annual Report 2007

4   FOOD AID & HIV/AIDS

❐ Every minute, a child under 15 dies of an AIDS-related illness. Every minute,
  another child becomes HIV-positive.
  Source: WFP HIV/AIDS unit, 2007

❐ HIV/AIDS directly impacts a person's ability to provide enough food to feed
  themselves or their families, directly compromising their household's food
  security.
  Source: WFP HIV/AIDS unit, 2007

❐ Less than one in five people at risk of becoming infected with HIV
  worldwide have access to basic prevention services.
  Source: WFP HIV/AIDS unit, 2007

❐ WFP and UNAIDS estimate that it costs an average of US$0.66 per day to
  provide nutritional support to an AIDS patient and his/her family.
  Source: WFP HIV/AIDS unit, 2007

❐ Children with HIV/AIDS may face as a result: poverty, malnutrition,
  inadequate access to social services, discrimination, stigmatisation, gender
  inequality and sexual exploitation.
  Source: WFP HIV/AIDS unit, 2007

❐ Nutritious food combined with antiretroviral drugs is essential to maintaining
  the immune system and helping prolong the life of someone with HIV.
  Source: WFP HIV/AIDS unit, 2007

❐ TB is the main cause of death among AIDS sufferers. WFP uses food aid to
  encourage patients to treat TB.
  Source: WFP Brochure, HIV/AIDS & Children: Bringing hope to a generation

❐ By 2020, the AIDS epidemic will have claimed one-fifth or more of the
  agricultural labour force in most southern African countries.
  Source: WFP HIV/AIDS unit, 2007

❐ Most households will never fully recover from the death of a parent, which
  means that the effects of HIV/AIDS are likely to be felt for generations to come.
  Source: WFP HIV/AIDS unit, 2007

5   FOOD & AGRICULTURAL PRODUCTION

❐ The concentration of hunger in rural areas suggests that no sustained
  reduction in hunger is possible without special emphasis on agricultural and
  rural development.
  Source: FAO, The State of Food Insecurity in the World, 2006

❐ Productivity-driven growth in agriculture can have a strong positive impact
  on the rural, non-farm economy by boosting demand for locally produced
  non-agricultural goods and by keeping prices low.
  Source: FAO, The State of Food Insecurity in the World, 2006

6   AID SPENDING

❐ In a 1970 UN Resolution, most industrialised nations committed themselves
to tackling global poverty by spending 0.7% of their national incomes
on international aid by 1975. Only Norway, Sweden, Luxembourg, the
Netherlands and Denmark regularly meet his target.
Source: DATA (Debt, AIDS, Trade, Africa) facts map, 2006–2007

❐ The 22 member countries of the OECD Development Assistance
Committee, the world's major donors, provided US$ 103.9 billion in aid in
2006 – down by 5.1% from 2005.
Source: Organisation for Economic Co-operation and Development, 2007

❐ The largest donors were the United States (US$24 billion), Japan
(US$18 billion), the United Kingdom (US$13 billion), Germany and France
(US$12 billion each), the Netherlands (nearly US$6 billion), Spain and Italy
(just over US$4 billion each) representing 80% of the total.
Source: Organisation for Economic Co-operation and Development, 2007

7   WFP FOOD AID

❐ Since it was founded in 1962, WFP has fed more than 1.4 billion of
the world's poorest people and invested more than US$30 billion in
development and emergency relief.

❐ WFP's largest operation in 2006 was Sudan which targeted 6.1 million
beneficiaries. The operation accounted for 20% of total direct expenditure.
Source: WFP Annual Performance Report 2007

❐ Partners distributed 90% of WFP's food in 2006.
Source: WFP Annual Performance Report 2007

❐ 56% of WFP's emergency operations in 2006 were related to disasters.
Source: WFP Annual Performance Report 2007[44]

And, from the *Observer* article cited above we derive the following relevant
statistics.[45]

❐ 93 million acres of corn were planted by US farmers in 2007, an increase of
20% on 2006. Of this, 76% was used for animal fodder, while about 22% was
used to produce five billion gallons of ethanol.

❐ In 1985, the average Chinese person consumed 20 kg of meat, but by 2007
that had increased to 50 kg – and, of course, there were many more Chinese
in 2007 than in 1985.

❐ The World Food Programme had, in 2007, a shortfall of US$500 million, in
attempting to meet the food needs of 89 million needy people.

❐ The world's total population now (2008) is about 6.6 billion, but by 2050 it is
predicted to reach 7.2 billion.

- [ ] The cost of wheat in 2008 was 130% of what it was in 2007.
- [ ] The world's richest 20% consumed 16 times as much food (measured in calories) as the poorest 20%. Such a gross inequity in food cannot be sustained if global health equity is to be a reality.
- [ ] The cost of pork in China increased 55% between 2007 and 2008, while the price of rice worldwide has risen 30% from 1 April 2008 to 1 May 2008.

All of this may prepare us to consider the issues of ethics and global justice, which form the subject of the next chapter.

REFERENCES

1 Blunn W. *The Anti-Empire Report.* Available at: http://members.aol.com/bblum6/aer57.htm (accessed 17 May 2008).
2 Ziegler J. Biofuels are a crime against humanity. Speech to the UN General Assembly 3 May 2008.
3 *UN Condemns Biofuels Growth.* Available at: http://english.aljazeera.net/news/europ/2008/04/200861503650109945.html
4 James J. *The End of Cheap Food.* Available at: www.countercurrents.org/james040807.htm (accessed 17 May 2008).
5 Elliott F, Smith L. *Rush for Biofuels Threatens Starvation on a Global Scale.* Available at: http://offthegridgirls.wordpress.com/2008/03/13/rush-for-biofuels threatens-starvation-on-a-global-scale/ (accessed 20 Mar 2008).
6 Wikler B. *Biofuels: the fake climate change solution.* Available at: http://lists.kabissa.org/pipermail/pha-exchange/msg03753.html (accessed 20 Mar 2008).
7 The Rush For Biofuels. Available at: www.timesonline.co.uk/tol/news/environment/article3500954.ece?token=null&offset=12 (accessed 19 May 2008).
8 The End of Cheap Food. Available at: www.economist.com/opinion/displaystory.cfm?story_id=1025205 (accessed 19 May 2008).
9 Rosenthal E. *Biofuels Deemed a Greenhouse Threat.* Available at: www.nytimes.com/2008/02/08/science/earth/08wbiofuels.html (accessed 19 May 2008).
10 Searchinger T, Heimlich R, Houghton, R, *et al. Biofuels Produce Greenhouse Gases Through Land Use Change.* Available at: www.celsias.com/2008/02/13/the-last-straw/ (accessed 20 Mar 2008).
11 The Nature Conservancy. *New Study Raise Major Questions on Biofuels.* Available at: www.nature.org/initiatives/climatechange (accessed 19 May 2008).
12 UN: Intergovernmental Panel on Climate Change Open Letter Sent to US President Bush and Speaker-of-the-House Nancy Pelosi Urging Reconsideration of Biofuels Policy. 2007.
13 Agence France Press. *WFP Chief Warns EU About Biofuels.* Available at: http://afp.

google.com/article/ALeqM5hpCFf3spGcDQUuILK5JFV–6NL1Dg (accessed 20 May 2008).

14 US Food and Agriculture Organization (FAO). *Foodcrops and Shortages*. Available at: www.fao.org/docrep/004/w0486e/w0486e11.htm (accessed 20 May 2008).

15 Edwards R, Smith K. *The Year of Global Food Crisis*. Available at: www.sundayherald.com/misc/print.php?artid=2104849 (accessed 20 May 2008).

16 World Food Programme (WFP). *WFP Warns of 'Silent Tsunami' of Hunger*. Available at: www.straitstimes.com/Latest%2BNews/World/STI (accessed 20 Mar 2008).

17 India Today. *Grain Stocks Plummet in India*. Available at: www.//india-today.com/btoday/20011014/trends.html–24k (accessed 20 Mar 2008).

18 Stewart H, Elliot L. *Darling Calls for Urgent Review of Biofuels*. Available at: www.guardian.10.uk/environment/2008/apr/13/food.climatechange-

19 BBC News. *Robert Zoellick, Head of World Bank, Tackles Food Shortage Emergency*. Available at: http://news.bbc.co.uk/2/hi/business/7344892.stm (accessed 20 Mar 2008).

20 Withers J. National Farmers' Union. *The Scottish Farmer's Leader*. 30 Apr 2008. pp. 11–13

21 Scott J. *How Can We Return Power to the People?* Available at: www.telegraph.co.uk/news/youview/1552209/How-can-we-return-power-to-the-people.html (accessed 20 Mar 2008).

22 Maynard R. *Organic Farming Can Save the World*. Available at: www.sundayherald.com/display.var.2104849.0.0.P (accessed 20 Mar 2008).

23 Lockhead R. *Food Waste Processing in Scotland*. Available at: http://news.scotsman.com/views/Article.aspx?articleid=3314405–103k (accessed 20 Mar 2008).

24 Mitchell D. *High Food Prices – A Harsh New Reality in the 2008 World Bank Report*. Available at: http://web.worldbank.org/WBSITE/EXTERNAL/COUNTRIES/AFRICAEXT/CDIVOIREEXTN/0,,contentMDK:21665883~menuPK:382613~pagePK:2865066~piPK:2865079~theSitePK:382607,00.html (accessed 20 Mar 2008).

25 IRIN. *CARE Refuses to Handle Monetised Food Aid From the US Government*. Reported online by Robert Koppenleituer (of the People's Health Alliance); Rkoppenleituer@t-online.de (accessed 20 Mar 2008).

26 Clay E. *The Iron Triangle to Support US Food Aid*. Available at: www.innews.org/report.aspx?Reportid=74257 (accessed 20 Mar 2008).

27 US Governmental Accountability Office (GAO). *US Farm Practices are Wasteful*. Available at: www.nytimes.com/2007/04/14/world/14food.html (accessed 20 Mar 2008).

28 Odo G. *CARE Turns Down US Food Aid*. Available at: www.nytimes.com/2007/08/16/world/africa/16food.htm (accessed 20 Mar 2008).

29 Ibid.

30 Barrett C., Maxwell D. *Food Aid after Fifty Years: recasting its rôle*. London: Routledge; 2005. pp. 71–80.

31 Ibid.

32 Minot N. *Income, Diversification and Poverty in the Northern Uplands of Vietnam.* Washington, DC: International Food Policy Research; 2006.

33 *The Iron Triangle to Support US Food,* op. cit.

34 Hoddinot J. *Monetised Food Aid Under Scrutiny.* Available at: www.lists.kabissa.org/lists/archives/public/pha-exchange (accessed 19 Mar 2008).

35 McKie R, Stewart H. *Hunger-Strikes-Riots – The Food Crisis Bites. Observer.* 13 Apr 2008. pp. 22–3.

36 US Food and Agriculture Organization (FAO). *FAO Forecasts Continued High Cereal Prices.* Available at: www.fao.org/newsroom/en/news/2007/1000697/index.html–35k

37 *Robert Zoellick, Head of World Bank, Tackles Food Shortage Emergency,* op. cit.

38 Paulson H. *The Food Crisis Bites.* Available at: www.guardian.co.uk/environment/2008/apr/13/foodclimatechange–76k (accessed 20 Mar 2008).

39 Linday, R. *Inside Haiti's Food Riots.* Available at: www:/English.aljazeera.net/NR/exeres/B81DE374–B2B5–4247–B002–CA2A9D2A5B01.htm (accessed 22 May 2008).

40 Bernard J. An agricultural student at that time in Haiti, but now living in the Dominican Republic. Personal correspondence. 16 May 2008.

41 Personal conversation with student demonstrator François Bernard.

42 Personal correspondence with Graham Petrie.

43 *The End of Cheap Food,* op. cit.

44 US Food and Agriculture Organization (FAO). *Hunger Facts.* Available at: www.wfp.org/aboutwfp/facts/hunger_facts.asp (accessed 22 May 2008).

45 McKie R, Stewart H, op. cit.

Chapter 9

The barrier of moral parochialism

ROOTS OF THE PROBLEMS

We have in previous chapters already addressed eight barriers to global equity in health. By and large, the very first one – neoliberalism – heavily undergirds the subsequent seven barriers. While it doesn't directly *cause* all of them, it certainly is a major factor in providing a rationale for their existence and this may be of some small comfort to those of us who would rather not think about the deeper issues, especially when it presents us with the possibility of having to change our lifestyles. However, economics (which John Maynard Keynes referred to as the 'dismal science') may be classified as a 'social science', but is certainly not a physical science. Unlike physics, chemistry and biology it is not governed by a framework of irrefutable natural laws, which – unlike social laws – we are free to break.

We *can* break most economic laws, and frequently do, because economic laws only arise in the context of human social constructs. Thus, whatever we may have said about neoliberalism, we cannot throw up our hands and say, 'It is the will of God', or – more likely – 'There is nothing people can do about it'. In fact, we *can* modify economic laws – such as 'neoliberalism' generally, or even such fundamental ideas as the 'profit matrix' or the 'Law of Supply and Demand'.

Obviously, such changes are easier to bring about in small communities than in larger ones because, with fewer people, agreement about a course of action is more easily secured. But what determines the 'size' of a community? The physical size of the geographical area occupied by a given community used to be reasonably useful way of describing community size when humans could only move about by walking or by other relatively slow methods of surface transport. For thousands of years in human history even bodies of water could quite effectively separate communities and thus allow once minor differences between them to become more marked over time.

But advances in communication and transport have changed all of that. Different languages still create reasonably unbreakable barriers between different communities, but the exigencies of a complex matrix of international trade, the spread of common cultural forms of music and food preferences, are rapidly making us all one community. If a 'community' can be defined as a group that is so well integrated in behaviour and economics that disruption to any part of it effectively disrupts the whole, then all of the earth's people are rapidly becoming a single community. And the spread of communication, transport and trade (to say nothing of spread of disease) is, moreover, making ours a very small – and even a very frail – global village. The 'frailty' of our global village has been becoming more obvious to most people since the beginning of this millennium, due to our increasing awareness of such environmental problems as global warming and desertification.

If we manage to last long enough, generations far in the future will almost inevitably have to enlarge our psychological grasp of 'our village' to embrace a much vaster ambit than the Earth and its biosphere and to even include other planets. But that is well beyond the scope of this book! The point being made here is that our very survival depends upon us learning to think, plan and act in global, rather than regional, terms. And it does no good simply to blame neoliberalism, but to switch to a more globally sustainable system.

Such a project, though, cannot merely be a set of rules governing people 'from without', so to speak, but must be based on what governs us 'from within'. Anyone who has had experience of bringing up children or even teaching groups of people of any age, becomes very much aware of the fact that people can 'know' the rules, and can appreciate their general validity, but are often more strongly motivated to behave according to more personal and temporary desires. Whether we call it 'conscience' or 'super-ego', it has its roots in the need to protect and enhance an identifiable group of people. The 'social isolate' has much less survival power, say, than the family unit.

Over time, this extended – for good practical reasons – to include the 'clan' or 'tribe' – what the Greeks described as the 'ethnos'. In certain parts of the world, clan warfare still plays an important and defining social rôle. Those of us who have lived and worked in many parts of the Third World are very familiar with the issue, but it is also not entirely absent from recent European experience. Think, for instance, of vendettas in some cultures or of 'family feuds' in some remote Appalachian communities in North America.

It is instructive to consider what has been effective in overcoming these. One factor is certainly education. As people become literate and are in a position to find out about other groups and how they interact with one another and with whatever circumstance may throw at them, they find themselves able to overcome their 'parochialism'. That is, education definitely tends to enlarge the 'parishes' which inform our social views.

Nowadays, for instance, there are comparatively few places where Protestants and Catholics feel they are doing God's will by harming each other – or by even thinking about their religious differences at all as they work within a larger community of tolerance to enjoy themselves, to make a living and generally to get by. When the author was working in India in 1954, he quickly found that the more educated the local people were, the less they were concerned about caste differences or – even more broadly – differences between Hindus, Muslims and Christians.

Racial difference marked by different skin colouration is a more difficult issue because the visual impact of the difference makes an impression before one has had time to speak to another person, or to otherwise experience their company at a less superficial level. This author has only recently lost most of his sight and already finds that a pleasant side effect of this is that it is often only in the context of conversation that he realises that the other person is not of the same race.

THE CONCEPT OF THE NATION STATE

But our 'parochialisms' are also determined by 'nation', as a result of the so-called 'Peace (or Treaty) of Westphalia'. The word 'nation' has been with us, certainly since the earliest beginnings of recorded history, and probably even earlier. But, until fairly late in the 16th century, 'nation' referred to an ethnic group. 'Nations' were defined, as often as not, by what the people looked like and by what language they spoke.

However, things took a decisively different turn with the various treaties and border definitions which were formally established as the monumentally destructive Thirty Years War came to an end with the 'Peace of Westphalia'. It had raged on and off among the European states since about 1580. That war had seriously depleted the treasuries of many European states and had reduced vast swathes of their populations to levels of poverty, degradation and disease that had not been experienced for almost a century. However, the treaty that eventually ended the conflict was not a single decisive political act, such as, for example, the 1918 Treaty of Versailles. Instead, it really referred to a series of separate truces and peace deals between pairs of warring states running from 1618 to 1647.

The most important impact of these agreements was that the word 'nation' became defined predominantly by geography rather than ethnicity. Thus each nation

– over time – negotiated and/or fought to establish internationally recognised borders. This has prevailed, with a few minor changes, from then until the present day. Thus, the old League of Nations and the modern United Nations used the geographically defined 'nations' as the basic units in trying to mediate a workable mandate for peaceful coexistence and an end to large-scale warfare. All of this is described by the present author in another book.[1]

But what concerns us in this context is the modern concept of 'nations' with which we now live. The particular border definitions, and the concept itself, constituted the basis of 19th century European nationalism and they were more deeply entrenched in human psychology by the First and Second World Wars. For most of us now our 'parish' is no longer narrowly defined by family, clan or tribe, but by nationality. Nationality, of course, is not solely a matter of borders, but has taken on a huge cultural significance. All of the major art forms – graphic arts, music, literature and so on – are very strongly nationally defined and experienced.

WHY THE UN CONCEPT MUST SURVIVE
Therefore, one supposes that we cannot easily do away with 'nations' and replace it with some kind of transnational loyalty to 'one world'. Surely, national cultural differences will continue to delight and enthral the human spirit everywhere. But increasingly it is also clear that we have to survive as a planet with one biosphere on which we all depend for life.

Whatever faults we can identify with the United Nations (UN), it is by far the best concept for global survival generally that we have ever contrived. The defects can be assigned to four broad categories – organisational (too rigidly tied to the power and interest of a small and powerful coterie of nations), contradictions between the 'rights' of nation states and of individual people, conflict between various UN agencies, and a reluctance to act and think beyond national state interests. These have all been dealt with at length in one of the author's previous books, as cited above.

But globalised neoliberalism would have a much more disastrous impact on the lives of millions were it not for UN power and its representation in the public mind with some sort of morality that transcends national interests. The power and voices of neoliberalism in promoting (largely through their control of global media) disenchantment with the UN, and even with the UDHR, are increasing in stridency. These forces are anxious to portray the UN as a fat, lazy, inefficient and flabby bureaucracy.

While deficiencies in the organisation need to be recognised and acted on, the last thing we need is for it to be phased out altogether and for corporate interests to hold sway. And if we look at the evidence dispassionately, the picture of the

UN so eagerly promoted by Fox News and similar agencies does not stand up to scrutiny.

The UN has almost 55 000 staff. This may seem large but actually it is only about the same size of the Birmingham City Council, and no more than that of the New York Police and Fire Departments. Yet the UN's duties and responsibilities are far broader and more diverse than either of these. The above points were made to the author in a personal communication from Sir Richard Jolly, a deeply knowledgeable, well published and experienced Professor of International Relations at City University of New York and presently active as an advisor to the United Nations Association.[2]

This author's view is that the UN could be a much better advocate of human rights and mediator of international peace than it is at present. This can largely be achieved with a few administrative and structural changes at the organisational level by making the Security Council open by regular elections by all General Assembly membership and eliminating the idea of Five Permanent Members and their power to veto decisions of the General Assembly. But no matter how fair we make the structure of the UN on paper, it would be as foolish to argue that we could render it so perfectly adequate to the task as to the argue that it should be done away with.

Rather, as Jolly points out, the challenge is to set forth goals for the UN which can gradually lead to a widening of the parochial boundaries set by narrow nation state agendas. As this author has shown in previous books, the UN has, since 1948, achieved impressive goals for global health through the work of such agencies as UNICEF and WHO. We cannot afford to give it up!

NEOLIBERALISM AND THE FOOD CRISIS

In the last chapter, we dealt with the food crisis and it is interesting to consider how the UN, for instance, could be even more effective in coping with the problem without being so shackled by neoliberalism. In May 2008 the *Morning Star* reported that under its new President (Raul Castro) Cuba has blamed neoliberalism for the global food crisis.[3] This was not merely an academic observation, but was made in the context of a meeting at which solutions to the problem, at least at a regional level, were put forward and enacted.

As the article in question reported, a meeting (Food Sovereignty and Security Summit) was convened in Nicaragua on 8 May 2008 to consider the possibility of finding a regional solution to the growing food crisis. The Cuban delegate was reported as stating: 'The food crisis is a structural problem generated by unsustainable neoliberal economic policies.'

At the meeting, Venezuela offered US$100 million towards establishing an oil-for-food fund, where Latin American and Caribbean nations agreed to unite to eliminate the disastrous impact that rapidly rising food prices would otherwise have on the poorest families in the region. This is a perfect example of people developing economic policies in accordance with their needs, rather than assuming that 'economic laws' are beyond human adjustment.

Venezuelan Foreign Minister Nicolas Maduro said: 'We will devise a formula based on the price of oil and the level of production that would allow for the creation of a special oil-for-food fund, taking into consideration the means and needs of each country.' He pledged $100 million to kick-start agricultural investment for the region. Regional leaders agreed to press private banks to direct at least 10% of their total lending to farms. As well, Caracas suggested the creation of a 'Latin-American tax' on flights by non-Latin American airlines and to fund regional agricultural production with assets expropriated from drug traffickers.

According to the UN, food prices have risen 57% in one year and far more in the case of basic foodstuffs. In 2008, some 100 million more people than in 2007 are facing serious food shortages around the world.

Cuban Vice President Esteban Lazo pointed out that, a few decades ago, many countries in the region grew their own rice and corn, 'but, following the neo-liberal recipes of the IMF, they liberalised the market and began to import subsidised US and European cereals, eradicating domestic production. With the rise in prices at the pace we've seen, a growing number of people can no longer afford to eat basic food products.' He observed that: 'It comes as no surprise, thus, that they should take to the streets to find whatever means they can to feed their children.'

Mr Lazo declared that the food crisis 'is a structural problem generated by today's international economic order.'

The International Trade Union Confederation (ITUC) agreed, noting in a statement that 'the factors behind soaring food and agricultural commodity prices are part of the same set of global policies which have resulted in massive global financial instability and intensifying climate change and these three current global crises must be tackled through root-and-branch reform and effective regulation.'

ITUC general secretary Guy Ryder said: 'Large parts of the global agricultural system are built upon poverty wages and violation of workers' fundamental rights and no durable solution to the crisis can be found unless the appalling worker rights record in global agriculture is addressed.'

THE MORAL IMPERATIVE OF INTERNATIONALISM

The cultural advantages conferred by national consciousness need not (and must not) prevent an awareness of planetary parochialism, based on the well-substantiated realisation that – whatever we do within our respective nations – we cannot solve national problems in ways that are inconsistent with planetary survival. This is the moral imperative to which we must now adjust. The point is made by Robert Archer and Lawrence Gustin at Georgetown University Law Centre in Washington, US.[4]

This article opens with the question: 'What moral responsibilities do nation states have for one another in the field of health and welfare of one another's citizens?' The question is a pivotal one if we take the view that human survival requires a greatly reduced global inequity in access to health. As we have extensively documented thus far, there exist massive inequalities in health globally, with the result that poorer countries shoulder a disproportionate burden of disease and premature death. While poor countries have by far the greatest ongoing health needs, they also have the least capacity to meet those needs. In addition to the pervasive and debilitating effects of endemic disease, developing countries are likely to suffer far more from the effects of acute health hazards, ranging from natural disasters and dislocations, to emerging infectious diseases.

Certainly, governments and philanthropic organisations have responded to highly visible natural disasters, droughts and famines, at least while the issue remains salient in the media. And there has been increased international assistance for high-profile health threats such as AIDS and pandemic influenza. Even factoring in these new investments, most OECD countries have not come close to fulfilling their pledges to donate 0.7% of Gross National Income per annum to Third World aid.

The question then arises: If states have the capacity to assist less developed states (while continuing to fulfil their obligations to the health of their own citizens), to what extent do they have a well-defined legal or ethical responsibility to do so? We claim that states have a responsibility to help because of international law, political commitments, ethical values and national interest. However, international law does not enable states to operationalise this responsibility in specific cases and in a transparent manner. As a result, transnational cooperation by states tends to be ineffectual and inconsistent, although states can and sometimes do act effectively when ethical and legal responsibilities and commitments align with self-interest.

The above confronts us, then, with a question that must be addressed before we even think about applying band-aid to the gaping wounds of the lack of access of millions to clean water, let alone to healthcare. Paul Colliers phrased the question thus: How do we rescue the bottom billion?[5]

One-sixth of the planet's population are facing disaster, and – in economic terms – are slipping further behind. As the reader is aware, neoliberalism was supposed to be the ultimate answer, as far as development for less developed countries was concerned. What has become obvious in the past decade, though, is a pattern of *some* Third World countries (India and China are good examples) becoming much richer than they had been, but their development is more than matched by a precipitous decline in the fortunes of those LDCs which were already the poorest.

Poor countries showing signs of growth, such as India and Brazil, are well on their way to pulling themselves out of poverty, but there are a billion people living in impoverished countries showing no signs of economic growth. Paul Colliers argues that many developing countries are doing just fine and that the real development challenge is the 58 countries that are economically falling behind and getting caught in one or more 'traps': armed conflict, natural resource dependence, poor governance, and geographic isolation. Colliers's proposed solutions might well constitute some kind of middle way between the dangers of 'development' being promoted for the benefit of First World corporations and gross exaggerations of its advantages by local politicians.

Colliers does offer a solution, but entirely within the context of a continued reliance on neoliberal financial orthodoxy. He suggests that the G8 nations put forward four main 'action committees' to address the needs of those 58 countries, especially those which are emerging (or which have just emerged) from a situation of civil war.

1   Direct Economic Aid Committee – Channelling financial aid for post-conflict reconstruction and regional infrastructure development.
2   Five international charters addressing:
    i   national resources
    ii   democracy
    iii   budget transparency
    iv   post-conflict politics
    v   international investment.
3   A trade policy to help the 'bottom-billion' compete with Asia.
4   Limited military interventions.

Although most of this is beneficial it represents benevolence entirely as determined by First World agencies, but without local input, such as statements of perceived needs and with no local involvement in drafting the five charters. The idea of a trade policy to help the poorer nations trade with Asia leaves no room for those nations to determine Asian policies on the trade. This author would see such a procedure as exemplifying what used to be called 'benevolent imperialism' and this would surely be disadvantageous to the 'bottom billion' should the G8 nations economies fall into a balance of payments problem. Above all, it becomes 'charity', not a 'shared human responsibility.'

It leaves entirely untouched the scope for action of neoliberal business enterprises and it is these very same enterprises, as the author has argued in previous chapters that keep the bottom billion on the bottom. In fact, it could fairly be said that corporate power is one of the strongest forces shaping our world. More than half of the top 100 economic entities today are private corporations. With their immense size comes commensurate influence, to the point where corporations are able to wreak social and environmental destruction, with few serious consequences felt by themselves. Yet, amazingly, this subject is too often essentially absent from any study of economics.

The conservative economic theory that dominates the profession is based on the core belief that as little as possible should interfere with businesses' pursuit of profit. This approach to economics ignores history, politics, poverty, the natural environment, and social class, among other inconvenient realities. Conservative economics would almost be laughable, were it not for the fact that this way of thinking helps prop up the worst excesses of capitalism.

This becomes very clear with respect to the way that the WTO operates. In theory, it is one of the most democratic organisations in the world. Every nation state can attend their policy meetings at which trading rules affecting all of them are decided. But the trick is that any nation's delegate can be accompanied by as many lawyers and experts on trade law as they wish. It all looks benignly democratic but, in fact, it represents the art and power of exclusion perfectly. What happens is that those who already 'have' gain more, while those who 'have not' end up with less. Why? Because at WTO meetings, when subcommittees are formed to consider particular trade issues, they meet in parallel sessions. The First World nations, especially the US, have a sufficient number of specialists in attendance to send one to every subcommittee.

In this way democracy is excluded by neoliberalism. The analogy has been made with the Marxist idea of 'class war'. And after 30 years of neoliberal policies, the class war on behalf of the richer nations is becoming daily more intense. In previous chapters the author has discussed Naomi Klein's book *Disaster Capitalism*. In that book, she used the metaphor of 'torture' to describe the impact of shock therapy on poor nations.

Henry Giroux and Chronis Polychroniou, in a contribution to the online journal *Analysis* early in 2008, analysed the situation particularly effectively.[6] They do not make the common mistake of assuming that neoliberalism only has a malign impact on the Third World while being cosily accommodated in the social context of the First World. To see how mistaken such a view would be one only has to consider, say, children's health – or even health and human rights generally – in the US. The author will deal with that issue below, but first let us address ourselves to Giroux and Poluchroniou's analysis of global neoliberalism.

They see the situation in terms of a class war launched by the rich against the poor. This class war – easily seen as a war by the controllers of money, against the working class – is creating a situation in which it is utterly impossible to conceive of any higher level of community organisation than clusters of alienated people fighting over the necessities of life. This really is the predictable end-state of a system based on competition and unguided by any kind of overarching moral imperative. It is parochialism that even falls below the parish level and where the individual is the only unit that counts.

Among 'liberal' thinkers the view is common that the disadvantages of neoliberalism are only to be found in Third World societies. At present, they are certainly more evident in that context, but as we shall see, neoliberalism has no national loyalties. It is utterly unprejudiced in who it exploits and hence is socially insidious. This is becoming increasingly evident in the most recent analyses of social damage in the US and in the other large, well-off, industrialist nations of the First World. Yet the media (largely owned and controlled by corporate interests) would still have us believe that with the advent of neoliberalism we are now privileged to be living in a gilded age in which everything is a commodity and anything is for sale.

As Giroux and Poluchroniou describe it, stories abound about the lifestyles of celebrities and billionaires who spend $50 000 to have their dogs groomed or hand over a mere $20 million to take a ride into space. At the same time, nothing is reported about the destructive power of corporations and market fundamentalism on every facet of life. Governments around the world, from neoliberal to social democratic ones, are promoting policies that transfer wealth from the many to the few and shaping in the process the conditions for ravaged and broken societies beset by poverty, unemployment, social malaise and discontent, crime and police brutality.

As social inequality drives the engine of a ravaging neoliberalism, the global marketplace wages a war against social citizenship, the social contract, and all vestiges of the public good. Various reports over the years by supra-governmental institutions, such as Social Watch, UNICEF, and UNDP have drawn attention to deteriorating socio-economic conditions around the world. Internationally renowned economists, such as Joseph Stiglitz and Paul Krugman, decry the undemocratic and unethical agenda of the neoliberal elite.

With power loosened from traditional modes of politics, public policy has been hijacked by global corporate elites and the state has been forced to abandon its comprehensive social welfare agenda in order to cater to the needs of the plutocrats. Wedded to the belief that the market should be the organizing principle for all political, social, and economic decisions, neoliberalism wages an incessant attack on democracy, public institutions, and non-commodified values. Privatisation, deregulation, commercialisation, and cuts in social spending rule the day and the prevailing mentality is that everything is for sale, and what is not for sale has no value as a public good or practice.

In the United States, George Bush repeatedly vetoes major spending measures that would have funded education, healthcare and job training programmes, but eagerly signs bills that increase Pentagon funding and strengthen the military-industrial complex, while transferring billions of public funds to the coffers of private firms and corporations.

In Central, South-eastern and throughout Eastern Europe, governments are vying to downsize the public sector and to privatise as many social services as they can get away with. Higher education itself is increasingly being replaced by the goals and values of the market. Governments under-fund tertiary education in order to open up the sector to private market forces – a recommendation long made by the World Bank – and seek to convert higher education into a form of training for the needs of corporate and digital capitalism.

There is a clear correlation between neoliberal policies and incarceration rates. As the strongest advocate of neoliberal policies, the United States incarcerates about eight times more of its people per capita than does any Western European country. The state under neoliberalism does not disappear as much as it gets reconstructed, largely as a repressive force for providing a modicum of safety for the rich and privileged classes while increasing its focus on the disciplining and displacing of those sub-populations and groups that pose a threat to the dominant social order.

As the state becomes 'hollowed out', so to speak, and public services are either cut or privatised, repression increases and replaces compassion as real issues – long-term unemployment, poverty, homelessness, youth violence, and drug addiction – are overlooked in favour of policies that favour discipline, containment and control.

Today's political-economic and social culture is reinforced by fear and insecurity about the present, and a deep-seated scepticism in the public mind, and for these reasons worry about the future leads to a more pessimistic outlook for the present. As the discourse of neoliberalism seizes the public imagination there is no vocabulary for political or social transformation, democratically inspired visions, or critical notions of social agency to enlarge the meaning and purpose of democratic public life. Ideas and freedom are associated through the prevailing ideology and principles of the market, and the public feels there is no alternative. Hope is foreclosed while a sense of quiet despair is regarded as 'realism'. What, then, explains the rise and dominance of neoliberalism and how do we challenge it?

The reasons for this historically unique and totally obscene one-sided class warfare, which has caused so much human suffering and destruction, are many and varied. They range from structural changes in advanced capitalist economies to the impact of the collapse of socialism; they vary from the distancing of power from traditional modes of politics, because of the impact of negative globalisation, to the emergence of militarised states; the celebration of a new social Darwinism, and an ongoing war against minorities of class and colour who have become the human waste products of globalisation. Moreover, the left appears to be suffering from a conceptual and political crisis plagued by deterministic thinking, on the one hand, and refusal to theorise the need for new forms of individual and social agency within the geography of transnational capitalism, on the other.

FROM MOTOWN TO NOTOWN

Examples abound. Consider, for instance, the state of the automobile industry in the US. As a result of such splendid instruments of neoliberalism as GATS, NAFTA and a host of other bilateral and multilateral 'agreements' (except that the affected employees and their union representations never agreed!) job security is becoming an outdated concept. To assume that this has no ethical or moral implications is a serious mistake, for it has gutted communities and has high-profiled a sense of pessimism in broad swathes across the US itself. Detroit – once called 'Motown' because it was the hub of the automobile manufacturing industry – could now more realistically be called 'Notown' because it is no longer a cohesive community.

As a result of Henry Ford's pioneering attempts in the early 20th century to organise a more efficient way of manufacturing cars (and other commodities), the term 'Fordism' entered commercial vocabulary as a descriptor of what represented a new stage of capitalism. It brought ethical changes with it, as it reduced workers to assembly line cogs. But neoliberalism has now further eroded even the small 'parish' of the factory. In fact, the latter has probably closed down.

How can these trends be addressed and remedied? Again we turn to Giroux and Polychroniou's analysis. As they point out, the reorganisation of the labour process – having shifted away from industrial capitalism to a post-Fordist, highly mobile form of production, often accompanied by violently opening up of the world's markets – has greatly transformed the relation between capital and labour. As a result of the revolutionary development brought about by the new technologies and information systems work relations, the labour process, and income distribution have been redefined and reshaped according to the commands and logic of global capital. The conflict between an industrial labour force and industrial capital no longer defines the basic relations in advanced capitalist society. The industrial labour movement has become quite weak and with the sharply increasing atomisation of working people, the balance between capital and labour has been radically altered.

In their analysis, they also point a finger at the corporate-owned media, as the author has in previous chapters. This has taken place in the context of the moral impoverishment of many intellectuals, by virtue of their growing refusal to speak out critically about the unjust social order, and to more energetically oppose this massive ideological triumph of neoliberalism.

Any real challenge to neoliberalism can only come through the reclaiming of a language of power, social movements, politics, and ethics. This calls for a discourse capable of examining the effects of the neoliberal order on labour, the environment, culture and all others of those spheres and spaces in which democratic identities and relations of power that are essential to viable forms of political agency. Educators and intellectuals must link learning to social change, recognising that every sphere of social life is open to political action.

In our societies, perhaps especially in the First World, an entire panoply of ideologies and social relations currently offered by consumerism must be challenged by producing new public spheres, places, and spaces that forge the knowledge, identifications, emotional investments, and social practices necessary to produce political subjects and social agents capable of extending and deepening the bases of radical democracy. The school, the workplace, the market, the cultural terrain must become infused with critical consciousness and critical and practical engagements with present social behaviours, institutional formations and everyday practices.

This, sadly, is most evident in our institutions of higher education. That entire arena of the formation of societal values cries out to be reclaimed as an ethical and political response to the demise of democratic public life. Higher education needs to reassert itself in the democratic project and society must come again to the realisation that learning is more than preparing students for employment. Citizenship must be appreciated as more than conspicuous consumption and being part of the cheap, banal entertainment provided by most of today's TV networks. Likewise, democracy is more than making choices at the nearest supermarket. Higher education is not only about issues of work and economics, but also has to concern itself with questions about justice, social freedom, and self-development. Higher education must principally be focused on seeking expression of a guiding social morality, a higher good, and express itself as a mission to expand the human imagination.

To confront the deadly politics of capitalist globalisation, a transnational democratic political movement must develop that not only recognises the changing nature of globalisation under the imperatives of capitalism, but also provides those forms of educated hope that offer the grounds for creating public intellectuals and social movements capable of linking education to critical agency, and linking learning to broader global considerations and social issues.

But this is none other than a call to recover from the corporate power structure and the bankers our sense of what it means to be a human – not just a Detroit car worker or even a US citizen – but a world citizen.

What this author, then, has argued so far is that neoliberalism has in many respects already privatised and alienated us to the degree that we have become complicit in dividing ourselves – race from race, and nation from nation. That makes it possible for it so easily to narrow the boundaries of our social parishes. The moral imperative is, as emphasised in the final chapter, to reassess our humanity and worth by expanding our parish to include all of the world's people. It is all too often the case that, when neoliberals use the phrases 'democratic' and 'individual rights', they undermine this idea.

REDISCOVERING 'DEMOCRACY'

That is, we need to overcome the tendency of neoliberalism to continually reduce the size of our parish – to privatise and alienate us – if we are ever able to overcome 'institutionalised' global inequities, and in the long term, to survive as a civilisation. The author uses the phrase 'institutionalised' advisedly, because we have been conditioned to believe that market forces (rather than ethics) decide all important issues and that therefore the global control of trade by the rules of neoliberal finance, is a 'given'.

These ideas, by their very nature, are alien to neoliberalism. The latter sees democracy as synonymous with free markets, while issues of equality, social justice, and freedom are stripped of any substantive meaning and are used to disparage those who suffer systemic deprivation and chronic punishment. Individual misfortune, like democracy itself, is now viewed either as an excess or as being in need of radical containment. As Giroux and Polychroniou so eloquently phrase it: 'Democracy, as both an ethical referent and a promise for a better future, is much too important to cede to a slick new mode of authoritarianism, advanced by advocates of neoliberalism and other fundamentalists.'

If we value the hard-fought-for Western idea of 'democracy' as a social ethic, transcending 'getting and doing what we want' and if it is to provide us with a theoretical framework, a practical means of achieving community purpose, social justice must be our goal. And if it is to be used in the interests of social justice, such as in a real and sustained renewal of the labour movement, the struggle for the social state, and the necessity to confront hierarchy, inequality, and power as they now prevail in an era of rampant neoliberalism, we must recognise that world peace is the only possible context for it.

Ultimately, then, the issue becomes a moral and ethical one if we are seriously to undertake any kind of broader project, which allows us to implement the 'routine' configurations of political democracy in matters of global representation, participation, and shared power. The stakes are too high to ignore such a task. We live in dark times and the spectre of neoliberalism and other modes of authoritarianism are gaining ground throughout the globe. We need to rethink the meaning of democratic politics, take risks, and exercise the courage necessary to reclaim the pedagogical conditions, visions, and economic projects that make the promise of a democracy and a different future worth envisioning and fighting for. These considerations now allow us to consider some of the practical impacts on First World life of neoliberalism's assault on the need for a global parish, as we consider changes to life expectancy figures for women to the US.

SHORTER LIVES FOR US WOMEN UNDER NEOLIBERALISM

In April 2008, the *Washington Post* ran an alarming article on changes in the US to the lifespan of women, and much of the following is drawn from it.[7] The item begins by observing that for the first time since the Spanish flu epidemic of 1918, life expectancy for a significant number of US women is falling. In fact, in nearly 1000 counties that together are home to about 12% of the nation's women, life expectancy is now shorter than it was in the early 1980s, according to a study published early in 2005. The downward trend is evident in places in the Deep South, Appalachia, the lower Midwest and in one county in Maine. It is not limited to one race or ethnicity but it is more common in rural and low-income areas. The most dramatic change occurred in two areas in southwestern Virginia (Radford City and Pulaski County), where women's life expectancy has decreased by more than five years since 1983.

The trend appears to be driven by increases in death from diabetes, lung cancer, emphysema and kidney failure. It reflects the long-term consequences of smoking, a habit that women took up in large numbers decades after men did, and the slowing of the historic decline in heart disease deaths. It may also represent the leading edge of the obesity epidemic. If so, women's life expectancy could decline broadly across the United States in coming years, ending a nearly unbroken rise that dates back to the mid-1800s.

'I think this is a harbinger. This is not going to be isolated to this set of counties, is my guess,' said Christopher J L Murray, a physician and epidemiologist at the University of Washington, and who led the study. It is being published in *PLoS Medicine*, an open-access journal of the Public Library of Science. Also quoted was Elizabeth G Nabel, director of the National Heart, Lung and Blood Institute of the National Institutes of Health: 'The data demonstrate a very alarming and deeply concerning increase in health disparities in the United States.'

The study found a smaller decline, in far fewer places, in the life expectancy of men in the USA. In all, longevity is declining for about 4% of males. The phenomenon appears to be not only new but distinctly American. 'If you look in Western Europe, Australia, Japan, New Zealand, we don't see this,' Murray said.

About half of all deaths in the United States are attributable to a small number of 'modifiable' behaviours and exposures, such as smoking, poor diet and lack of exercise. Although it is impossible to know exactly what is going on in the 1000 counties, Murray thinks it 'would be a reasonably obvious strategy' to target them for aggressive public health campaigns.

Life expectancy, of course, is not a direct measure of how long people live. Instead, it is a prediction of how long the average person would live if the death rates at the time of his or her birth lasted a lifetime. For that reason, life expectancy can dip or rise abruptly. The death rate from the Spanish flu was so high, especially among the young, that life expectancy fell by about seven years in 1918. But it rebounded quickly when the epidemic was over.

In general, though, it takes huge forces to drive down life expectancy over longer periods. The AIDS epidemic has done so in some African countries. In the early 1990s, the social disruption following the collapse of the Soviet Union decreased life expectancy of Russian men by six years and of women by three years; this was an unprecedented decline in a modern industrialised nation. In the study, Murray and collaborators at the Harvard School of Public Health (as cited in the *Washington Post* article) examined mortality and cause-of-death data for the United States from 1961 through 1999. They divided the country into 2068 units, including cities, counties or combinations of counties.

Across that four-decade period, average life expectancy nationwide increased from 66.9 years to 74.1 years for men and from 73.5 years to 79.6 years for women. From 1961 to 1983, life expectancy went up everywhere for both sexes. This was largely because the death rate from heart attacks, which had been rising for half a century, began to fall in the late 1960s. There were two reasons. Huge numbers of people lowered their chances of having a heart attack by modifying 'risk factors,' such as smoking, hypertension and high cholesterol. Improvements in medicine – coronary care units, use of aspirin and beta-blocker drugs, and various surgical procedures – greatly increased survival in patients with heart disease. About two-thirds of the longevity gained over the past four decades has come from the decrease in cardiovascular deaths.

These changes were so dramatic that even the poorest and least healthy groups benefited. In fact, counties with low life expectancy in 1961 had steeper rises over the next dozen years than counties that started out with high life expectancy. Overall, the drop in heart attack deaths more than offset rising mortality from cancer, emphysema and diabetes during this period.

By the early 1980s, however, the rapid gains were coming to an end. The low-hanging fruit on the tree of heart attack prevention and treatment had been picked. Further strides tended to happen mostly in places where people were already healthy and long-lived. As a consequence, the rise in longevity began to stagnate in places with the least-healthy people. In those counties, life expectancy increased by only one year (from 74.5 to 75.5) between 1983 and 1999, while in the healthiest places, life expectancy of women had reached 83. It was during this interval that women's life expectancy fell in nearly 1000 counties in the USA. If one adds counties where it rose only insignificantly, then 19% of

American women – nearly 1 in 5 – are now experiencing stagnating or falling life expectancy.

The trend was far less pronounced for men. That is because they entered the 1980s with higher death rates from heart attacks than women, and thus gained more from better prevention and better treatment. In the 1990s, however, AIDS and homicide began to take large tolls, depressing male life expectancy in some places.

Murray's team, which also included Ari B Friedman of Harvard and Sandeep C Kulkarni of the University of California at San Francisco, used Internal Revenue Service data to check whether high levels of migration, or migration of people with particularly high or low incomes, might explain the discrepancy between the 1000 counties and their neighbours. They found no evidence for it.

Unlike some European countries, the United States does not collect health information other than birth and death statistics at the local level. Instead, there are national, state and regional surveys of people's health, behaviour and access to medical care. Trends those studies have picked up shed light on what is happening in the 1000 counties.

Obesity has risen markedly in the past two decades, with women more affected than men. About 33% of women are now obese, compared with 31% of men. Extreme obesity is more than twice as common in women (7%) than in men (3%).

Being overweight greatly increases the risk of developing Type 2, or 'adult-onset,' diabetes. A national survey in 2002 found that 85% of diabetics were over-weight or obese.

In recent years, the prevalence of high blood pressure has been increasing in women, as well; this is partly the result of weight gain. In 1990, 42% of women older than 60 had hypertension; by 2000 it was 51%. (In men, the trend is still dropping, as it has been for several decades.)

'This is a story about smoking, blood pressure and obesity,' said Majid Ezzati, of the Harvard Initiative for Global Health, a co-author of the paper.

But she could also have said that it is a story about how neoliberalism uses advertising to isolate people from one another, to emphasis the 'glories' of private ownership, of gaining competitive advantages over others and pandering to self-indulgence through consumerism at all levels. This is all used shamelessly by advertisers, both to create feelings of inadequacy and loneliness and to then offer 'solutions' by purchasing something. The supermarket becomes a metaphor for our times, not a place to meet and relate to neighbours, but a place to 'buy' a feel-good factor and to compete with others as well as to gradually undermine both one's psychological and physical health while doing so.

The industry of popular culture is replacing that of ideology. Nowhere more can this be seen than in the influence that advertising and propaganda has gained over us. We all have lived long enough to witness the absolute victory of advertising and propaganda.

Advertising is, of course, the notorious enemy of promise. It is nakedly capitalist and as far away from human rights as can be possibly be imagined – for everything, as well as everybody and every principle clear to us, is for sale. Advertising soothes our pain, our anguish of loneliness and of ignorance, especially the pain of wanting without knowing what is wanted. No wonder advertising and propaganda are popular; 'they show us the road ahead', they are thus not part of the problem; they solve things the easy way.

Advertising does not brainwash us, it stains our brains! It is based on the belief that ignorance, if backed up by sufficient dollars, becomes wisdom. Through it, knowledge exercises power over us from on high. On issues that matter in the world (for instance human rights), 'Mall America' and the aspirations of the 'gym generation' lead to the distraction of our contemporaries. Uncertainty is at the heart of what we are; nothing is written in stone, and everything can crumble, we are told. This, again, is an ethical issue and one that can only be overcome by seeking a larger, mutually supportive parish and thus to enlarge our own moral parochialism.

In this author's view, it would not be surprising if US people, with their typical verve and audacity, were to lead the world out of this isolating loss of our humanity. And, he would also argue that it will be the health issue that prompts the turn-around. For in the US mounting healthcare costs are becoming a major factor in bankrupting its citizens and/or driving them to despair with worry. If that is the trigger, it will be the healthcare system as a whole which becomes overhauled. It is now confusing, chaotic, with no over-all national control and needs to be taken out of the hands of business and to be taken over by government, because government (in a democracy, like that in the US) is ultimately responsible to voters and taxpayers, rather than to a small coterie of stockholders.

COULD THE US LEAD THE WAY TO REFORM?

This, in turn, could have a much wider impact on life in the US by energising people to look at other areas of their life that are dominated by corporate interests. Having thereby released so much scope for democratic action in their own society, it would not be long before that influence was felt beyond the country's borders and throughout the world. These views and possibilities are addressed further in the final chapter.

We did come close to this scenario under President Bill Clinton's administration. There had been mutterings long before he became President, to the effect that the US badly needed a national health service of some sort and, no doubt, these mutterings had a cumulative impact on political thinking over the years.

Then, in 1992, Bill Clinton put the call for universal healthcare at the centre of his programme. But, once president, his closeness to Wall Street and his intellectual dependence on Robert Rubin, also of Wall Street, and whom he appointed as Secretary of the Treasury, made him leery of antagonising the insurance industry.

It was President Clinton's unwillingness to confront the insurance companies that led to his failure to honour his commitment to work toward a universal healthcare programme. The type of reform President Clinton called for was a health insurance-based model called 'managed care', in which insurance companies remain at the centre of the process. An alternative approach could have been to establish a publicly funded healthcare programme (which was favoured by the majority of the population) that would cover everyone, providing medical care as an entitlement for all citizens and residents. This could have been achieved, such as by expanding the federal Medicare programme to cover everyone. To do so, however, would have required neutralising the enormous power of the insurance companies with a massive mobilisation of the population against them and in favour of a comprehensive and universal healthcare programme. Neoliberalism in the US was too well-entrenched to allow that to happen, at that time, but it is this author's view that this marks a temporary set-back only.

President Clinton's loyalty to Wall Street prevailed. His administration's top priorities were reduction of the federal deficit (at the cost of reduced public social expenditures) and approval of NAFTA (without amending President George HW Bush's proposal, which Clinton had inherited, and refusing to address the concerns of the labour and environmental movements). These actions antagonised and demoralised the grassroots of the Democratic Party. Clinton lost any power to mobilise people for the establishment of a universal healthcare programme. This frustration at the grassroots level, and especially among the working class, also led to the huge abstention by the Democratic Party base in the 1994 congressional elections and the consequent loss of the Democratic majority in the House, the Senate, and many state legislatures. At the root of this disenchantment with the Clinton administration was its unwillingness to confront the insurance companies and Wall Street. Could that happen again? We may well know, even before this book is published!

The trends at the global level also encourage belief that a moral response may gradually be attaining ascendancy over neoliberalism. This is reflected in a recent release by PAHO (Pan American Health Organization).[8]

At the heart of the right to the highest attainable standard of health lies an effective and integrated health system, encompassing healthcare and the underlying determinants of health, responsive to national and local priorities, and accessible to all.

The Human Rights Council, in its decision 2/108, requested the Special

Rapporteur on the right of everyone to the enjoyment of the highest attainable standard of physical and mental health, to identify and explore the key features of an effective, integrated and accessible health system from the perspective of the right to health, bearing in mind the level of development of countries. Their report is a response to that request.

There is a growing recognition that a strong health system is an essential element of a healthy and equitable society. In any society, an effective health system is a core social institution, no less than a fair justice system or democratic political system. However, according to a recent publication of the World Health Organization, health systems in many countries are failing and collapsing.

The narrowing parochialism dictated by neoliberalism must be addressed as an ethical issue even more urgently than as an issue of efficiency or cost. As things stand now, even medical science is being undermined to serve the needs of neoliberalism, and in this, Big Pharma, as previously discussed, is highly implicated. Consider, for instance, the area of public health and the growing science of epidemiology. Neil Pearce,in a recent article in the *International Journal of Epidemiology*, showed how and to what degree epidemiological research was being hijacked in the interests of Big Pharma.[9] Indeed, corporate influences on epidemiology have become stronger and more pervasive in the last few decades, particularly in the contentious fields of pharmacoepidemiology and occupational epidemiology. For every independent epidemiologist studying the side effects of medicines and the hazardous effects of industrial chemicals, there are several other epidemiologists hired by industry to attack the research and to debunk it as 'junk science'.

In some instances these activities have gone as far as efforts to block publication. In many instances, academics have accepted industry funding which has not been acknowledged, and only the academic affiliations of the company-funded consultants have been listed. These activities are major threats to the integrity of the field, and its survival as a scientific discipline. There is no simple solution to these problems. However, for the last two decades there has been substantial discussion on ethics in epidemiology, partly in response to the unethical conduct of many industry-funded consultants. Professional organisations, such as the International Epidemiological Association, can play a major rôle in encouraging and supporting epidemiologists to assert positive principles of how science should work, and how it should be applied to public policy decisions, rather than simply having a list of what not to do.

And, of course, a by-product of the imposition of neoliberalism across a wide spectrum of inequalities can obviously only exacerbate the situation. That is, it is intended to (and will) put the 'haves' in an even stronger position, and put the 'have-nots' further down the queue. This is not only particularly disastrous when applied to health, and to access to healthcare, but also unambiguously easy to document.

As Keith Moser at the London School of Hygiene and Tropical Medicine has demonstrated, health inequities (both between and within countries) persist and for almost all diseases and general health problems.[10] Between countries, both average life expectancy and child mortality figures have shown a considerable improvement only in the wealthier countries, but a continuing decline in most less developed nations. This has been so, even when most countries' progress on redressing health inequities is uneven – because their internal economics are dominated by neoliberalism – and the data has not always been available over time. Michael Marmot of University College in London, from analysis of 22 countries, for which relevant data was available, established that only 5 of them had reduced health inequities in childhood mortality across income from 1995 to 2000.[11]

EXACERBATING CLASS WAR AGAINST THE POOR

Before moving onto the closing section of this chapter, let us examine one example of the impact of neoliberalism on the health of the already disadvantaged – the very people who a system guided by ethics would treat with the greatest consideration.

On 28 March 2008, the Johannesburg *Star* ran a story about a new policy (enacted in the name of business efficiency) by which the Johannesburg City Council ceased making access to free supplies of clean water to those earning less than US$1.00 per day. The *Star* headline screamed: 'TARIFF INCREASE ESCALATES THE WAR ON THE POOR' and told how the regular supply of free basic water (FBW) to the destitute was to be stopped. What people, unfamiliar with the situation there before this policy was enacted, would not realise is that the new measures were not imposed suddenly. There was plenty of prior committee work, but the local NGO Anti Privatisation Forum (APF) was not consulted about the proposal.[12]

The shock headline in the *Star* that the City of Johannesburg is doing away with its Free Basic Water (FBW) policy is not as abrupt as the newspaper proclaims. Tariff hikes for basic services hit the poor hardest and the 85% increase in the price of water announced in the 28 March edition would certainly necessitate 'illegal' connections for poor households. Enquiries to the office of the mayor by the Coalition Against Water Privatisation in response to the *Star*'s article have shown, however, that the plug hasn't been entirely pulled on free water. But what the story confirms more than anything else is that the commodification of water has indeed made water users vulnerable to arbitrary increments.

According to the Coalition's mayoral source, the tariff increases are to take effect on 1 July 2008. These increases in the costs of water, electricity, sanitation and refuse removal will be open to public comment. While the APF and the Coalition Against Water Privatisation have not received any information or seen contracts about the proposals, such action can only invite the escalation of struggle for access to basic resources by the poor. All Johannesburg households will get 10 kL FBW per household per month, but unlike the current 6 kL FBW allocation, this will fall away if you use more than 10 kL. If you use 11 kL or more it will be as though there was no FBW at all and you will be paying at the rate of R2.50 for every kilolitre from 0 up to 6kL; and R4.40 per kL from 6kL to 10kL. For every kilolitre from 10kl to 15kl you'll pay R5.90, and so on, in stepped tariffs. At May 2008 rates, 15R = 1UK£ (approx).

The indications are that poor households will also be induced to accept prepaid meters under the new tariff regime. The *Star* reported that tariffs charged to households using a prepaid meter will be lower than those tariffs applied to credit-metered consumption. Accordingly, R3.40 will be charged per kilolitre in the 7–10kL range for prepaid water users, and R4.00 per kilometre consumed in the 11kL–15kL range. If the *Star*'s report is accurate on differential tariffs for prepaid and credit meters, the FBW policy will become all the more a cynical ploy to get poor users to cut their consumption. Research conducted by the APF in Phiri in Soweto in 2006, after prepaid meters were introduced, showed that each household consumed, on average, between 8.7 and 15.3 kiloliters of water per month. The pressure to limit consumption to the 10kL threshold, therefore, will become stricter and will confirm secondary findings of the research that water users will flush the toilet less, bath less regularly and thus increase levels of poor health and stress in the household. One cannot help but suggest that a morally based system would take human dignity into account!

To soften the blow for poor households, a revamped indigency register will accompany the increased tariffs. Not only is the present system hopelessly inadequate and inaccessible (if ever proof was needed then one only has to look at the one-fifth of poor households that are presently on the register), but the humiliating means-testing that goes along with registering as an indigent requires that the poor – in other words, those least able to do so – register themselves. The City plans a big publicity campaign to publicise the indigency register, but there are no guarantees that the changes to the registration process will be made before the proposed changes to the FBW policy and tariff increases. The registration of indigent households is only a flimsy cover for the City's unwillingness to do what they know they should be doing – namely, providing adequate and accessible free basic services to the poor.

It is not surprising to the APF that there are these proposed increases by the municipality since the 2002 privatisation of City management. Johannesburg Water, City Power and Pickitup are run as municipal business entities regulated by their profitability. From the onset in 2000 of the neoliberal, micro-economic plan, the APF has mobilised affected communities against the privatisation of basic services. The tariff hikes proposed by the City are only the latest salvo in the war against the poor. This transpires in a context in which more than 50% of the community is dependant on government grants and more than 40% is unemployed. The APF rejects tariff increases as they overlook these harsh realities and measure need according to profitability.

From all of the information so far in this chapter, one surely can only conclude that neoliberalism, especially in its close involvement with advertising and the media, has already weakened the moral bases for effective and harmonious community life throughout the world, not least in the more economically favoured parts of it, and that a precondition for reducing the global health inequity gap, is to address the moral and ethical issues. To make the point more emphatically, I will not apologise for closing this chapter with reference to a timely book by an American thinker – the sort of person who will hopefully be very much involved in helping us address neoliberalism intelligently and creatively. The man in question is Morris Berman and the book is *Dark Ages America – The Final Phase of Empire*.[13]

DARK AGES AMERICA – CAN THE WORLD SURVIVE IT?

Berman begins his sombre book with a comment to the effect that anybody who had voted for the incumbent President, George W Bush, would find his book incomprehensible. On that point this author would disagree because people vote the way they do because the choices they are given are largely illusory. But Berman goes on to comment that more of his countrymen are worrying about what appears to be the USA's 'terminal decline'.

As he sees it, the 'American Empire' was already in its twilight phase when Ronald Reagan, with a bland disregard of history, declared his election as president as 'Morning in America'! Twenty-odd years later, under the 'boy emperor' George W Bush (as Chalmers Johnson refers to him), the US have entered the Dark Ages in earnest, pursuing a short-sighted path that can only accelerate its decline. For what we are now seeing are the obvious characteristics of the West after the fall of Rome: the triumph of religion over reason; the atrophy of education and critical thinking; the integration of religion, the state, and the apparatus of torture – a troika that was for Voltaire, the central horror of the pre-Enlightenment world; and the political and economic marginalisation of our culture. Of course, the Dark Ages were not uniformly 'dark' – as any informed historian would argue – and neither is America completely dark. Space does not permit this author to give this book the attention it deserves except to strongly recommend it to the reader, but he would like to briefly consider Berman's comments about torture in the context of describing the moral crises we must overcome.

Torture, of course, is prohibited under the Geneva Convention. Generally speaking, some European countries, the UK and the US can be said to have adhered to it and – as a matter of course – eschewed the practice. Of course, there were exceptions. British servicemen known to the author claimed to have tortured prisoners during the Malaya Emergency and some US and some Australian servicemen were strongly suspected of torturing prisoners during the Korean War. But such activity was generally held to be disgraceful, and not only was it not often spoken of, but it was never government policy. Multitudes of ordinary US, British and Australian citizens even believe that it could never have occurred.

What about the situation now?

Today, especially since the attack on the World Trade Centre in New York in 2001, the idea of using torture, of even legalising it, has crept back – after decades of virtual silence – into everyday conversation. Our newspapers have even carried photographs of it being done by US service personnel and there is, in official circles, even serious debate as to how much fear or suffering one may legitimately inflict on another person without calling it 'torture'.

As Berman says in his book, we associate the use of torture with the Dark Ages (Were no prisoners tortured in prisons by the British in Northern Ireland?) and he asks, rhetorically, whether the USA has returned to using it with full public knowledge? Does not America have its own gulag in Afghanistan and Guantanamo Bay?

He points out that the US not only condones torture carried out in other countries, but is perfectly open in using the 'evidence' derived from such procedures to condemn prisoners in its own courts. In fact, the US now routinely transfers suspects to Saudi Arabia, Egypt, Syria and Morocco to secure information obtained through torture as a basis for conviction back in the US. Indeed, there is even evidence suggesting that the UK has cooperated in these extraordinary renditions.

Of course, the torture used in these places does not stop at waterboarding, but includes starving prisoners, hanging them from the ceiling, subjecting them to electric shocks, forcing objects up their recta, tearing their fingernails out, and fracturing their spines. It seemed, though, as time went on, that US officials were willing to be pretty brutal themselves. Since Abu Ghraib, there have been periodic revelations in the press about American-led torture being worse, and more widespread, than previously thought. Articles began appearing with headlines such as 'The US Military Archipelago', or 'Secret World of US Interrogation'. Phrases used in these unflinching reports include 'worldwide constellation of detention centres', 'elaborate CIA and military infrastructure,' and 'global detention system run by the Pentagon'.

America has been transformed 'from a country that condemned torture and forbade its use to one that practices torture routinely.' Americans began torturing prisoners after 9/11 and never really stopped. For example, the near drowning of suspects, or waterboarding, a technique long used in Latin American dictatorships, is now common to us. Yet there was no outcry over any of this, and the few congressional hearings that took place were 'distinguished by their lack of seriousness'. And what should we make of all of this in light of the post-2004 election outcome? Alberto Gonzales, the man who wrote the legal briefs justifying the use of torture, is now, in Orwellian fashion, Head of the Department of Justice! Add to this the substantial evidence that many of these practices are a standard feature of the domestic prison system, and America's return to the Dark Ages would seem to be complete.

HAS THE US MARGINALISED ITSELF?

Although torture is a theme that Berman addresses at length, it was not his only basis for arguing that US civilisation has entered a new Dark Ages. He quotes, for instance, the fact that the US's infant mortality figures are among the highest in the more developed nations and that the WHO categorises the US's health service as only the 37th best in the world.

He concludes that, by many of its recent actions, the US has marginalised itself from the world community and can no longer be regarded as a serious civilising influence. Again, this author is not that pessimistic, feeling that books like Berman's will stimulate a spirit of moral renewal among educated US citizens. Anyone familiar with American culture cannot write off this jewel in the crown of human greatness so easily.

Berman goes on to say:[14]

> The American legal system, at one time the world standard, is now regarded by many other nations as outmoded and provincial, or even barbaric, given our use of the death penalty. That we have lost our edge in science to Europe, that our annual trade deficit (half a trillion dollars) reveals a nation that is industrially weak, and that the US economy is being kept afloat by huge foreign loans ($4 billion a day during 2003)? What do you think will happen when America's creditors decide to pull the plug, or when OPEC members begin selling oil in euros instead of dollars? The Boston Globe actually compared our habit of borrowing against the future to that of ancient Rome, and an International Monetary Fund report of 2004 concluded that the United States was 'careening toward insolvency.' Meanwhile, while America is spending hundreds of billions of dollars on phoney wars, the money is piling up in Europe and Asia, and in 2003 China finally supplanted the United States as the number one destination for worldwide foreign investment, with France weighing in as number two. Almost any of our domestic economic problems, writes the *Washington Post*, 'is a greater threat to the economy than virtually any imaginable form of terrorism.' And in response, we do nothing about it.

Rome in the late-empire period is the obvious point of comparison here, and it is important to remember that it did not so much fall as fall away as it became socially and economically nonviable, as its military was finally strained to the breaking point by what has been called 'imperial overstretch.' Rome simply became irrelevant on the world stage. Power eventually flowed to the Eastern (Byzantine) Empire, and the revival of Europe, when it began in the eleventh century, occurred elsewhere, to the north. As for the United States, all that awaits it on the domestic front is bankruptcy and popular disaffection; internationally speaking, we'll be looking at second- or third-rate status by 2040, if not before. History is no longer on our side; time is passing us by, and the star of other nations is rising as ours is sinking into semidarkness.

As far as the impending collapse of the US's hegemony in world affairs is concerned, Berman sees the events of 9/11 as some kind of 'coup de grace'.

If all of this has been under way since the 1960s or 1970s, it is clear that something as horrific as the 9/11 attack might well have been anticipated. In the wake of that event, civil liberties were severely compromised, the already huge gap between rich and poor was rendered even more extreme, and the USA began to behave like a rogue nation, acting as a law unto themselves. The nation's whole posture has been one of dealing with symptoms, crushing external manifestations; sophisticated analyses of the underlying causes of terrorism – let alone of how they might address these – have a hard time becoming part of public dialogue. Phraseology such as: 'They hate freedom' or 'They are jealous of us', does not exactly qualify as sophisticated. So 9/11 has entered US national mythology as a day on which the United States, a decent and well-meaning nation, was attacked by crazed fanatics hell-bent on destroying its way of life. All indications are that this is how it will be remembered – but possibly only by Americans!

Berman is convinced that it will definitely not become the day on which they began to reflect on their own fanaticism, on how they were living, and on how historically, they had treated the peoples of the Third World. He argues that it is not likely that such a day of self-examination will ever come to pass. It will, in short, serve the very blindness that brought it on, and that is doing the US in. Whatever the outcome of the war on terrorism, or its war on America, one could argue that the terrorists are already winning, in that they have managed to 'push us further along the downward trajectory we were already on'.

This author, however, is much more optimistic about the USA's eventual rôle, and it is US writers such as Berman that reinforce his view. It should be clear to the reader that Berman's book should not be regarded as simply one 'American' exhorting his erring countrymen – although it is that – for it constitutes a warning to all of us. This consideration of his comments constitutes an appropriate close to our listing and analysis of some of the barriers we must overcome if we are to seriously move toward tomorrow and close that global health gap. Until we do, we live in peril.

In the last chapter, we shall briefly recall the barriers identified in previous chapters, and how we might go about considering alternative approaches to rediscovering our common humanity and making the world a safer and happier place for generations to come.

REFERENCES

1 MacDonald T. *Health, Human Rights and the United Nations: inconsistent aims and inherent contradictions.* Oxford & New York: Radcliffe Publishing; 2008. pp. 9–11.

2 Personal correspondence with Sir Richard Jolly, 2008.

3 Neoliberalism to Blame for Food Crisis. *Morning Star.* 9 May 2008. p. 3.

4 Archer R, Gustin L. The duty of state to assist other states in need: ethics, human rights and international law. *J Law Med Ethics.* 2007; 35: 526–27.

5 Colliers P. *The Bottom Billion: why the poorest countries are failing and what can be done about it.* Oxford: Oxford University Press; 2007.

6 Giroux H, Polychroniou C. *The Scourge of Global Neoliberalism and the Need to Reclaim Democracy.* Available at: http://onlinejournal.com/artman/publish/article_2959.shtml (accessed 25 May 2008).

7 *Life Expectancy Drops for Some US Women.* Available at: http://tinycurl.com/316bz5 (accessed 26 May 2008).

8 PAHO. *Promotion and Protection of all Human Rights.* Available at: EQUIDAD@listserv. patio.org (accessed 25 Mar 2008).

9 Pearce N. Corporate influences on epidemiology. *Int J Epidemiol.* 2008; 37: 46–53

10 Moser K. *Inequity in Death Rates Increases.* Available at: www.Ishtm.ac.uk/news/2005/ deathrates.html-8k (accessed 26 May 2008).

11 Marmot M. *Only Five out of Twenty-Two Countries Reduce Health Inequities Among Children.* Available at: www.who.int/social_determinants/strategy/en/Marmot-social%20 (accessed 26 May 2008).

12 Anti-Privatisation Forum [letter]. *Star* 24 Mar 2007. p. 11.

13 Berman M. *Dark Ages America.* Available at: www.bullnotbull.com/archive/dark–ages–america.html (accessed 27 May 2008).

14 Berman M. *Dark Ages America: the final phase of empire.* New York: WW Norton; 2006. p. 2.

Chapter 10

What can we do now?

IMPROVE AND USE THE UN

Our corporate-owned media delight in telling us that the United Nations is a defunct organisation that has passed its sell-by-date and should be discarded. They point to its various spectacular failures to adequately defend human rights in Rwanda, Darfur, Kenya and Myanmar, to the venality and outright corruption of various members of its staff, its bloated inefficiency and so on. But even a cursory examination of the UN's record of achievement will quickly show – as pointed out in the preceding chapters – that much of this anti-UN campaign is prompted by the well-founded belief that the UN, its agencies and rules, impede and restrict the global thrust of neoliberalism.

The fact is that the UN had certain defects (not evident to its founders at the time) built into the way it was established. These have become more evident in the six or so decades of its life, and now amount to a well-marked pattern of internal contradictions and inconsistencies. These, indeed, have been exhaustively described in the author's *Health, Human Rights and the United Nations*.[1] But if we are to surmount the barriers to global equity in access to healthcare, we desperately need the UN. It is our only, and best, defence against unrestrained neoliberalism. What is required, then, is to remedy the structural defects in the UN, *not to abolish it*.

It is the UN which has given us the Universal Declaration of Human Rights (UDHR) and it is the UDHR which has enshrined health as a basic human right, where the word 'basic' simply means 'non-negotiable'. Moreover, the WHO (established in 1948), has as its first mandate, to defend and promote that basic right. From 1948 on, it has pursued this mandate by running an impressive array of immunisation programmes worldwide, mediating research in various aspects of public health and epidemiology, and establishing clinics and health training centres.

In 1978, at Alma-Ata, the WHO held a conference at which it developed and approved the now famous Alma-Ata Declaration (AAD). As described in the author's book, cited above, it was the AAD that first made it the basis of WHO philosophy that 'health' was to be treated more as a social/economic phenomenon than a purely biomedical one.[2] That is, whether an individual is healthy or not generally depends more on whether or not he/she is content, at ease with his/her community, fulfilled in his/her employment, and adequately housed more than on various clinical or biomedical criteria. The implication of this realisation means that health has to be recognised as a political issue, and it is this realisation that has led public health professionals today to lay such stress on what they call 'the social determinants of health'.

That is why the continuing gross inequity in access to health globally cannot be resolved by the most inspired and diligent medical research, elaboration of new vaccines and understanding of the rôle of genetics in such grave conditions as Alzheimer's disease on their own. These things can only be effective within the context of a political framework and a social philosophy than can effectively accommodate them. And we need a transnational body with the authority to be both an advocate and a mediator with respect to the exercise of such politics. That, indeed, is the function of the World Health Organization and of such agencies as UNICEF.

But, as indicated very strongly in one of the author's later books, neither the WHO nor the UN are adequately meeting this challenge.[3] As previous chapters of this book have made abundantly clear, the present worldwide financial power of neoliberalism has become a major obstacle to the UN and their agencies. Various thinkers, including this author, have over the years suggested alternative approaches which could allow the UN to become more effective in making a reality of the UDHR.

Jeffrey Sachs, for instance, writing in *Scientific American*, suggests ten resolutions which, if adopted by the WHO (and hence the UN) could ensure the right to health globally and at a very modest cost.[4] As he points out, at the launch of the WHO in 1948, the world's governments agreed that health is a basic human right 'without distinction of race, religion, political belief, economic or social condition'. Then, at Alma-Ata three decades later, the WHO adopted an ambitious proposal for achievement of health for all by the year 2000 (HFA2000). As pointed out by the author this was never achieved, prompting Kofi Annan (then Secretary General of the UN) to draw up eight of what he called 'Millennium Development Goals' (MDGs) to be achieved by 2015.[5] These were not intended to replace the HFA2000 targets (of which there were 38) but to bring us to the point at which we could realistically begin to prepare for them. However, as the author shows, there is virtually no prospect that we will even achieve the MDGs!

THE GLOBAL FUND COULD BECOME UN-INCORPORATED

Originally called the Global Fund to Fight AIDS, Tuberculosis and Malaria (GFATM) the body is now more often simply called the 'Global Fund' as its arena of action has widened since its inception.[6] The Global Fund is not a UN agency, but there is little reason as to why it cannot become so. Indeed, it was first proposed by Kofi Annan in 2001, while he was General Secretary of the UN. It officially came into being as an independent public/private partnership in 2002. Although international in organisation, staffing and funding, it is (as of now) a Swiss non-profit foundation.

Around fifty countries have pledged money to the GFATM so far. Many of these are wealthy Western or Middle Eastern nations, although pledges have also been received from countries directly affected by AIDS, TB and Malaria. Uganda for example has pledged $2 000 000 to the Fund, while Burkina Faso has given $75 000. The biggest single donor country is the US, whose donations make up around 33% of the funds pledged every year.

It is already highly coordinated with the UN as the following indicates. The Fund is governed by an international board of nineteen voting members and four non-voting members. Voting members include government representatives from donor and recipient countries as well as representatives from affected communities, private sector businesses, philanthropic foundations and NGOs. Representatives of UNAIDS and the WHO also participate as ex-officio (non-voting) members, as does the World Bank, and these serve as the Global Fund's trustees. The Board is assisted by committees that advise on ethics, policy and strategy, finance and auditing, and management of the portfolio. A large group of stakeholders known as the Partnership Forum also meet twice a year to review progress and provide advice and suggestions to the Fund's board.

Over 120 different nations, from Afghanistan to Zimbabwe, have benefited (or will benefit) from Global Fund money. The full list, along with detailed progress reports, can be found on the Global Fund website. In January 2007, about 55% of the money was going to sub-Saharan African nations, 25% to East and South Asia, the Middle East and North Africa, 10% to Latin America and the Caribbean and 10% to Eastern European and Central Asian countries.

To receive money, a country's government (or even an individual organisation) will need to make a grant application. The GFATM has a policy of only giving money to those who apply for it, unlike some other funding programmes (such as President Bush's PEPFAR, the President's Emergency Plan For AIDS Relief scheme) which actively seek out suitable recipients and offer them money. This means that in theory, funding is available to anyone who needs it. The only restriction the Fund has is the amount of money available in their central bank account. There are, for example, no 'quotas' as such on how much money is spent on each disease. This is governed strictly by need, allowing greater flexibility in tackling the most urgent crises.

In November 2007, around 58% of funding was being spent on HIV and AIDS, 24% was being used to fight Malaria and 17% was going on Tuberculosis programmes with the remainder being spent on general health system strengthening. The amount given to joint TB and HIV programmes has increased significantly over the last few years, reflecting the close link between the two diseases (those with HIV are far more likely to develop TB).

An important part of any country's funding application process is the negotiations that take place with their Country Coordinating Mechanism (CCM). In every country that wishes to receive funding from the Global Fund, a CCM will be set up to help organise and submit grant applications to the Fund and monitor their implementation. A CCM will generally be made up of a broad range of representatives from government agencies, NGOs, local community and faith-based organisations, individuals working in the field and private sector institutions.

When the grant is approved and the money arrives, it is given to the principal recipient (PR), which is basically the body that is legally responsible for distributing it or using it to tackle HIV, Malaria or TB in the country designated. The PR is often a government department or agency, but it can be a local public or private organisation, and several different PRs may exist within one country. The day-to-day administration of the fund is mediated by a Secretariat of 70 people based in Geneva, Switzerland. The description which follows is derived from the Fund's own publicity material.

The board of the Global Fund does not have the power to dictate who should donate money nor how much should be donated, but it does issue guidelines on how much will be needed to maintain funding and to approve new grants. Major developed countries are expected to meet a proportion of this estimate dependent on their GDP, though pledges are essentially made on a 'goodwill' basis (with the obvious political kudos that this may bring). This allows the funding level estimates to be increased in the event of an emergency.

The Fund also now has a system based on regular periodic replenishments, which enables more accurate forecasting of available resources over the coming years. This replaces a more 'ad hoc' and flexible system of replenishment that was used in the early years to attract new donors who may otherwise have been wary about committing large sums to an untested scheme. To implement the new system, special 'replenishment conferences' are now held on a regular basis, facilitating debate about the Fund's needs and encouraging potential new donors to enter into discussion and offer pledges.

The Global Fund goes to great lengths to make sure that the money given in grants actually reaches the right people. To make sure this happens, every PR is allocated a local fund agent (LFA). The LFA is an independent organisation contracted by the Secretarial to administer and verify the correct allocation of the funding.

Grants are usually made on a two-yearly basis. At the end of that period, an assessment is made as to how wisely the funding has been used so far. If the results are positive, the grants can be renewed for up to five years. The entire process is more in keeping with what one would expect of a non-profit public body, such as the UN, than of a public-private enterprise. In fact, bodies like the IMF could do worse than to learn from Global Fund procedures.

In the early years of the Fund's operation, pledges were not made to any set schedule. In the first year of the Fund's operation, most countries pledged a large amount sufficient for several years of funding. Any extra resources that were necessary were then negotiated on an ad hoc basis. However, this method eventually led to the appearance of funding gaps (where the amount of money held by the Fund was less than the total needed to fully finance grants) so in 2005, a new system was implemented. The first three 'Voluntary Replenishment Conferences' were held in Stockholm, Rome and London. These conferences enabled donors to see the extent to which the Fund would need to be replenished in 2006 and 2007, and to pitch their pledges accordingly. Donations for 2008 and beyond were negotiated in three similar meetings in 2007.

Partly because the need to so vigorously check the bona fides of the organisations receiving grants, complaints have sometimes been made over the slowness of its response. But in some countries this need to check, especially in poor countries that lack facilities for organising administrative means of monitoring and paperwork involved, can cause long delays. It is also a problem in countries that already have highly bureaucratic governmental processes in place. In June 2004, for example, India was allocated $140 million dollars for HIV and AIDS treatment, yet for over a year the grant remained unsigned and no money was disbursed. During this time, around 80 000 people are believed to have died from AIDS in India. The problems have since been resolved, but for this to happen, funding had to be cut, and a new management team brought in to administer the money. Unfortunately, the problems encountered in India are not unique, and a number of other countries, including Kenya and Uganda, have struggled to quickly and efficiently distribute the large sums they have received from the Global Fund.

The Global Fund is not designed as an implementing organisation, and as such, it cannot intervene directly to facilitate the distribution of funds. However, in August 2005, the GFATM did announce the launch of a new Early Alert and Response System (EARS) to help overcome some of the problems with slow implementation. EARS is designed to be a support mechanism that will alert everyone involved in a particular grant project to any potential hold-ups. Action can then be taken by the government of the country concerned, or another 'facilitator'. In the case of India (mentioned above) this facilitator was the Clinton Foundation, a US globally deployed charitable funding body.

From what has been said about the Global Fund so far, the reader will be able to see why it is ideally structured to deal with the 10 proposals that follow. But as the following lines suggest, it could be far more effective as a UN agency in its own right. As such, it could more adroitly fight off the inroads of neoliberalism, which the IMF and the World Bank have not been able to do as effectively as might be wished.

Many of the countries that receive Global Fund grants are also countries that are covered by the World Bank and International Monetary Fund's Heavily Indebted Poor Countries (HIPC) scheme. HIPC was set up in 1996 as a way of helping countries out of the crippling external debt they acquired by accepting extensive loans from the World Bank and IMF in the 1970s, 80s and 90s. The scheme works on a conditional basis. That is, in order to receive debt relief, a country has to agree to meet certain economic and financial criteria as outlined by a personalised 'Poverty Reduction Strategy Paper' (PRSP). The problem lies in the fact that this PRSP contains 'targets' for spending on public services that can effectively become 'limits' if more money than is budgeted for comes into a country.

One such example is Uganda. When the country received several large grants from the Global Fund a few years ago, it sparked arguments between the health and finance ministries who, not wishing to go against IMF guidelines, refused to increase the country's healthcare budget to take into account the value of the grants. Had the Ugandan Health Ministry agreed to accept the full value of the grants at the rate intended, it would have effectively pushed a massive amount of money out of the department's existing budget for healthcare. Although this does not sound like a problem in principal, the money given by the Fund was specifically intended for AIDS, TB and malaria, meaning all other areas of healthcare would have suffered extensive budgetary cuts.

The World Bank and the IMF have officially denied the active limitation of healthcare budgets in Uganda and elsewhere. However, many governments still impose restrictions because they believe it is the only way to maintain a good relationship with their debtors. The reasoning behind this strategy is that rapid exchanges of foreign cash can quickly increase the value of a nation's currency and therefore the price of its exports. This, say many finance ministers, could adversely affect competitiveness and displease the IMF. But, as the 2004 UNAIDS report on the Global AIDS epidemic states: 'The short-term inflationary effects of increased and additional resources applied in tackling the HIV epidemic pale in comparison with what will be the long-term effects of half-hearted responses on the economies of hard-hit countries.'

Sachs' proposals, which follow, will now seem much more feasible and provide a way of overcoming some of the obstacles to global equity in access to health discussed in previous chapters.[7] They are eminently practical and would fit in with WHO's mandate and the AAD in particular.

SACHS' TEN PROPOSALS:

1 Affluent countries should devote 0.1 % of their gross domestic product to healthcare for low-income countries. With a rich world GDP of US$35 trillion, that would create a fund of roughly US$35 billion a year; this is enough for US$35 per capita in added health services for the roughly one billion people who need them.

2 Half the increase should be channelled through the Global Fund to Fight AIDS, Tuberculosis and Malaria. The Global Fund has proved to be a highly effective institution, with minimal bureaucracy and maximum impact. It has supported the distribution of approximately 30 million antimalaria bed nets; helped to get nearly one million Africans on antiretroviral treatment and helped to cure more than two million people of TB.

3 Low-income countries should devote 15% of their own national budgets to health. Consider a poor country where the average income is US$300 a year. The total national budget might be around 15% of GDP, or roughly US$45 per capita. 15% of that figure devoted to health would come to just US$6.75 per person per year: not enough to provide adequate basic healthcare on its own, but combined with US$35 per capita from donor aid, it would do the job.

4 The world should adopt a plan for comprehensive malaria control, aiming to bring malaria mortality nearly to zero by 2012 through comprehensive access to antimalaria bed nets, indoor spraying where appropriate, and effective medicines when malarial illness arises.

5 The rich countries should follow through on their long-standing and achievable commitment to ensure access to antiretrovirals for all HIV-infected individuals by 2010.

6 The world should fill the financing gap of roughly US$3 billion a year for comprehensive TB control; this is another area where known and long-proved interventions are highly effective, but chronically underfunded.

7 The world should honour, for just a few billion dollars a year, the access of the poorest of the poor to sexual and reproductive health services, including family planning, contraception and emergency obstetrical care.

8 The Global Fund should offer roughly US$400 million a year for comprehensive control of several tropical diseases (mainly worm infections), which occur in virtually the same regions in which malaria is rampant.
9 The Global Fund should open a new financing mechanism to bolster primary healthcare, including – most importantly – the construction of clinics and the hiring and training of nurses and community health workers.
10 Using recent breakthroughs in medicine and public health, the expanded health systems in the poorest countries should be equipped to handle noncommunicable diseases that have long been neglected but which are treatable at low cost: in other words, hypertension, cataracts and depression.

These simple steps could save the lives of nearly 10 million adults and children a year, at a cost that would be nearly unnoticeable to the world's wealthiest nations. These measures would also slow, rather than accelerate, population growth in impoverished regions, thereby easing the economic and environmental strains that bulging populations are imposing on them. Health for all is not only the moral imperative it was at the launch of the World Health Organization 60 years ago, it is also the best practical bargain on the planet.

The reader will recall that, at the 2005 G8 Summit at Gleneagles, the 8 richest nations of the world agreed to devote 0.7% of their GDPs (7 cents out of every US$10.00!) to aid programmes, and that really *would* have made poverty history. To date, none of them have met that target, although a few countries who are *not* in the G8 (e.g. Norway) have done so. But if the G8 nations did increase its aid in this way, it would more than meet the costs of Sachs' ten proposals.

BRINGING EXISTING CORPORATE POWER TO HEEL

But, as we have seen, it is corporate power which holds the whip hand over much of what the UN and its other agencies are able to do. It is true that some alternative suggestions for a more efficient and fairer way to run the world would argue that corporate power would have no place in such a dispensation. Perhaps this is true, but in the meantime corporations do need to be bound by explicit rules governing human rights. This is perfectly consistent with the UDHR and provides yet one more example of the scope still left for the UN to more effectively exercise its influence in the UN's mandated defence of human rights.

This was well and explicitly stated by Peter Fuchs and Lionel Plank for the NGO Corporate Watch, on the need to enact legislation 'with teeth' to keep corporate commercial interests in line with the UN's UDHR.[8] Under UN rules, this is binding on all member states and has been from the UN's beginning in 1944. An edited and abbreviated version of their recommendation follows:
1 Corporations must be held to account on human rights.

2   Corporations must not be allowed to decide on rights implications of proposed policies without the oversight of civil authorities.
3   Corporate Social Responsibility (CSR) must be explicitly defined in each case.
4   Ideally, CSR (sometimes called 'social accountability') must be monitored by non-corporate civil society agencies.
5   Laws governing corporate action must be clear and explicit – no marketing of harmful products and tight controls on advertising content.
6   Voluntary codes should not in themselves be regarded as adequate.
7   Grassroots political input must be rigorously insisted upon in enforcing CSR.
8   'Market forces' cannot be relied upon to guarantee fair or equitable outcomes.

And, of course, one of the closest links between neoliberalism and the widening health equity gap is provided by the pharmaceutical industry, as detailed in Chapter 4.

Biochemical and physiological research has led to, and continues doing so, a huge array of spectacular pharmaceutical breakthroughs and have thus played a major rôle in improving the quality (and length) of people's lives. But, as Michael Santoro puts it, 'The industry has delivered miracles, but in recent years they have been throwing it all away by putting personal profit on a far higher plane than responsibility to suffering humanity'.[9] Many instances of this have been detailed in Chapter 4.

Public opinion is rightly rather cynical about drug companies and their claims to social concern. This is reflected in increasing complaints about overcharging and use of TRIPS. These tendencies are particularly strong in the US because it is so widely known that such things do not prevail to the same extent next door, in Canada. As well, there is much critical public comment about unethical practices in testing drugs on people in LDCs and pressures brought to bear on scientific journals to report favourably on results so obtained.

Pharmaceutical advertising definitely has a bad reputation, replete with accounts of 'bribes' (in the form of free lunches and expensive trips to conferences, and so on) offered to physicians as inducements to use their products. Particularly disgraceful has been the tone of the debate over the rôle of Big Pharma in marketing antiretrovirals to Third World countries, as discussed in Chapter 4. It is unarguable that this has often given the general public a negative view of biomedicine generally, and has been seized upon by alternative therapies (e.g. homeopathy) to promote their own unproven nostrums.

While it is true that many life-enhancing pharmaceuticals have resulted from Big Pharma's efforts, many people cannot afford to access them, especially in the Third World. Contrast this with such high-profile First World conditions where GPs are offered a panoply of markedly similar treatments eagerly endorsed by a well-funded market, with the Third World, where only very few options are available for scourges such as malaria. As unsolicited advertisments on our computer screens make evident, Big Pharma promotes erectile dysfunction remedies much more vigorously than it does ailments leading to large numbers of deaths.

If we look for the root cause of this distorted alignment of effort, we are confronted by such questions as: How big is the gap between profits and public health? What must we do to bridge this gap? How do we balance the intellectual property rights of pharmaceutical corporations with the basic human right to health?

As we know, private enterprise can do a marvellous job of stimulating creativity and innovatory approaches that can capture the public imagination, but what is perhaps not so widely understood is that it can also restrict access to important products. Nowhere is this truer than in the pharmaceutical industry, where it not only can (and does) restrict access but also distorts medical priorities of both nations and individuals.

Santoro points out that it is now incumbent on the pharmaceutical industry to become far more transparent and to increase communication and cooperation with health promotion community advocates and with stakeholder groups. It must be seen as part of public health enterprise. In that way, both the industry itself and the general public will come to see it more as part and parcel of various popular health advocacy groups, NGOs and local hospitals, all engaged in a drive to prevent disease and to improve health, than as a highly secretive money-making parasite.

But, as suggested above, it is unrealistic to assume that corporations driven first and foremost by the neoliberal competitive ethos and a 'profits before people' policy can self-regulate their behaviour. There has to be a series of controlling and accountability mechanisms. One way of achieving this in the UK, for example, is to have representatives of the firm concerned to actually be present at one of the regularly convened GP/patient group meetings. Minutes of these are held in local authority offices. The second suggestion will be far more difficult to implement, but is vital. It recognises, after all, that the health and welfare of citizens cannot remain effectively determined by semi-arcane commercial interests alone, but must be more broadly accountable.

As Santoro states:[10]

> Inaction is not an option for the pharmaceutical industry. The void from the absence of cooperation and partnership with stakeholder groups will be filled ineluctably by increased government regulation, including the spectre the industry probably fears most – price controls. The loser in this eventuality will not be just the pharmaceutical industry, which will inevitably be less profitable. Society,

too, will lose because the heavy hand of government regulation and bureaucracy, although sometimes necessary, can rarely function as efficiently and creatively as coalitions of diverse groups, including government, working together. Therein lies the moral imperative for change in the pharmaceutical industry – the hope for a future where society continues to enjoy a steady stream of drugs to improve health and well-being and where these fruits are broadly distributed among rich and poor, and throughout the globe.

PREVENTING WAR

The first rôle envisioned for the UN, when it was established, was to prevent international conflict. That it has not succeeded is obvious, because we have had almost continuous warfare since 1945. But it has played a paramount rôle in preventing war between the large industrial nations and in preventing (so far) nuclear war.

Although it may strike the reader as excessively cynical to suggest that perhaps the reason for the lack of a nuclear war since those first two atomic bombs were used on Japan in 1945, is that there is no clear way of making a financial profit out of it. It is (so far) too difficult to restrict the range of its effects, both geographically and over time. The distribution of radiation fallout, after the initial detonation, is determined by such a complex matrix of meteorological factors that it is virtually impossible to predict which areas will be affected and how badly. In the same way, what we have learned – not only from the Hiroshima and Nagasaki blasts, but also from subsequent above-ground nuclear tests – about the genetic implications of nuclear radiation has not been reassuring.

Corporate involvement in the nuclear power industry is already considerable and, as the author's research on the issue reported in a previous book shows, it has strong financial reasons for wanting to avoid a nuclear war.[11] Indeed, the IAEA (International Atomic Energy Agency) a UN agency, was shown in that book to not only be a proponent of the construction of nuclear power stations for such domestic purposes as electricity generation, but to have elaborated various methods for restricting research into and discussion about the negative effects of nuclear radiation.

But, even if we ignore nuclear war, corporate interests are only too happy to get involved. And this is not a recent phenomenon. From the late 1800s, US capitalism has been intimately involved with warfare as business in its own right. A well-known account of that was given by the late Major General Smedley D Butler who, after retirement from a working lifetime as a professional soldier in the US Army, had time to reflect on the deeper meaning of what he had been doing. His remorse and honesty led him to make the following comment, quoted by Leo Huberman and Paul Sweazy:[12]

I spent thirty-three years and four months in active military service as a member of this country's most agile military force – the Marine Corps. I served in all commissioned ranks from Second Lieutenant to Major-General. And during that period, I spent most of my time being a high class muscle-man for Big Business, for Wall Street and for the Bankers. In short, I was a racketeer, a gangster for capitalism . . .

Thus I helped make Mexico, and especially Tampico, safe for American oil interests in 1914. I helped make Haiti and Cuba a decent place for the National City Bank boys to collect revenues in . . . I helped purify Nicaragua for the international banking house of Brown Brothers in 1909–1912. I brought light to the Dominican Republic for American sugar interests in 1916. I helped make Honduras 'right' for American fruit companies in 1903. In China in 1927 I helped to see to it that Standard Oil went its way unmolested.

During those years, I had, as the boys in the back room would say, a swell racket. I was rewarded with honours, medals, and promotion. Looking back on it, I feel that I could have given Al Capone a few hints. The best he could do was to operate his racket in three city districts. We Marines operated on three continents. (*Common Sense*, November, 1935.)

The passing decades have changed little, except the technology, as evidenced by another quote, this time by the US author, Thom Hartman.[13] He has written extensively on the issue of corporate power and, specifically, the link between war, neoliberalism and oil. But his message is very similar to Major General Smedley Butler's, and both suggest (perhaps unwittingly) a solution:

I thought of it as dinosaur blood when it dripped on my hand this morning, and it made me wonder how the US war strategy would change if Saddam made a small recalibration in his business practices.

Of course, the gasoline that spilled as I refilled my rental car this morning at the Washington airport – and the refined kerosene that will fuel the plane I'll fly in today – is far more ancient than even the spectacular Tyrannosaurus Rex bones discovered north of here. They vanished around 65 million years ago, but the fossilized plants and bacteria that made my gasoline are 300 to 400 million years old. By the time dinosaurs ruled the Earth, pretty much all of the oil production of the planet was finished. Strange, when you consider it in those terms, that we'd base a nation's foreign policy on a limited supply of fossils older than the dinosaurs.

But Saddam Hussein has a goodly supply of those fossils under the soil of Iraq – the second largest supply in the world, and perhaps a supply even larger than Saudi Arabia's, which has been draining much faster and much longer. And he has hundreds of miles of shared borders with Saudi Arabia, Kuwait, and Iran – where much of the rest of the oil in the region is held.

Which led me to wonder: How would things change if Saddam, tomorrow, were to say, 'I've decided to put my oil reserves up for auction to the highest corporate bidder, and, like many other oil-producing nations, all I want is a commission from the oil company that wins the auction.'

Once the stampede was over, I'll bet the US would discover that there are dozens of dictators in the world more vicious than Saddam. Robert Mugabe of Zimbabwe, for example, has engineered a cynical strategy of racial exploitation that has pushed six million of his citizens into famine today. Burma's ruling junta has turned that nation into a slave-labour camp, where torture, executions, and terror are daily fare. And in North Korea, the policies of dictator-for-life Kim Jong-Il have turned a formerly fertile and prosperous land into a concentration camp where people are forced to eat grass to survive, and anybody who questions the great leader's brilliance is executed. There is no shortage of 'evil' leaders of nations – the list could go on for pages.

Of course, none of these nations have oil.

But if Saddam were to invite in the oil companies who – through the corporate theft of human rights – have captured control of many of the policies of the United States Government, I suspect many things would change even in our thoughts about oil-rich Middle Eastern countries.

While profit is a fine value for a corporation to hold, it's not the prime value of humans and it's definitely not one of the values that drive or preserve democracy.

If we are to save our world from a profit-frenzy driven Armageddon, if we are to restore democracy to our American republic, we must first get corporations out of government, so our politicians can once again become statesmen.

Great words indeed, and he is one who suggests as a solution the expelling of corporate influences from US Government at all levels. But there is a more immediate solution, and that is education. If that sounds too simple and too idealistic, consider the following:

For every international war we have ever learned about in school (unless it is a war so remote from our own national feelings that the truth can be told) we were given 'reasons' for the conflict that perhaps seemed reasonable until or unless we learned the appropriate language and ended up living and working in one or both of the countries concerned. There we would also run across (usually in their own school history texts!) 'reasons for the war'. But the 'reasons' were often not only different in each of the two countries, but many of the 'reasons' in each case, could be categorised as 'moral', in that some ethical good was at stake and the country's soldiers were called forth to fight – perhaps to suffer and even die – for the moral issue concerned.

Investigating further, two things would no doubt become obvious:

1 The 'reasons' given in each case fitted in most conveniently with prevailing national trading and other financial interests.

2 Either the real 'reasons' usually have no moral basis at all or these 'reasons' could have been resolved by discussion.

The fact that large numbers of people keep being willing to accept the most out-landishly ridiculous reasons for blowing up each other's homes, hospitals, and places of worship, to say nothing of inflicting wide-scale death and the most appalling levels of suffering on the people of the countries attacked, suggests one of three things:

1 People have short memories.

2 People, on the whole, are stupid.

3 People everywhere are not being properly educated.

In the UK people speak of the 'dodgy dossier', which was said to have been used as a basis for the British government lining up with the US to invade Iraq. But, by and large, the British people eventually accepted it as a 'mistake' of some kind and did not effectively oppose their government's actions. Corporate interests kept them entertained, and morally supine, by various media distractions, while the shops were full of exciting and interesting things thereby allowing them to exercise their right to gain solace through retail therapy!

One of the advantages of effective education is that it enables the person to gradually see a pattern, to understand connections between ideas and events. And it involves the learner in the process. It might not always be the best way of equipping the person to rack up the highest grades in frequently staged exams, but it would equip them to understand other people, to recognise our various common needs and to enjoy life. It is not a particularly effective way to get people to be willing to risk their lives and health to inflict death or injury on 'foreigners'. Indeed, given the speed and frequency with which people are increasingly mobile, there soon won't be much use for that word 'foreigner'!

In other words, the barrier to global health equity imposed by war – with war itself usually imposed by appeal to some form of distorted economic theory, from which only a select few benefit and of which neoliberalism is a good example – is best overcome by much more of our resources being spent on education and healthcare. Recall the figures from Chapter 5 and 6. Our wars, wherever they take place, are prodigiously expensive. If only a small fraction of that money were directed to health, education and other social services, war would become less and less easily posited as a necessity. And along with that, people would begin to see just how small and unrepresentative was the cluster of people benefiting from such wars. Put it another way, as war becomes less of a hallmark of human history and endeavour, so will neoliberalism.

That cannot be allowed to remain as some kind of lofty hope or a pious ideal, for unless we make it a reality, civilisation and all of its values will fade away like a dream or the lifting of the morning mist.

Again, a strengthened and more assertively confident UN can be the mediator of such a turnabout in human events. War, after all, violates international law and international law is unambiguous in providing a clear recourse to situations which threaten to lead to war. Under international law, such a matter can be taken to the Security Council which itself cannot initiate a war. The launch of the coalition attack on Iraq, as discussed in Chapters 4 and 5, is a good example.

Indeed, it is in the context of the Iraqi war that we can perhaps most easily appreciate the cogency of better education as the most effective means of surmounting warfare as a barrier to global equity in health. Some of the issues of the US involvement in Iraq have been effectively addressed by Michael Albert and Stephen Shalom in an article published on the internet.[14] For, as well as the Iraq War being a gross violation of international law, there are at least four other rational arguments against the legitimacy of ever having mounted it. These are:

1   A putative aggressor has not been unambiguously identified. The *New York Times* even stated (20 September 2001): 'Law enforcement officials have little solid evidence tying the attacks in New York to Mr Bin Laden's group.' The basis for rational human conduct and a precondition for logical global interaction between peoples and nations is the rule of law. If this is so, and if we, as world citizens, are committed to law and justice, then when crimes such as the 9/11 attacks are committed, we are not permitted to act on the basis of 'hunches' or on the face of media-induced frenzy about assumed Islamic global ambitions. We have no basis, if we regard the rule of law seriously, for imposing punishment or especially a collective punishment that inflicts suffering on far more people than the supposed culprits. We should demand proof. We need to reject vigilantism. We need to reject guilt by association. This is elementary and incontestable, except when fear and the drums of war cloud our consciousness. In the case of September 11, though an Islamic or Middle Eastern connection seems clear, there are many extremist groups that might have been responsible. To rush to punitive judgement, much less to war, before responsibility has been determined, violates basic principles of justice. Guilt should be proven, not merely suspected.

2   The war in Iraq, even before it was launched, had virtually no chance of eliminating even those we had been led (by hunches fed by corporate-owned media)

to believe responsible for the atrocity of 9/11. If Bin Laden and his cohorts had been responsible for the 9/11 events, why would they have waited for the US military to eliminate them? And now they are, of course, even harder to find. The war we are waging in Iraq has virtually ensured that its primary victims would be ordinary uninvolved people and not the prime suspects.

3   The Iraq War has perverted the moral argument. If it is immoral to disrupt the US economy by such outrages as the 9/11 attacks; how can it be moral to respond by killing hundreds of thousands of innocent people who happen to live in the country in which the leaders of that attack might be hiding? Ignorance is a close ally of immorality in war. Take steps to abolish ignorance worldwide and war will likely vanish with it.

4   US citizens were told that the war would make their country safer. It is clear now that the opposite is true. Had their media (and that in the EU and elsewhere) been truly a servant of their people, the argument about national security would have been nowhere near as compelling because, with better and more balanced information (more education, in other words) they would have asked the basic questions; 'Why on earth were we attacked in this way? What could possibly persuade individual people, full of life and the potential for joy, to willingly sacrifice themselves as suicide bombers or as pilots of aircraft doomed to bloody destruction?' Answers to these questions can never justify what those criminals did, but asking the question as a basis for rational counter-measures would have led educated minds to realise that counter violence, especially violence even less specifically targeted than the attacks in New York had been, was about the most counter-productive action conceivable.

In considering these questions, which we now must do in any case because the war hasn't worked, we would have realised the causes of the 9/11 attack are complex and deeply psychological. They were certainly sustained by deep feelings of insult, anger and frustration at the West's (and the US's especially) rôle and actions in the Middle East. This author, for instance, watched appalled as friendly and apparently 'moral' Palestinian adults cheered in the streets when the World Trade Centre attack was announced on the radio. Again, back in 1956, he was equally horrified at Israeli expressions of joy in a cinema when shots of blown-up Palestinian villages and banana groves, scattered with dead and wounded parents and children, flickered onto the screen at an international meeting in Sydney.

When the coalition forces attacked Iraq, unquestionably *some* military personnel were killed, but so were a far larger number of ordinary, uninvolved people.

We, all of us, who stood by and allowed our Blairs and Bushes to lie to us and to send our soldiers to injury and death, and their families to despair, have not yet even started to pay in any real sense for the folly we have committed. And by 'pay',

I am not referring to the billions of pounds it is costing us to wreck Iraq, Gaza, and so on. I am referring to the future we have now ensured for our children of further hate, uncertainty, intolerance and even worse wars. There is no question in this author's mind that such a debt unquestionably hangs over us, but the only sure way of making sure that we will never face it again is a thorough and systematic campaign of action to make our views known to our politicians, holding them much more aggressively to account than we have in the past, and a determination to play a much more prominent rôle in deciding what we want of our media. Education, real insights into how our brothers and sisters in other cultures see things – how they pray, sing and think and raise their children – are the sorts of issues that we need our media to address.

All of that will require a conscious determination to seek moral solutions, indeed to seek out the moral dimensions to the many problems we will face. It is high time that we insisted on assuming the responsibility for running our communities, our countries and our entire global village. Moral parochialism is an indulgence we can no longer afford. It is with that in mind, then, that we attempt to find effective ways of overcoming the two remaining factors identified in previous chapters as barriers to global access to health. These are, of course, what this author has referred to in a previous chapter as 'health imperialism' (including recent inequities in the way that the global availability of healthcare is presently so badly distorted) and, likewise, the current and accelerating crisis of a global food shortage. Let us address health imperialism first.

IMPERIALISM IN HEALTHCARE

To set the scene for what follows, an insight into the economic context is vital. Current neo-colonial situations are characterised by a gradient of power in which direct political dependency is replaced by a perpetuation of economic dependency. Multinational corporations and the governments of countries that support them strive to control markets in resources, finances, and goods in poorer countries. In a continuation of colonialism, these countries are used as a reservoir of cheap labour and raw materials, often without making any contribution to a diversified economic and social structure. Countries like Switzerland, which never had colonies, are still tied to these (neo)colonial relationships of power and exchange. Currently, they take form in the worldwide privatisation of drinking water or the rôle of the Swiss chemical industry in the trade of pharmaceutical and agrochemical products. Even projects for developmental aid turn out to be conflict-ridden and paradoxical ventures that produce relationships of economic dependence in a globalised world economy, although they seek to decolonise.

All forms of imperialism, of course, produce victors, but the fact that millions of people suffer and die in different parts of the world because imperialism (as the author has described in Chapter 7) has interfered with the world distribution of healthcare workers is a particularly gross example of it. In the spring of 2008, the General Secretary of the United Nations, Ban Ki-Moon, graphically drew attention to this when addressing the first ever world forum on the problem in Kampala, Uganda on the morning of 4 March 2008.[15] The conference went on until 7 March. He opened his comments by stating that almost 60 nations – most in Africa – face such an acute shortage of health workers that even basic healthcare is inaccessible to millions. He went on to argue that such a state of affairs cannot continue if even some of the Millennium Development Goals are to be met. He emphasised the cruciality of working globally – not just nationally – to address the situation.

Paramount in the discussions was the issue of poaching medically qualified people from the Third World to meet staffing needs for First World medical facilities.

Rich countries are poaching so many African health workers that the practice should be viewed as a crime, a team of international disease experts assert in an article published by British medical journal, the *Lancet*.[16] More than 13 000 doctors trained in sub-Saharan Africa are now practising in Britain, the United States, Canada and Australia, leaving behind colleagues with impossible caseloads. African nurses and pharmacists are also sought after by the clinics and chemist shop chains, offering better pay and legal assistance with immigration, said the experts, who include the heads of several pharmacy and medicine schools in Africa. 'The resulting dilapidation of health infrastructure contributes to a measurable and foreseeable public health crisis,' the article said. 'The practice should therefore be viewed as an international crime.'

At the meeting addressed by Ban Ki-Moon in Kampala, the delegates at that initial meeting of the Global Forum on Human Resources in Health endorsed a 'Global Agenda for action' on the alarming imbalances in availability of health workers because of the poaching described in Chapter 7. One component of that agenda was a pledge to 'accelerate negotiations on an international code of practice to more rationally control the international dispersal of health workers'. The first step was taken on 31 March 2008, with the launch of a three-week online global dialogue convened by the Health Worker Migration Policy Initiative. The above-cited *Lancet* report commented:

'The objective of the global dialogue is laudable. It provides a unique opportunity for anyone affected by the vast complexities of health worker migration, on effective strategies to retain health workers where they are needed most, and on what the key principles of a global code of practice should be. But is another code of practice really required?'

However, as explained in Chapter 7, although the problem is a serious one that will continue to lead to unnecessary suffering and loss of life if not urgently addressed, it is not easily resolved. Medical staff are not simply recruited by First World agencies from Third World countries, they are often only too glad to go! No one forces them, but circumstances such as low and erratic pay, poor technical support and outright corruption, often act as 'push' factors, while the comparatively high salaries in the First World, the chances of further professional training and better working conditions are persuasive 'pull' factors.

A pivotal solution may well lie in that aforementioned Global Agenda for Action, started at the Kampala meeting. But the degree of its success would be bolstered by the sort of solutions in First World attitudes mentioned above with respect to a more energetic public ownership of the media and its use for greater opportunities for global awareness.

Recently, of course, the global lack of access to food has featured heavily in the media. Just before considering that, though, it is worthwhile reminding ourselves that even under the constraints of neoliberalism, the moral issues are being addressed and can continue to be.

SOCIAL ENTREPRENEURISM

Morally fruitful approaches to enhancing community life, often at the very local level, have been emerging in what social scientists refer to as 'social entrepreneurism'. This phenomenon includes a variety of innovatory applications of existing capitalist structures and can involve venture development programmes, non-profit enterprises, and affirmative action agenda in business. At the centre of such actions lie many of the moral apprehensions mentioned in the previous chapter.

The people who plan and carry out such approaches to social inequity can be seen as social entrepreneurs, in that they act as social mediators in much the same way that many business professionals currently act as financial mediators. They attempt to use traditional business skills, but to apply them consciously, more with an eye to potential social benefit than to personal financial gain. We can classify such approaches in two broad categories: 'not-for-profit' and 'for profit'.

Examples of not-for-profit initiatives include campaigns for housing (especially in major urban areas) involving organised squatting of unused properties for housing homeless people, and food acquisition by reclaiming packaged foodstuffs put out just prior to their sell-by dates in the skips behind supermarkets. There is scope for a considerable admixture of idealism and creativity in organising such schemes and they are already being energetically pursued by groups of committed (usually, but not always, young) people in such cities as London and New York in the First World, and similarly in large Third World cities.

With respect to 'for profit' ventures, there are many examples. In these, financial profit is to some degree a guiding incentive, but with a 'delay' factor built in, so that such social goods as providing training for young people who have fallen through various statutory protection nets can be provided in the interim. Some major corporations now carry out such programs, regarding them as what might be called 'enlightened capitalism'. In this way, homeless – or otherwise disadvantaged people – can be trained for employment and acquire other social skills.

Both of these categories, but especially the first, could well lend themselves to the sort of social attitudes that any significant change from neoliberalism requires.

HUNGER AS A POLITICAL ISSUE

The author once ran across a cartoon, the provenance of which he has unfortunately lost track. It showed a ragged half-starved little child saying to an international aid worker: 'Sir. I'm hungry.' To which the aid worker replies: 'I'm sorry, but I am forbidden to discuss politics!'

The current global food crisis confronts us all with such a political issue. As the author suggested in Chapter 8, a variety of causes can be listed as being responsible. As well, the hand of neoliberalism is evident to some degree in all of these. But one case that is not so often listed with the others is the direct rôle of neoliberalism, and the degree to which the WTO has been so heavily implicated.

In the above, the author is alluding to the creation of a global market in food stuffs, allowing people, if they are sufficiently wealthy, to dine without reference to local climatic factors – strawberries in mid-winter Canada, tropical food stuffs anywhere – courtesy of rapid (and hugely atmospheric carbon generating) international air transport. Another factor which renders all of this possible is neoliberalism, enshrined in WTO trading regulations, which have opened the world to 'free trade' through such political mechanisms as GATS and GATT.

This has given rise to all sorts of anomalous situations – such as being able to produce sugar in Belgium, say, from sugar beets, more cheaply that it can be produced from sugar cane in Jamaica, Trinidad or Cuba. Of course, as we know, this can only be done on the basis of wealthy First World countries being able to provide their farmers (in the US or the EU) with agricultural subsidies, for instance, the US state of Mississippi is able to produce cotton more cheaply than it can be produced in Burkina Faso. The anomaly resides in the fact that soil conditions and meteorological conditions in Burkina Faso are absolutely optimum for cotton production. It is about the only export that that poor country has, and it produces it in profusion and of a higher quality than it can be produced naturally anywhere else in the world.

Yet, in Mississippi, with the US Government providing subsidies, cotton farmers can afford the enormous expense of nitrate fertilisers in abundance, thus producing cotton and being able to sell it at a price that Burkina farmers could not do without bankrupting themselves. And under the free trade rules insisted upon by the WTO, and by application of GATT, that is exactly what happens. As Burkina Fasso farmers are undermined and put out of business, stockholders in the First World suddenly become enormously wealthy.

The same, of course, goes for sugar (countries such as Jamaica being the natural home of sugar cane and cane sugar only costing a third as much to produce as beet sugar in Europe) and now for a whole range of food crops, especially grains. The neoliberals have the market sown up, and although adversely affected by such factors as global warming and changing dietary habits of millions of Asians, they can continue to garner spectacular profits, while most people are experiencing shortages.

The British newspaper, *The Independent*, recently ran a well-balanced article on the global food crisis and some of the information that follows is derived from it.[17]

Large multinational agribusinesses, protected by agricultural subsidies in their own countries, and by GATS and by GATT under WTO regulation, are both generating the food crisis and, at the same time, making enormous profits out of it. Prices of wheat, corn and rice have all increased hugely, reducing many of the world's poor to starvation. Yet Monsanto reported, in February 2008, that its profits had doubled over the same period in 2007. Similar sudden profits have been reported by other transnational agricultural corporations.

In the face of this bonanza, the FAO reports that 37 countries are in urgent need of food. All over the world, food riots are breaking out. In Haiti, participants in these riots have even been killed by police trying to restore order.

The Independent's article, referred to above, quoted Benedict Southworth, Director of the World Food Movement, as saying that the profits being made out of this are 'immoral'. As we have seen in previous chapters, the soaring prices in food and fertilisers ties in with increasing use of biofuels as a world commodity and the increase in the consumption of meat. This has been associated with greatly increased transport costs and rises in the price of oil have guaranteed further scope for neoliberalist 'winner takes all' policies. For instance, from January through March of 2008, Shell and BP, between them, recorded profits of 14 billion pounds (3 million pounds an hour!).

The Head of the UN's World Food Programme has called the food crisis: 'A silent tsunami which knows no borders and that is sweeping the world'. It may 'know no borders', but it is having a particularly malign impact on the Third World. In many developing countries, for instance, the consumers in the lowest 25% of the income range routinely spend 75% or more of their income on food, and now they are faced with rapidly increasing food prices. Without remedial action, starvation for them is the next step. But rising food prices are part of a wider range of price rises, and this represents a natural outworking of neoliberal competition policies.

Indeed, powerful corporate and banking interests are making profits by linking the prices of energy, industrial raw materials and food stuffs. In economic terms, the causative forces include rapid economic growth in some Third World countries (especially in Asia), increasing demand for energy, the weakness of the US dollar and global inflating pressures.

The real issue is not the rise in food prices – market prices, after all, go up and down. We would be foolish indeed to try to prevent that phenomenon. While some of the underlying causes relate to policy errors (unthinking support for mass production of biofuels for export, for example), and these should be corrected, the focus should bear principally on the causes of food vulnerability. It is this that makes food price volatility costly in terms of deepening hunger and poverty.

Two institutions in particular were discarded in the period of dogmatic liberalisation from the 1980s. First, state banks were rushed to privatisation. While this yielded some benefits by addressing some inefficiencies, it also generally led to sharp falls in rural lending of the sort that helped smooth consumption across volatile harvests, and provide investment funds for basics such as seed and fertiliser. Second, agricultural marketing boards were dismantled. While these again had often not functioned perfectly, they had nonetheless provided an important degree of stability and improved access to markets for marginal producers who typically sell little into the market, but for whom that little can be pivotal in determining whether they can continue and prosper over time.

One solution with respect to rational food provision, that also produces a reduced carbon footprint, is what this author, in a previous publication referred to as 'Localised Fair Trade'.[18] It could involve the world's surface being divided up into various climate/agricultural zones so that that countries within any one zone are likely to produce many of the same commodities – say, sugar and coffee – and thus, under a system of globalised free trade, to keep cutting each other's sales by direct competition for First World markets. But they could all belong to a 'Trade Differential Group', which would reach an agreement as to which of them would emphasise which products to trade. In the same way, they could divide up the First World markets between the various areas producing similar products. Within each region, their trade with one another could exploit their differences and involve methods for protecting their key First World trading products. To make the system work, of course, the WTO would have to become an arbiter of regional fair trade, rather than an enforcer of free trade. This, in fact, would bring it into line with Keynes's original vision of a WTO at the Bretton Woods meetings in 1944–48. Its current rôle, as an enforcer of strategies that enrich First World corporations, to the detriment of the health of people in the Third, would diminish accordingly.

The world as a whole can, and usually does, produce much more food than is required to feed all of us now, and even a predicted global population of about 9 billion by 2050. Localised (Regional) Fair Trade could greatly reduce the carbon footprint imposed by unimpeded free trade by the various regions agreeing ahead of time on how to move quantities the least distances. There would also be ample scope in such an enterprise for individual and local community activity in learning to eat more locally. This aspect of solution-finding once again raises the idea of a social morality, informed by science, and closely linked with insights into environmental variables.

The advantages of Regional Free Trade, of course, is that 'regions' (although defined at any one time) geographically, are not rigidly fixed, as are national frontiers, but can be varied by the relevant committees in response to climate changes and in such a way as to permit maximum flexibility for effective trade.

CREATING A MORE SUSTAINABLE WORLD

It is appropriate to end this book with a very brief comment on what we can do, both as governments and individuals, to make the world a sustainable place for human life. The author realises that this presupposes that we will indeed overcome the barriers referred to in this book – and others – and support the WHO as it moves to definitively reduce the global health equity. My optimism is based on many things, but not least, the conviction that the human race will not allow itself to be written off, either by war or unsustainable politic-economic systems.

In the book cited above, the author discusses solar energy, for instance, and the radical variations possible for generating energy from it.[19] These range all of the way from individuals using solar panels to heat their water, if not their homes, to entire communities deriving all of their electricity that they require from huge banks of mirrors situated in fields thousands of miles away. This is not the sort of thing that neoliberal interests can really get excited about because massive fortunes, if they are to be made from it, would be too difficult to centralise in such a way that control could be vested in the hands of a few powerful people. Also, the technology required is relatively low tech, so that probably vast fortunes are not to be made from it. Corporate power is much more anxious for us to go nuclear!

But consider the following potential application of solar energy, suggested in an online essay by an Australian, David Clarke.[20] As he observes, one problem with solar energy has been that not only do you only have it when the sun shines, but also any electricity produced thereby either has to be used immediately or be stored in prohibitively expensive batteries. However, scientists are gradually getting around this problem.

Figure 10.1 needs to be consulted here. One solution being researched at the Australian National University is to use large dish solar collectors to heat ammonia gas (NH_3) to a sufficient temperature for it to 'break up' into its constituent nitrogen

(N_2) and hydrogen (H_2) gasses. These gasses can then be piped to wherever energy is required and, as needed, the nitrogen and hydrogen are recombined to form the original ammonia, with the release of the original solar energy in the form of heat. This process is shown symbolically in the graphic below:

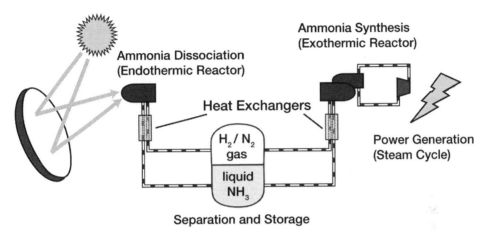

FIGURE 10.1. Source: ANU Department of Engineering's Internet site.

In chemist's symbols, the reaction is: $2\,NH_3 + Heat \rightleftharpoons N_2 + 3\,H_2$.

Clarke's writings on the subject include a number of other highly innovatory approaches, as well as interesting variations on some of the other more well-known sources of sustainable energy.

But in closing, the writer can do no better than to reflect on the thoughts of another Australian, the geneticist and immunologist, GJV Nossal as he takes up the author's oft repeated comment on our world's status as a 'global village', with all that implies.[21] As the reader will see, his view on morality and survival strongly reflects the tone of this volume.

The world is now truly a global village, a world where communication is so rapid and intensive that both the good and the bad things that happen anywhere are registered within minutes around the globe. This intensifies the emotions generated by major inequities. Greater social justice in the world can only be achieved by a more substantial engagement of the richer countries with the poorer, and moreover on a full partnership basis. This is desirable, not only on humanitarian grounds, but out of naked self-interest. Many trillions of dollars spent on armaments cannot ensure security, as the suicide bombers have shown. What I am urging in the longer term is a kind of global Marshall Plan, but centred on 'soft' infrastructure, including education, health, good governance and independent justice systems.

Some signs have emerged in the health field that real progress is possible at a price tag which the world can support. We are, however, talking about billions rather than millions of dollars. Government and United Nations agencies are not the only players. Some of the most successful programmes have involved private sector-public sector partnerships. Foundations and high net worth individuals are important, but so are ordinary citizens. There will be huge transfers of wealth as the baby boomers bequeath their savings to their relatively modest number of children. Surely some of this can be harnessed. In the last analysis, money alone will not be enough. Things will only change if we, the rich, recognise in fullest measure, the worth, the dignity and the ineffable potential of every single one of our fellow human beings. Manning Clarke said that 'the great Australian dream of social equality and mateship was bleeding to death in the jungles and paddy-fields of Vietnam.'[22] His somewhat tragic view of the human condition might have led him to believe that my dream of social equality and mateship around the world is hopelessly naïve. Perhaps so, but I do not think he would have opposed my trying to promulgate it.

REFERENCES

1 MacDonald T. *Health, Human Rights and the United Nations: inconsistent aims and inherent contradictions?* Oxford & New York: Radcliffe Publishing; 2007. pp. 22–3.
2 Ibid. pp. 166–81.
3 MacDonald T. *Sacrificing the WHO to the Highest Bidder.* Oxford & New York: Radcliffe Publishing; 2008.
4 Sachs J. Primary health for all. *Sci Am.* 2007; **297**(6): 14–15
5 MacDonald T. *The Global Human Right to Health.* Oxford & New York: Radcliffe Publishing; 2007.
6 *The Global Fund to Fight AIDS, Tuberculosis and Malaria.* Available at: www.avert.org/global-fund.htm (accessed 28 May 2008).
7 Primary health for all, op. cit.
8 Fuchs P, Plank L. Corporations need clear, binding human rights rules. *Corporate.* 2007; **34**. Available at: www.humaninfo.org/avive.Number69 (accessed 28 May 2008).
9 Santoro M. *Charting a Sustainable Path for the Twenty-first Century Pharmaceutical Industry.* Cambridge: Cambridge University Press; 2005.
10 Santoro M, Gorrie T. *Ethics and the Pharmaceutical Industry.* Cambridge: Cambridge University Press; 2007. p. 39.
11 *Sacrificing the WHO to the Highest Bidder,* op. cit., pp. 154–78.
12 Huberman L, Sweezy P. *Cuba: anatomy of a revolution.* New York: Monthly Review Press; 1960: pp 16–17.
13 Hartman T. *The Dinosaur War – to protect corporate profits.* Available at: www.commondreams.org/views02/1011–05.htm (accessed 29 May 2008).

14 Albert M, Shalom S. *Five Arguments Against War.* Available at: www.zmag.org/
fiverargs.htm (accessed May 28, 2008).

15 Moon B-K. Health-care workers, the 'true lifesavers' must be supported. Speech given
to the UN, 4 Mar 2008. Available at: www.who.int/mediacentre/en (accessed 29 May
2008).

16 A global dialogue on a global crisis. *Lancet.* 2008; **371**(9619). Available at: www.
thelancet.com/journal/article/P115014067360860496/fulltext (accessed 29 May
2008).

17 Lean G. *Multinationals Make Billions in Profit Out of Growing Global Food Crisis.* 4 May
2008. Available at: www.independent.co.uk/environment/green-living/multinationals-
make-billions-in-profit-out-of-growing-global-food-crisis-820855.html (accessed
May 29, 2008).

18 *Health, Human Rights and the United Nations,* op. cit., pp. 166–79.

19 MacDonald T. *Third World Health: hostage to First World Wealth.* Oxford & New York:
Radcliffe Publishing; 2005: pp. 19–31.

20 Clarke D. *Towards a More Sustainable World.* Available at: www.geocities.com/
daveclarkecb/Sustain.html (accessed 30 May 2008).

21 Nossal G. *Towards a Fairer World: historic trends in global health reform.* Fifth Annual
Manning Clark Lecture, Department of Pathology at the University of Melbourne.
3 Mar 2004. Available at: www.manningclark.org.au/papers/Healthreform.html
(accessed 29 May 2008)

22 Ibid.

Index

Rosenthal, Elizabeth 209
Rumsfeld, Donald 134–5, 140
RWE (water company) 61–2
Ryder, Guy 242

Sachs, Jeffrey 265, 270–1
SAGUAPAC (Bolivia) 73
Santoro, Michael 272–4
SAPs *see* Structural Adjustment Policies (SAPs)
Schifferes, Steve 131–2, 133
Schultz, J 63
Scott, Cheryl 198
Scott, John 215–16
Searchinger, Timothy 209–10
security concerns, impact on 'community' 42–4,
    143–4
Segerfeldt, Frederik 70
SEMAPA (Bolivia) 63–4, 69–70
Serbia
    Bosnian war 28–9
    US attacks 147–8
Shah, Anup 98
share ownership 17
Sheeran, Josette 210–11
Shell 284
The Shock Doctrine (Klein) 29, 41–2
Silverstein, Ken 104
Singapore 40
Smith, JW 99
Smith, K and Edwards, R 213
smoking, and lifespan 251
social change
    key actions
        changing WTO's role 285–6
        G8 initiatives 244
        Global Fund role enhancement 266–70
        improve UN effectiveness 264–6
        reigning in corporate power 271–5
        role of social entrepreneurs 282–3
        Sach's ten proposals 265, 270–1
        to healthcare 'imperialism' 280–2
        war prevention strategies 274–80
    rediscovering democracy 250–1
    role of citizenship education 249–50
    role of the US 254–7
social entrepreneurism 282–3
social insurance funding schemes 189–91
socio-economic inequalities
    and gated communities 38
    impact of global neoliberalism 245–8
    moral imperatives 242–8
solar energy 286–7
South Africa
    HIV/AIDS 91–4
        Communist Party views 93–4
        use of generic anti-AIDS drugs 90–1
    impact of neoliberal policies 257–9
Southworth, Benedict 284
soya oils 224
Spino, Mike 116
Sri Lanka
    healthcare funding 189
    post-tsunami aid management 25, 34, 35–6

SSRIs, marketing activities 101–2
Stephen, Andrew 133–5
Stiglitz, Joseph 106–7, 132–5, 146
Structural Adjustment Policies (SAPs) 4–5, 26–7
Suez (water company) 61–2
Sun Belt 74–5
surveillance technologies 41
sustainable energy initiatives 27–8

Tauzin, Billy 96
tax systems 9, 11–12
    and 'Non-Doms' 21–2
terrorist threats, public attitudes 42–4
Tesfachew, Taffere 223
Thatcher, Margaret
    and neoliberalism 8, 10, 15–17
    and the trade unions 16
Third World Health: hostage to first world wealth
    (MacDonald 2005) 146
Third World Network (TWN) 89–90
Thirty Years War 127–8
Tibet 147–8
TINA (there is no alternative) 10
torture, public attitudes 42–4, 143–4, 259–61
trade unions, constraints and restrictions 6
Trade-Related Aspects of International Property
    Rights (TRIPS) 89–91, 104–7, 200–1
trading agreements
    and food shortages 284–6
    Latin American models 49
    US-led neoliberal models 22–3
        FTAA investor protections 74–5
        NAFTA 74–5
    water privatisation and control 70–1
Trident missile systems 9, 153
TRIPS *see* Trade-Related Aspects of International
    Property Rights
Trovan 114–16
tsunami aid management 25, 34

UDHR *see* Universal Declaration of Human Rights
Uganda, grant management problems 269–70
Ukraine, and Chernobyl 165
UN Conference on Trade and Development
    (UNCTAD) 20–1
    on rise of privatisation 21
UN Intergovernmental Panel on Climate Change
    215
UNICEF, child welfare rankings 13
United Kingdom
    impact of neoliberalism 16–17
    post-9/11 conflicts, costs 138
    use of biofuels 207
United Nations 240–1
    improving effectiveness 264–6
    on neoliberalism 32–4
United States
    experiences of neoliberalism 18–20
    health of individuals 13
    healthcare
        financing 194–6, 254–5
        staff recruitment 174–7
    income distribution trends 18–19